PERCEPTUAL CONSEQUENCES OF COCHLEAR DAMAGE

OXFORD PSYCHOLOGY SERIES

Editors

1. *The neuropsychology of anxiety: an enquiry into the functions of the septohippocampal system*
   Jeffrey A. Gray
2. *Elements of episode memory*
   Endel Tulving
3. *Conditioning and associative learning*
   Nicholas J. Mackintosh
4. *Visual masking: an integrative approach*
   Bruno G. Breitmeyer
5. *The musical mind: the cognitive psychology of music*
   John Sloboda
6. *Elements of psychophysical theory*
   Jean-Claude Falmagne
7. *Animal intelligence*
   Edited by Lawrence Weiskrantz
8. *Response times: their role in inferring elementary mental organisation*
   R. Duncan Luce
9. *Mental representations: a dual coding approach*
   Allan Paivio
10. *Memory, imprinting, and the brain*
    Gabriel Horn
11. *Working memory*
    Alan Baddeley
12. *Blindsight: a case study and implications*
    Lawrence Weiskrantz
13. *Profile analysis*
    D. M. Green
14. *Spatial vision*
    R. L. DeValois and K. K. DeValois
15. *The neural and behavioural organization of goal-directed movements*
    Marc Jeannerod
16. *Visual pattern analyzers*
    Norma V. Graham
17. *Cognitive foundations of musical pitch analysis*
    C. L. Krumhansl

18. *Perceptual and associative learning*
    G. Hall
19. *Implicit learning and tacit knowledge*
    A. S. Reber
20. *Neuromotor mechanisms in human communication*
    D. Kimura
21. *The frontal lobes and voluntary action*
    R. E. Passingham
22. *Classification and cognition*
    W. Estes
23. *Vowel perception and production*
    B. S. Rosner and J. B. Pickering
24. *Visual stress*
    A. Wilkins
25. *Electrophysiology of mind*
    Edited by M. Rugg and M. Coles
26. *Attention and memory: an integrated framework*
    N. Cowan
27. *The visual brain in action*
    A. D. Milner and M. A. Goodale
28. *Perceptual consequences of cochlear damage*
    B. C. J. Moore

Perceptual Consequences of Cochlear Damage

BRIAN C. J. MOORE

Department of Experimental Psychology,
University of Cambridge

OXFORD PSYCHOLOGY SERIES
NO. 28

OXFORD NEW YORK TOKYO
OXFORD UNIVERSITY PRESS
1995

Oxford University Press, Walton Street, Oxford OX2 6DP

Oxford New York
Athens Auckland Bangkok Bombay
Calcutta Cape Town Dar es Salaam Delhi
Florence Hong Kong Istanbul Karachi
Kuala Lumpur Madras Madrid Melbourne
Mexico City Nairobi Paris Singapore
Taipei Tokyo Toronto
and associated companies in
Berlin Ibadan

Oxford is a trade mark of Oxford University Press

Published in the United States
by Oxford University Press Inc., New York

A catalague record for this book is available from the British Library

Library of Congress Cataloging in Publication Data
Moore, Brian C. J.
Perceptual consequences of cochlear damage / Brian C. J. Moore. — 1st ed.
(Oxford psychology series; no. 28)
Includes bibliographical references and index.
1. Hearing disorders. — 2. Cochlea—Pathophysiology. — 3. Hearing–Physiological aspects.
I. Title. II. Series.
RF291.M66 1995 95–18523
617.8′—dc20

ISBN 0 19 852330 0

Typeset by Pure Tech India Ltd, Pondicherry
Printed and bound in Great Britain by
Biddles Ltd, Guildford and King's Lynn

Preface

Over the last ten to fifteen years there has been a revolution in the understanding of the mechanisms of sound analysis in the normal cochlea. Along with this, the mechanisms associated with cochlear hearing loss are also much better understood. However, these improvements in understanding have been mainly in terms of physiological mechanisms. This book emphasizes the *perceptual* changes associated with cochlear hearing loss and relates these to the underlying physiological mechanisms. The book is intended to provide a theoretical framework for understanding and interpreting the perceptual changes. The results obtained with hearing-impaired subjects have important implications for theories of normal perception, especially in relation to loudness, temporal processing and pitch perception. The data and theories surveyed are used as a conceptual framework for discussing the difficulties of speech perception experienced by the hearing impaired, the limitations of current hearing aids, and the design of new signal-processing hearing aids that can compensate more effectively for the perceptual effects of cochlear damage.

The book is aimed at a rather broad audience. Cochlear hearing loss is the commonest type of hearing loss in adults, and it affects a large proportion of the population, so the subject area is of general interest. The potential audience includes: psychologists and physiologists interested in basic mechanisms of hearing and hearing impairment; audiologists and audiological scientists; otologists; hearing aid dispensers; and audio engineers, especially those working in the hearing-aid industry, or in audio systems for hearing-impaired persons. Although not primarily intended as a student text, the book might well be used for graduate courses in departments of Psychology, Speech and Hearing Science, and Audiology. The book assumes some prior knowledge about sound. For example, it assumes familiarity with the decibel and the concept of the spectrum of a sound. Those unfamiliar with these concepts should consult textbooks such as B. C. J. Moore (1989) *An Introduction to the Psychology of Hearing*, 3rd Edn (Academic Press, London) or W. A. Yost (1994) *Fundamentals of Hearing* (Academic Press, San Diego).

The book aims to present both data and concepts in an integrated way. The main goal is to convey a general understanding of the perceptual changes associated with cochlear hearing loss, and of the difficulties faced by the hearing-impaired person. The reader should come away with an impression not only of what happens, but also of why it happens.

Appreciation of the perceptual consequences of cochlear damage can be helped by listening to simulations of these consequences; examples of such simulations are described in chapter 7. A compact disc (CD) containing simulations of different aspects of cochlear damage can be obtained by writing to the author at: Department of Experimental Psychology, University of Cambridge, Downing Street, Cambridge CB2 3EB.

The cost of the disc is 12 pounds sterling or 20 US dollars. Payment should be enclosed with the order. The disc also illustrates the effectiveness of various types of amplification and compression in compensating for the effects of cochlear damage.

I would like to thank the colleagues and research students who commented promptly and forthrightly on the drafts of chapters that I circulated among them. They include Joseph Alcántara, Thomas Baer, Steve Borrill, Shigeto Furukawa, Brian Glasberg, Stefan Launer, Andrew Oxenham, Marina Rose, Michael Stone, Deborah Vickers and Magda Wojtczak. I would also like to thank Ian Cannell, Brian Glasberg and Deborah Vickers for assistance in producing figures.

Cambridge B. C. J. M
December 1994

Contents

1 The physiology and function of the normal and damaged cochlea

Introduction

Hearing loss caused by damage to the cochlea (inner ear) is probably the most common form of hearing loss in the developed countries. Its most obvious symptom is a loss of ability to detect weak sounds. However, it is also accompanied by a variety of other changes in the way that sound is perceived. Even if sounds are amplified (for example by a hearing aid) so that they are well above the threshold for detection, the perception of those sounds is usually abnormal; the person with cochlear damage reports that the sounds are fuzzy, unclear, muffled and distorted. A common complaint is difficulty in understanding speech, especially when background sounds are present. One of the main aims of this book is to give an account of the perceptual changes accompanying cochlear damage, and to relate the perceptual changes to changes in the physiology of the cochlea.

Cochlear damage can arise in many ways, for example by exposure to intense sounds or to ototoxic chemicals (such as certain antibiotics, drugs used to treat high blood pressure or solvents), by infection, by metabolic disturbances, by some forms of allergies and as a result of genetic factors. These agents can produce a variety of types of damage to the cochlea, and, to complicate matters further, the damage may not be restricted to the cochlea. For example, an infection may produce damage at several sites in the auditory system including the auditory nerve and higher centres in the auditory pathway. In addition, cochlear hearing loss is sometimes accompanied by conductive hearing loss, a reduced efficiency of sound transmission through the outer and/or middle ear. This may be caused by wax (cerumen) in the ear canal, damage to the eardrum produced by infection or trauma, damage to the ossicles in the middle ear (see below), or fluid in the middle ear caused by infection. A conductive loss results in an attenuation of sound reaching the cochlea, so that all sounds appear quieter than normal. However, that is the main perceptual consequence of a conductive loss; unlike cochlear damage, it does not generally result in marked distortions or abnormalities in other aspects of sound perception. Conductive hearing loss can often be treated by drugs (to cure infections) or surgery.

Although hearing loss can involve structures other than the cochlea, it is common for the most serious damage to occur within the cochlea. This is probably true for the majority of cases of presbyacusis, the hearing loss that is associated with aging. Furthermore, it is common for the damage to be largely confined to certain specific structures within the cochlea. Hence, this book will concentrate on the situation where the hearing loss arises primarily from damage to the cochlea. Henceforth, when the phrase 'hearing impairment' is used, it should be taken to imply hearing impairment caused by cochlear damage. However, it should be borne in mind that, while it is relatively easy to produce 'pure' cochlear damage in animal models, such 'pure' damage may be relatively rare in hearing-impaired humans.

In the last twenty years there has been a considerable increase in understanding of the physiology and function of the normal cochlea. Along with this has come improved understanding of the changes in function that are associated with cochlear damage. This chapter starts by briefly reviewing the structure and function of the normal peripheral auditory system. It then goes on to consider the changes that occur when the cochlea is damaged.

Structure and function of the normal peripheral auditory system

The outer and middle ear

Figure 1.1 shows the structure of the peripheral part of the human auditory system. It is traditionally considered as composed of three parts, the outer, middle and inner ear. The outer ear is composed of the pinna and the auditory canal or meatus. The pinna and meatus together create a broad resonance which enhances sound levels at the eardrum, relative to those at the entrance to the ear canal, over the frequency range

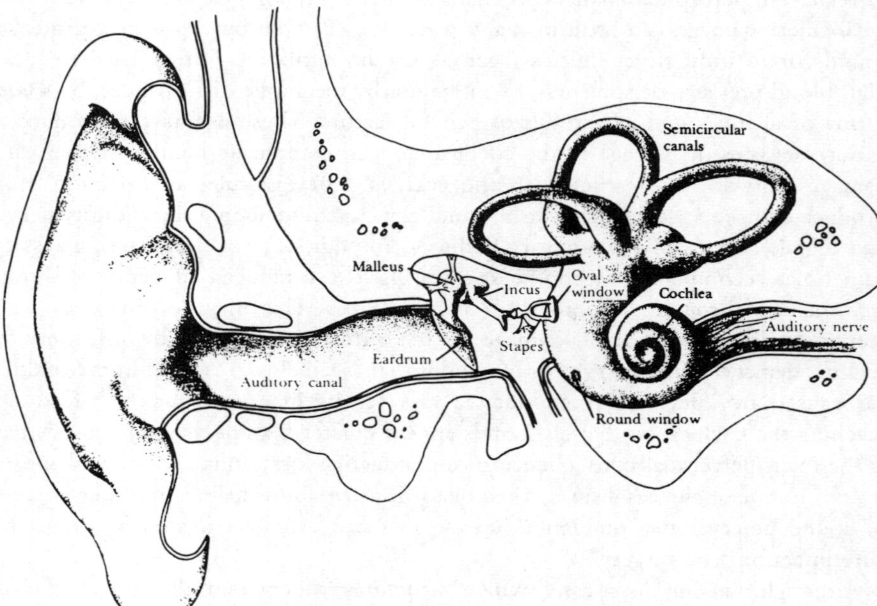

Fig. 1.1. Illustration of the structure of the peripheral auditory system showing the outer, middle and inner ear. Redrawn from Lindsey and Norman (1972).

from about 1.5 to 5 kHz. The maximum boost is typically about 12 dB in the region around 2.5 kHz. When a hearing aid is fitted so as to block the meatus, this broad resonance is reduced in magnitude and may be shifted to higher frequencies, and this has to be taken into account when fitting hearing aids. The pinna significantly modifies the incoming sound at high frequencies. Specifically, when the sound contains a broad range of frequencies, the pinna introduces a complex pattern of peaks and notches into the spectrum. This pattern varies systematically with the direction of the sound source relative to the head, and the spectral changes thus provide important information about sound location (see chapter 6 for more details).

Sound travels down the meatus and causes the eardrum, or tympanic membrane, to vibrate. These vibrations are transmitted through the middle ear by three small bones, the ossicles, to a membrane-covered opening in the bony wall of the spiral-shaped structure of the inner ear—the cochlea. This opening is called the oval window. The three bones are called the malleus, incus and stapes, the stapes being the lightest and smallest of these and the one which actually makes contact with the oval window.

The major function of the middle ear is to ensure the efficient transfer of sound from the air to the fluids in the cochlea. If the sound were to impinge directly onto the oval window, most of it would simply be reflected back, rather than entering the cochlea. This happens because the resistance of the oval window to movement is very different to that of air. This is described as a difference in acoustical impedance. The middle ear acts as an impedance-matching device or transformer that improves sound transmission and reduces the amount of reflected sound. This is accomplished mainly by the 27:1 ratio of effective areas of the eardrum and the oval window, and to a small extent by the lever action of the ossicles. Transmission of sound through the middle ear is most efficient at middle frequencies (500–4000 Hz).

The ossicles have minute muscles attached to them which contract when we are exposed to intense sounds. This contraction, known as the middle ear reflex or acoustic reflex, is probably mediated by neural centres in the brain stem, but its anatomical basis is not fully known. The reflex can be triggered by sound of any frequency, but it reduces the transmission of sound through the middle ear only at low frequencies. It may help to prevent damage to the delicate structures inside the cochlea. However, the activation of the reflex is too slow to provide any protection against impulsive sounds, such as gun shots or hammer blows.

It is relatively easy to determine when the reflex is activated by measuring the reflection of sound from the eardrum using an 'impedance audiometer'. The lowest sound level that will activate the reflex is known as the 'acoustic reflex threshold' (ART) and many impedance audiometers can measure it automatically. The ART can be useful in confirming that a hearing loss is primarily cochlear in origin. In such a case, the ART usually has a value close to normal, around 90 dB HL (HL stands for 'hearing level'. It is used when a sound level in decibels is expressed relative to the average absolute threshold of young normally hearing people for the sound in question). If a conductive loss is present, both the absolute threshold for detecting sounds and the ART are elevated, by about the same amount.

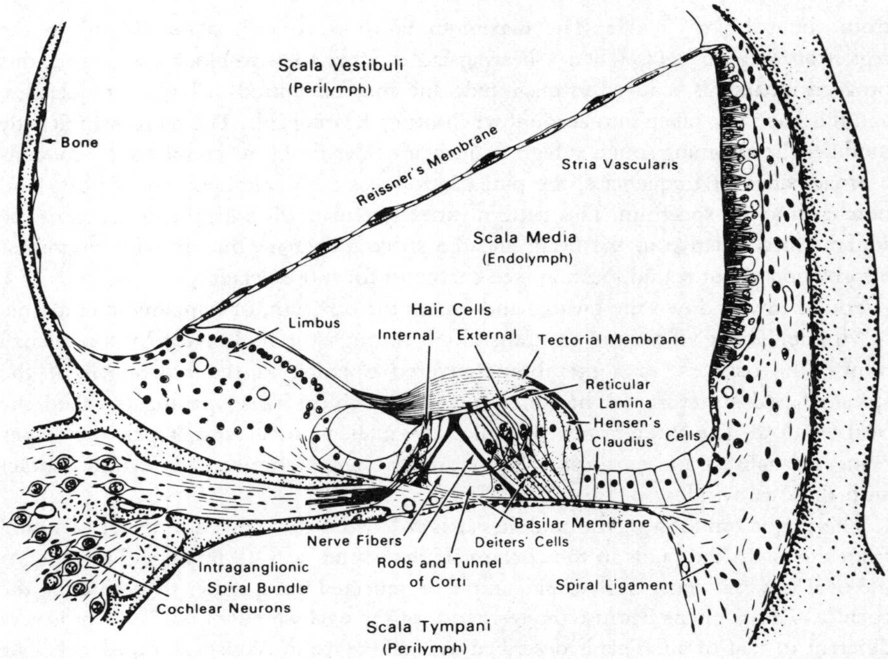

Fig. 1.2. Cross-section of the cochlea, showing the basilar membrane, Reissner's membrane, and the organ of Corti which lies between the basilar membrane and the tectorial membrane. Redrawn from Davis (1962).

The cochlea, the basilar membrane and the organ of Corti

The inner ear is also known as the cochlea. It is filled with almost incompressible fluids, and it also has bony rigid walls. It is divided along its length by two membranes, Reissner's membrane and the basilar membrane (BM; see Figure 1.2). The start of the cochlea, where the oval window is situated, is known as the base; while the other end, the inner tip, is known as the apex. It is also common to talk about the basal end and the apical end. At the apex there is a small opening (the helicotrema) between the BM and the walls of the cochlea, which connects the two outer chambers of the cochlea, the scala vestibuli and the scala tympani. Inward movement of the oval window results in a corresponding outward movement in a membrane covering a second opening in the cochlea—the round window. Such movements result in turn in movement of the BM (see below for details).

A second membrane, called the tectorial membrane, lies above the BM, and also runs along the length of the cochlea. Between the BM and the tectorial membrane are hair cells, which form part of a structure called the organ of Corti (see Figures 1.3 and 1.4). They are called hair cells because they appear to have tufts of hairs, called stereocilia, at their apexes. The hair cells are divided into two groups by an arch known as the tunnel of Corti. Those on the side of the arch closest to the

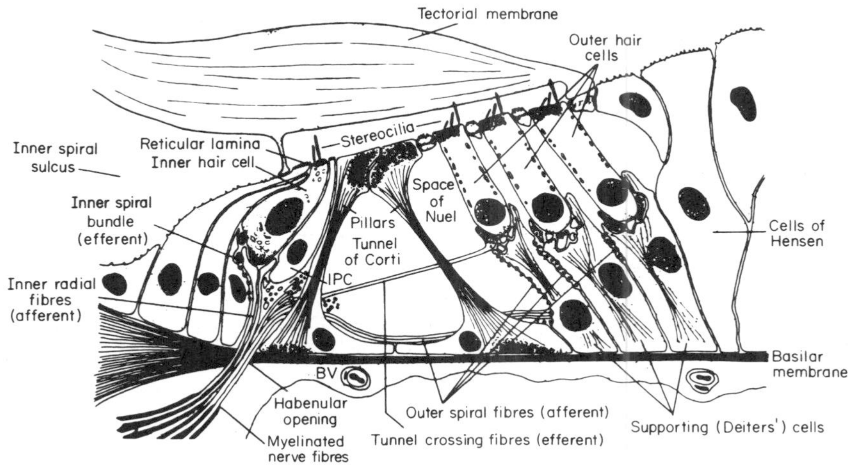

Fig. 1.3. Cross section of the organ of Corti as it appears in the basal turn of the cochlea. Adapted from Ryan and Dallos (1984).

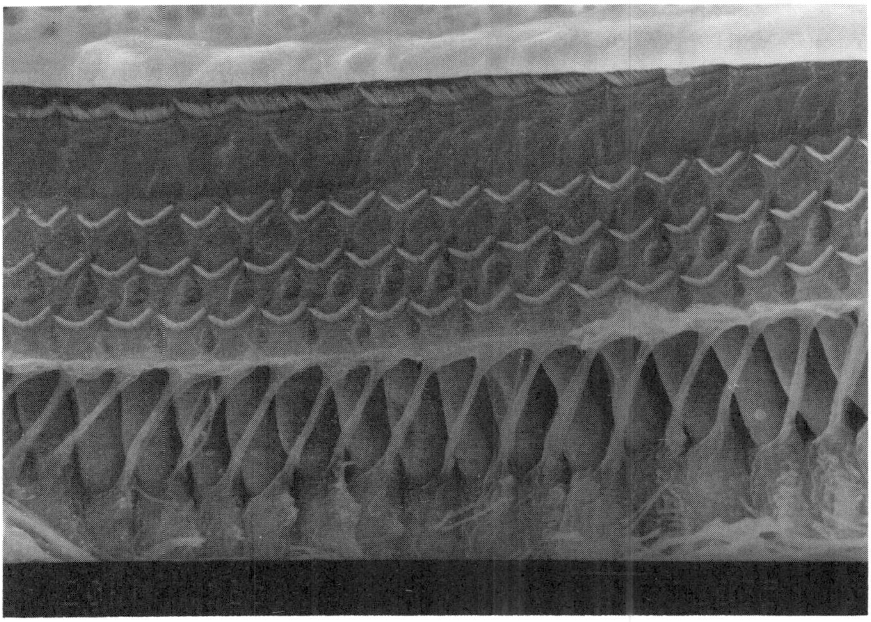

Fig. 1.4. The organ of Corti viewed from the top, the tectorial membrane having been removed. The stereocilia of the IHCs form a single row visible towards the top of the figure. The stereocilia of the OHCs form three rows. The 'sausage-like' structures are the bodies of the OHCs. The electronmicrograph was supplied by Dr. Andrew Forge of the Institute of Laryngology and Otology, University College London Medical School.

outside of the cochlea are known as outer hair cells (OHCs), and they are arranged in three rows in the cat and up to five rows in humans. The hair cells on the other side of the arch form a single row, and are known as inner hair cells (IHCs). The stereocilia on each OHC form a V or W-shaped pattern, and they are arranged in rows (usually about three) that are graded in height, the tallest stereocilia lying on the outside of the W or V. The stereocilia on each IHC are also arranged in rows graded in height, but the arrangement is more like a straight line or a broad arc. There are about 25,000 OHCs, each with about 140 stereocilia protruding from it, while there are about 3500 IHCs, each with about 40 stereocilia.

The tectorial membrane, which has a gelatinous structure, lies above the hair cells. It appears that the stereocilia of the OHCs actually make contact with the tectorial membrane, but this may not be true for the IHCs. The tectorial membrane appears to be effectively hinged at one side (the left in Figure 1.3), so that when the BM moves up and down, a shearing motion is created between the BM and the tectorial membrane. As a result the stereocilia at the tops of the hair cells are displaced. It is thought that this opens ion channels, modulating the standing flow of current though the IHCs, and resulting in a receptor current. This current then leads to a receptor potential, which leads in turn to the release of neurotransmitter and the generation of action potentials in the neurones of the auditory nerve. Thus the IHCs act to transduce mechanical movements into neural activity.

There are many details of the transduction process which remain poorly understood. However, it now seems clear that the IHCs and OHCs have very different functions. The great majority of afferent neurones, which carry information from the cochlea to higher levels of the auditory system, connect to IHCs; each IHC is contacted by about 20 neurones (Spoendlin 1970). Thus, most, if not all, information about sounds is conveyed via the IHCs. The main role of the OHCs may be actively to influence the mechanics of the cochlea; the consequences of this are described below. There is even evidence that the OHCs have a motor function, changing their length and shape in response to electrical stimulation (for a review, see Pickles 1988).

It is likely that the action of the OHCs is partly under the control of higher centres of the auditory system. There are about 1800 efferent nerve fibres which carry information from the auditory system to the cochlea, most of them originating in the superior olivary complex of the brain stem. Many of these efferent fibres make contact with the OHCs, and thus can affect their activity. It appears that even the earliest stages in the analysis of auditory signals are partly under the control of higher centres.

Tuning on the basilar membrane

When the oval window is set in motion by an incoming sound, a pressure difference occurs across the BM. The pressure wave travels almost instantaneously through the incompressible fluids of the cochlea. Consequently, the pressure difference is applied essentially simultaneously along the whole length of the BM. This causes a pattern of motion to develop on the BM. The pattern does not depend on which end of the cochlea is stimulated. Sounds which reach the cochlea via the bones of the head rather than through the air do not produce atypical responses.

The response of the BM to stimulation with a sinusoid of a specific frequency takes the form of a travelling wave which moves along the BM from the base towards the apex. The amplitude of the wave increases at first and then decreases rather abruptly. The basic form of the wave is illustrated in Figure 1.5, which shows the instantaneous displacement of the BM (derived from a cochlear model) for two successive instants in time, in response to a 200-Hz sinusoid. This figure also shows the line joining the amplitude peaks, which is called the envelope. The distance between peaks or zero-crossings in the wave decreases as the wave travels along, and the envelope shows a peak at a particular position on the BM.

The response of the BM to sounds of different frequencies is strongly affected by its mechanical properties, which vary progressively from base to apex. At the base it is relatively narrow and stiff, while at the apex it is wider and much less stiff. As a result, the position of the peak in the pattern of vibration differs according to the frequency of stimulation. High-frequency sounds produce a maximum displacement of the BM near the base, while low-frequency sounds produce a maximum near the apex. Figure 1.6 shows the envelopes of the patterns of vibration for several different low-frequency sinusoids (data from von Békésy 1960). Although it is now known that responses on the BM are more sharply tuned than shown in this figure, the figure does illustrate the important point that sounds of different frequencies produce maximum displacement at different places along the BM, i.e. there is a frequency-to-place transformation. If two or more sinusoids with different frequencies are presented simultaneously, each produces maximum displacement at its appropriate place on the BM. Thus, in effect, the cochlea behaves like a frequency analyser, although with a less than perfect resolution.

A number of different methods may be used to specify the 'sharpness' of tuning of the patterns of vibration on the BM. Most of the recent data are based on measurements of the responses of a single point on the BM to sinusoids of

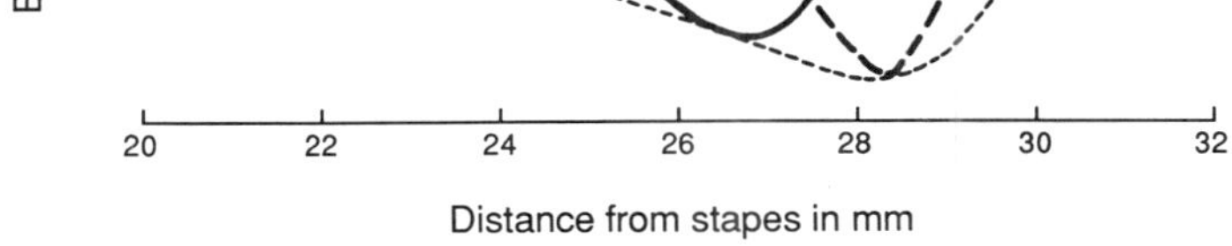

Fig. 1.5. The instantaneous displacement of the cochlear partition at two successive instants in time, derived from a cochlear model. The pattern moves from left to right, building up gradually with distance, and decaying rapidly beyond the point of maximal displacement. The short-dashed line represents the envelope traced out by the amplitude peaks in the waveform. Redrawn from von Békésy (1947).

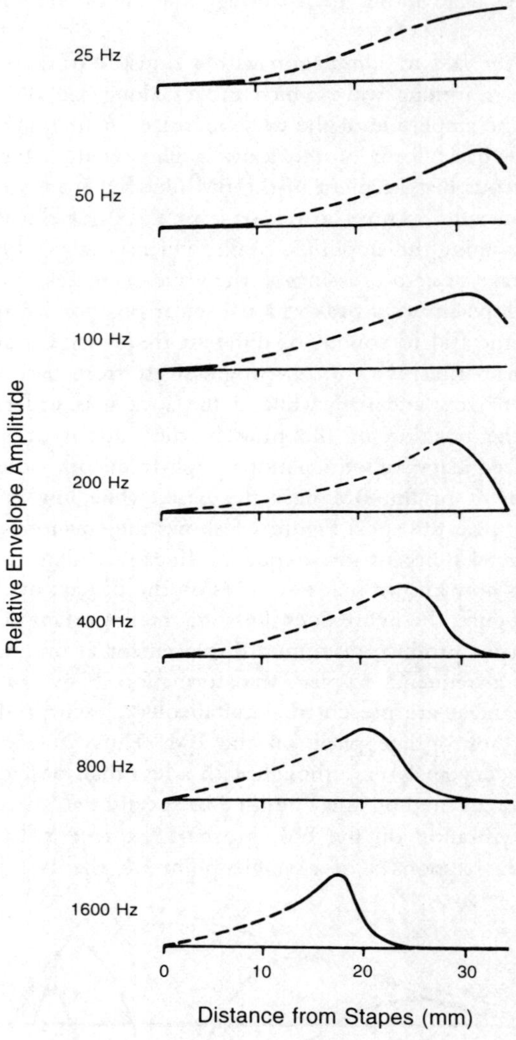

Fig. 1.6. Envelopes of patterns of vibration on the basilar membrane for a number of low-frequency sounds. Solid lines indicate the results of actual measurements, while the dashed lines are von Békésy's extrapolations. Redrawn from von Békésy (1960).

differing frequency. Each point on the BM can be considered as a bandpass filter with a certain centre frequency or characteristic frequency (CF) and bandwidth, and with certain slopes outside the passband. Thus measures such as the 3-dB bandwidth, and slopes in dB/octave, can be applied to the responses of specific points on the BM. Often it is difficult to measure the 3-dB bandwidth accurately, and a measure taken further down from the passband is used. The commonest measure is the 10-dB bandwidth, which is the difference between the two frequencies at which the response has fallen by 10 dB. It is sometimes useful to use the relative bandwidth, which is the bandwidth divided by the CF. The reciprocal of the relative bandwidth gives a measure of the sharpness of tuning, known as Q. A large Q value indicates a sharply tuned filter. Normally it is assumed that the 3-dB bandwidth is used to define Q. However, it is quite common in measurements of BM responses, and neural responses (see later), to use the 10-dB bandwidth. In this case the measure of sharpness of tuning is described as Q10 dB.

Most of the pioneering work on patterns of vibration along the BM was done by von Békésy (1960). His technique involved the use of a light microscope and stroboscopic illumination to measure the vibration amplitude at many points along the BM in human cadaver ears. For practical reasons his measurements were limited to the apical end of the BM, so that he measured mainly low-frequency responses. The 'tuning curves' found by von Békésy were rather broad, with Q10dB values of about 1. However, there are a number of difficulties associated with the technique used by von Békésy. Firstly, the vibration amplitudes had to be at least of the order of one wavelength of visible light, which required very high sound levels—about 140 dB SPL. The sharpness of tuning on the BM is now known to reduce with increasing sound level. Secondly, the frequency analysing mechanism is physiologically vulnerable, so that cadaver ears give markedly atypical responses. We now know that the active mechanism mediated by the OHCs ceases to function after death; indeed its operation can be adversely affected by even moderate trauma.

Recent measurements of BM vibration, using different techniques in living animals, have shown that the BM is much more sharply tuned than found by von Békésy. One technique uses an effect called the Mössbauer effect. A radioactive source of gamma rays, of very small mass and physical dimensions, is placed upon the BM. Changes in the velocity of this source, produced by motion of the BM, can be detected as a change in the wavelength of the emitted radiation. This is an example of a Doppler shift, and is the same in principle as the shift in pitch that can be heard when a vehicle with a siren approaches a person and then moves away; the pitch appears to drop. The sensitivity of this method increases with increasing frequency; at 1000 Hz a peak deflection of about 20 nanometres (nm) (1 nm is a ten millionth of a centimetre) can be measured, while at 10 kHz the limit is about 2 nm. Thus this method has been used mainly at high frequencies, where sound levels much lower than those used by von Békésy can be utilized. A second technique involves placing a small mirror on the surface of the BM and shining a laser beam onto the mirror. The interference between the incident and reflected light can be used to determine the motion of the mirror; hence the name 'laser interferometry'. A third technique involves placing glass microbeads on the BM and measuring the Doppler shift of laser light reflected from the beads, a technique called 'Doppler-shift laser velocimetry'.

Results using these techniques in live animals have shown that the sharpness of tuning of the BM depends critically on the physiological condition of the animal; the better the condition, the sharper is the tuning (Khanna and Leonard 1982;

Sellick *et al.* 1982; Leonard and Khanna 1984; Robles *et al.* 1986; Ruggero 1992). Nowadays, the physiological status of the cochlea is often monitored by placing an electrode in or near the auditory nerve, and measuring the combined responses of the neurones to tone bursts or clicks; this response is known as the compound action potential (AP or CAP). The lowest sound level at which an AP can be detected is called the AP threshold. Usually, the BM is sharply tuned when the AP threshold is low, indicating good physiological condition.

An example is given in Figure 1.7, which shows the input sound level (in dB SPL) required to produce a constant velocity of motion at a particular point on the BM, as a function of stimulus frequency (Sellick *et al.* 1982). This is sometimes called a 'constant velocity tuning curve'. At the start of the experiment, when AP thresholds were low, a very sharp tuning curve was obtained (solid circles). As the condition of the animal deteriorated, the tuning became broader, and the sound level required to produce the criterion response increased markedly around the tip.

It is now clear that in a normal, healthy ear each point on the BM is sharply tuned, responding with high sensitivity to a limited range of frequencies, and requiring higher and higher sound intensities to produce a response as the frequency is moved beyond that range. Q10 dB values are typically in the range 3–10. It also seems likely that the sharp tuning and high sensitivity reflect the active

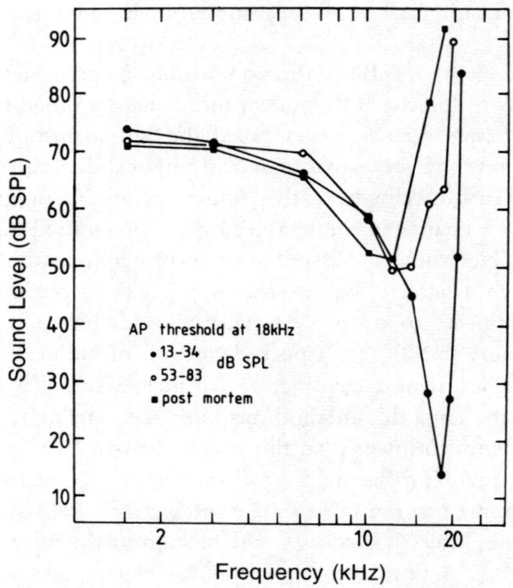

Fig. 1.7. Tuning curves measured at a single point on the basilar membrane. Each curve shows the input sound level required to produce a constant velocity on the basilar membrane, plotted as a function of stimulus frequency. The curve marked by solid circles was obtained at the start of the experiment when the animal was in good physiological condition. Redrawn from Sellick *et al.* (1982).

process; that is, they do not result simply from the mechanical properties of the BM and surrounding fluid, but depend on biological structures actively influencing the mechanics (Pickles 1986, 1988; Yates 1986). The most likely structures to play this role are the OHCs.

The nonlinearity of input–output functions on the BM

Recent work has also shown that the BM vibration is nonlinear; the magnitude of the response does not grow directly in proportion with the magnitude of the input (Rhode 1971; Rhode and Robles 1974; Sellick *et al.* 1982; Ruggero 1992). This is illustrated in Figure 1.8, which shows what are referred to as input–output functions of the BM for a place with a CF of 8 kHz (from Robles *et al.* 1986). A series of curves is shown; each curve represents a particular stimulating frequency, indicated by a number (in kHz) close to the curve. The output (velocity of vibration) is plotted on a log scale as a function of the input sound level (in dB SPL). If the responses were linear, the functions would be parallel to the dashed line. Two functions are shown for a CF tone (8 kHz), one (at higher levels) obtained about one hour after the other. The slight shift between the two was probably caused by a deterioration in the condition of the animal.

While the function for the CF tone is almost linear for very low input sound levels (below 20 dB) and approaches linearity at high input sound levels (above 90 dB), the function has a very shallow slope at mid-range levels. This indicates a compressive nonlinearity; a large range of input sound levels is compressed into a smaller range of responses on the BM. The form of this function can be explained, at least crudely, in the following way. At low and medium sound levels the active physiological mechanism amplifies the response on the BM. The amplification may

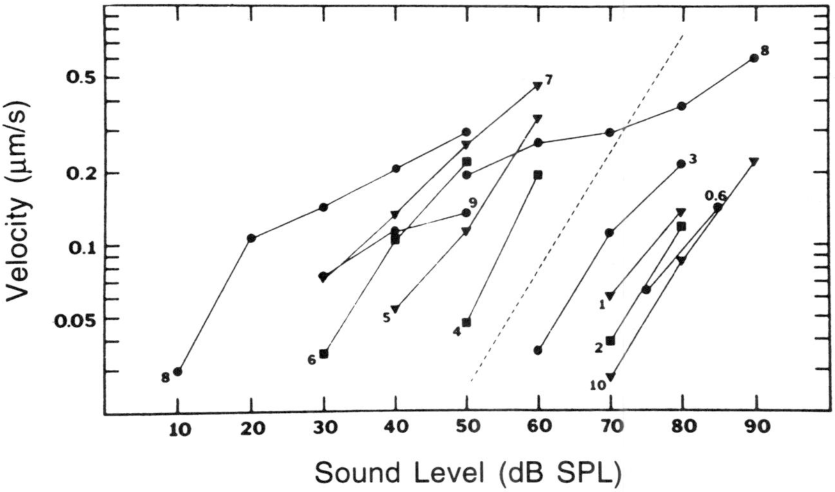

Fig. 1.8. Input–output functions for a place on the BM with CF = 8 kHz. The stimulating frequency, in kHz, is indicated by a number close to each curve. The dashed line indicates the slope that would be obtained if the responses were linear (velocity directly proportional to sound pressure). Redrawn from Robles *et al.* (1986).

be as much as 40–50 dB. At very low sound levels, below about 20 dB, the amplification is roughly constant. As the sound level increases, the amplification progressively reduces. Thus the response grows more slowly than it would in a linear system. When the sound level is sufficiently high, around 90 dB SPL, the active mechanism is unable to contribute any amplification, and the response becomes linear.

The nonlinearity mainly occurs when the stimulating frequency is close to the CF of the point on the BM that is being monitored. For stimuli with frequencies well away from the CF, the responses are more linear. Hence the curves for frequencies of 7 and 9 kHz (close to CF) show shallow slopes, while the curves for frequencies below 7 kHz and above 9 kHz show steeper (linear) slopes. Effectively, the compression occurs only around the peak of the response pattern on the BM. As a result, the peak in the pattern flattens out at high sound levels, which partly accounts for the broad tuning observed by von Békésy. The nonlinearity decreases as the physiological condition of the cochlea worsens, and after death the responses are linear. This suggests that the active process responsible for sharp tuning and high sensitivity on the BM is also responsible for the nonlinearity.

Responses to complex sounds

All of the results described so far were obtained with sinusoidal stimuli. While there are some disagreements about the details of patterns of vibration, it is now beyond doubt that pure tones produce patterns with single maxima, whose positions on the BM depend upon frequency. In other words, there is a frequency-to-place conversion. The situation with other types of sounds is somewhat more complex. Consider first the case of two sinusoids, of different frequencies, presented simultaneously. The kind of pattern that occurs depends on the frequency separation of the two tones. If this is very large, then the two tones produce two, effectively separate, patterns of vibration. Each produces a maximum at the place on the BM which would have been excited most had that tone been presented alone. Thus the response of the BM to a low-frequency tone of moderate intensity is essentially unaffected by a high-frequency tone, and vice versa. In this kind of situation the BM behaves like a frequency analyser, breaking down the complex sound into its sinusoidal components. When the two tones are relatively close in frequency, however, the patterns of vibration on the BM interact, so that some points on the BM respond to both of the tones. At those points the displacement of the BM as a function of time is not sinusoidal, but is a complex waveform resulting from the interference of the two tones. When the two tones are sufficiently close in frequency, there is no longer a separate maximum in the pattern of vibration for each of the component tones; instead there is a single, broader, maximum. Thus, in a sense, the BM has failed to resolve the individual frequency components.

It is of interest to consider the pattern of responses on the BM to a harmonic complex tone, such as a voiced vowel or an instrument playing a note. The position of the BM which is excited most by a given frequency varies approximately with the logarithm of frequency, for frequencies above 500 Hz. Further, the relative bandwidths of the patterns of vibration on the BM in response to sinusoidal stimulation are approximately constant in this frequency range. This means that the frequency separation necessary for the resolution of two tones is proportional to centre frequency. For a harmonic complex tone, the frequency separation between adjacent harmonics is constant (and equal to the fundamental frequency). Thus the patterns of vibration for the higher harmonics overlap much more than those for the lower harmonics. A perceptual consequence of this is that individual low harmonics can often be 'heard out' as separate tones, while higher harmonics cannot be individually heard. These factors play a crucial role in the perception of complex tones, as will become apparent in chapter 5.

Two-tone suppression

Experiments using two tones have revealed another aspect of nonlinearity on the BM, namely two-tone suppression. The effect is analogous to an effect that was first discovered from measurements of the responses of single neurones in the auditory nerve (see below for details). The response to a tone with frequency close to the CF of the place on the BM being studied can be reduced by a second tone with a higher or lower frequency (Rhode 1977; Patuzzi *et al.* 1984; Ruggero *et al.* 1992). The effect is illustrated in Figure 1.9 for a 'probe' tone of 8.8 kHz (close to the CF) and a suppressor tone at 10.6 kHz. Ruggero *et al.* (1992) provided a detailed comparison of the properties of mechanical two-tone suppression on the BM and two-tone suppression measured in the auditory nerve. They concluded that all of the properties match qualitatively (and mostly quantitatively), and that

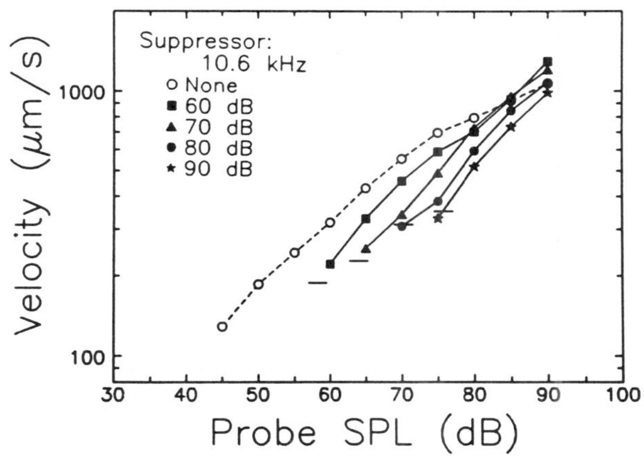

Fig. 1.9. An example of two-tone suppression for a place on the BM with CF = 8.6 kHz. The dashed curve with open circles shows an input–ouput function for an 8.8-kHz tone alone, referred to as the 'probe'. The solid curves show input–output functions when a suppressor tone was added to the probe. The suppressor was presented at each of several overall levels, from 60 to 90 dB SPL, as indicated by the key in the figure. Redrawn from Ruggero *et al.* (1992). The solid curves are truncated at the level where the suppressor led to an increase in response rather than a decrease.

two-tone suppression in the auditory nerve probably originates from two-tone suppression on the BM. Like the other nonlinearities observed on the BM, two-tone suppression is physiologically vulnerable, and is reduced or abolished by damage to the cochlea, especially damage to the outer hair cells (see below for details).

Combination tone generation

Yet another aspect of BM nonlinearity is the generation of distortion products, also known as combination tones. When two tones are presented simultaneously, and their frequency separation is not too great, their response patterns overlap on the BM. It appears that, at the point of overlap, distortion products are generated that behave like additional sinusoidal tones. For example, if the two primary tones presented to the ear have frequencies f_1 and f_2 ($f_2>f_1$), the distortion products may have frequencies such as $2f_1–f_2$ and $2f_2$-f_1. The distortion products appear to propagate along the BM to the locations tuned to their own frequencies (Robles *et al.* 1991). Like the other nonlinearities observed in BM responses, the nonlinear generation of combination tones only occurs when the cochlea is in good physiological condition; cochlear damage results in their reduction or abolition.

Human listeners can sometimes hear these additional tones. The one with frequency $2f_1$-f_2 is especially easy to hear. It is audible even for relatively low levels of the primary tones when frequency f_2 is about 1.2 times frequency f_1 (Smoorenburg 1972a,b).

Cochlear echoes

Evidence supporting the idea that there are active biological processes influencing cochlear mechanics has come from a remarkable phenomenon first reported by Kemp (1978). If a low-level click is applied to the ear, then it is possible to detect sound being reflected from the ear, using a microphone sealed into the ear canal. The early part of this reflected sound appears to come from the middle ear, but some sound can be detected for delays from 5 to 60 ms following the time of presentation of the click. These delays are far too long to be attributed to the middle ear, and thus they almost certainly result from activity in the cochlea itself. The reflected sounds are known as 'evoked oto-acoustic emissions' although they have also been called 'Kemp echoes' and 'cochlear echoes'.

Although the input click in Kemp's experiment contained energy over a wide range of frequencies, only certain frequencies were present in the reflected sound. Kemp suggested that the reflections are generated at points on the BM, or in the transduction mechanism, where there is a gradient or discontinuity in the mechanical or electrical properties. The response is nonlinear, in that the reflected sound does not have an intensity in direct proportion to the input intensity. In fact, the relative level of the reflection is greatest at low sound levels; the echo grows about 3 dB for each 10 dB increase in input level. This nonlinear behaviour can be used to distinguish the response arising from the cochlea from the middle ear response; the latter behaves in a linear manner. Sometimes the amount of energy reflected from the cochlea at a given frequency may exceed that which was present in the input click. This has led Kemp and others to suggest that the echo reflects an active process of biological amplification. Indeed, many ears emit sounds in the absence of any input and these can be detected in the ear canal (Zurek 1981). Such sounds are called 'spontaneous oto-acoustic emissions', and their existence indicates that there is a source of energy within the cochlea which is capable of generating sounds.

Cochlear echoes can be very stable in a given individual, both in waveform and frequency content, but each ear gives its own characteristic response. Responses tend to be strongest between 500 and 2500 Hz, probably because transmission from the cochlea back through the middle ear is most efficient in this range. Cochlear echoes can be measured for brief tone bursts as well as clicks, and it is even possible to detect a reflected component in response to continuous stimulation with pure tones. The echo response to a particular component in a stimulus can be suppressed if the ear is stimulated more strongly at a neighbouring frequency, an effect analogous to the mechanical two-tone suppression described earlier. By presenting neighbouring tones at a variety of frequencies, and adjusting their levels, it is possible to map out contours of equal suppression. These contours have the same general shape as tuning curves on the BM. This lends strong support to the notion that the echoes are generated within the cochlea.

Cochlear echoes are usually only observed in ears which are in good physiological condition. Thus human ears with even moderate pathology of cochlear origin usually show no detectable echoes. The echo is also abolished in ears which have been exposed to intense sounds or to drugs which adversely affect the operation of the cochlea. In the former case, the echo may return after a period of recovery. This suggests that the echo is linked to a physiologically vulnerable process, just like the process which is responsible for the sharp tuning and high sensitivity of the BM. The measurement of cochlear echoes provides a sensitive way of monitoring the physiological state of the cochlea, and is now being commonly applied in clinical situations, especially for assessing cochlear function in the very young.

When the ear is stimulated with two tones, a cochlear echo may be detected at the frequency of one or more combination tones, particularly $2f_1$-f_2. This confirms that the combination tone is present as a mechanical disturbance in the cochlea, probably as a travelling wave on the BM. The level of the combination tone, relative to the level of the primary tones in the ear canal, can be reversibly reduced by exposing the ear to a fatiguing tone of 80–90 dB SPL at a frequency near or slightly below the primary frequencies. Again this indicates that the nonlinear aspect of cochlear function is physiologically vulnerable.

Sometimes the transient stimulation used to evoke a cochlear echo induces a sustained oscillation at a particular frequency, and the subject may report hearing this oscillation as a tonal sensation. The phenomenon of hearing sound in the absence of external stimulation is known as tinnitus. It appears that tinnitus may arise from abnormal activity at several different points in the auditory system, but in a few cases it corresponds to mechanical activity in the cochlea.

In summary, while the exact mechanism by which the cochlear echo is generated is not understood, there is agreement that it is connected with active processes occurring inside the cochlea. These processes have a strong nonlinear component, they are biologically active, they are physiologically vulnerable and they appear to be responsible for the sensitivity and sharp tuning of the BM.

Neural responses in the normal auditory nerve

Most studies of activity in the auditory nerve have used electrodes with very fine tips, known as microelectrodes. These record the nerve impulses, or spikes, in single auditory nerve fibres (often called single units). The main findings, summarised below, seem to hold for most mammals.

Spontaneous firing rates and thresholds

Most neurones show a certain baseline firing rate, called the spontaneous rate, in the absence of any external stimulus. Liberman (1978) presented evidence that auditory nerve fibres could be classified into three groups on the basis of their spontaneous rates. About 61% of fibres have high spontaneous rates (18 to 250 spikes per second); 23% have medium rates (0.5 to 18 spikes per second); and 16% have low spontaneous rates (less than 0.5 spike per second). The spontaneous rates are correlated with the position and size of the synapses of the neurones on the IHCs. High spontaneous rates are associated with large synapses, primarily located on the side of the IHCs facing the OHCs. Low spontaneous rates are associated with smaller synapses on the opposite side of the hair cells. The spontaneous rates are also correlated with the thresholds of the neurones. The threshold is the lowest sound level at which a change in response of the neurone can be measured. High spontaneous rates tend to be associated with low thresholds and vice versa. The most sensitive neurones may have thresholds close to 0 dB SPL, whereas the least sensitive neurones may have thresholds of 80 dB SPL or more.

Tuning curves and iso-rate contours

The frequency selectivity of a single nerve fibre is often illustrated by a tuning curve, which shows the fibre's threshold as a function of frequency. This curve is also known as the frequency-threshold curve (FTC). The stimuli are usually tone bursts, rather than continuous tones. This avoids effects of long-term adaptation, and also makes it easier to distinguish spontaneous from evoked neural activity. The frequency at which the threshold of the fibre is lowest is called the characteristic frequency (CF). Some typical tuning curves are presented in Fig. 1.10. On the logarithmic frequency scale used, the tuning curves are generally steeper on the high-frequency side than on the low-frequency side. It is generally assumed that the frequency selectivity in single auditory nerve fibres occurs because those fibres are responding to activity at restricted regions of the BM. In other words, a single nerve fibre is assumed to derive its output from a particular part of the BM. Experiments tracing single neurones whose tuning curves had been determined

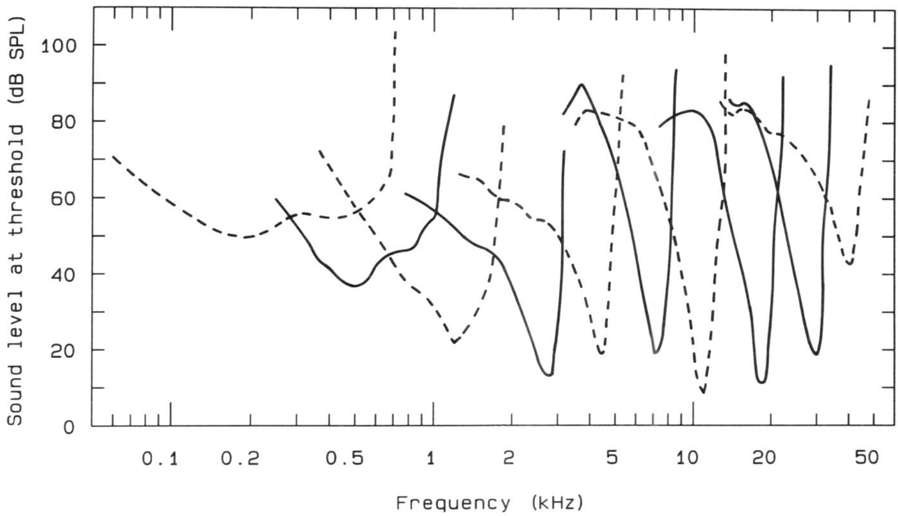

Fig. 1.10. A sample of tuning curves (also called frequency-threshold curves) obtained from single neurones in the auditory nerve of anaesthetized cats. Each curve shows results for one neurone. Dashed and solid lines are used to aid identification of individual curves. The sound level required for threshold is plotted as a function of the stimulus frequency (logarithmic scale). Redrawn from Palmer (1987).

directly confirm this supposition (Liberman 1982). Furthermore, CFs are distributed in an orderly manner in the auditory nerve. Fibres with high CFs are found in the periphery of the nerve bundle, and there is an orderly decrease in CF towards the centre of the nerve bundle (Kiang *et al.* 1965). This kind of arrangement is known as tonotopic organization and it indicates that the place representation of frequency along the BM is preserved as a place representation in the auditory nerve. It appears that the sharpness of tuning of the BM is essentially the same as the sharpness of tuning of single neurones in the auditory nerve (Khanna and Leonard 1982; Sellick *et al.* 1982; Robles *et al.* 1986).

In order to provide a description of the characteristics of single fibres at levels above threshold, iso-rate contours can be plotted. To determine an iso-rate contour the intensity of sinusoidal stimulation required to produce a predetermined firing rate in the neurone is plotted as a function of frequency. The resulting curves are generally similar in shape to tuning curves, although they sometimes broaden at high sound levels.

Rate versus level functions

Figure 1.11 shows how the rate of discharge of an auditory nerve fibre changes as a function of stimulus level. The stimulus was a sinusoid at the CF of the unit. The general shape of the curve is typical of most auditory nerve fibres, although there is considerable variability in both the spontaneous firing rate and the maximum firing rate. Notice that above a certain sound level the neurone no longer responds to increases in sound level with an increase in firing rate; the

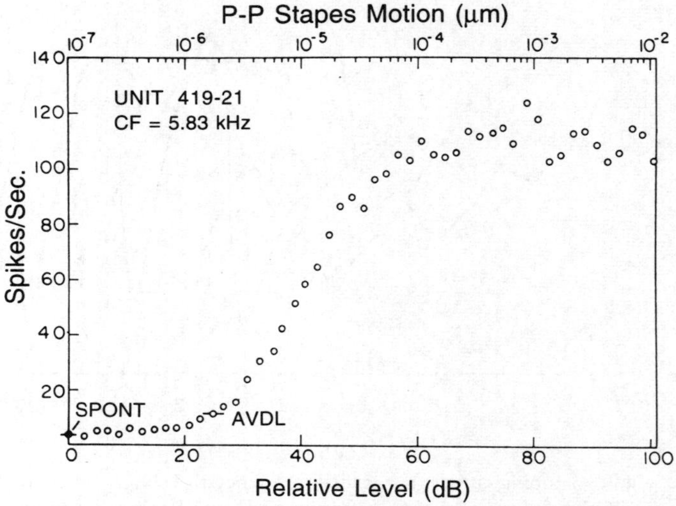

Fig. 1.11. An example of how the discharge rate of a single auditory nerve fibre varies as a function of stimulus level, for a stimulating tone at the CF of the neurone. The threshold of the neurone is the lowest sound level at which there is a detectable change in firing rate and is indicated by the letters AVDL (audio visual detection level). The sound level is specified in dB with an arbitrary reference level. The level at the point marked AVDL corresponds to about 2 dB SPL. Redrawn from Kiang (1968).

neurone is said to be saturated. The range of sound levels between threshold and the level at which saturation occurs is called the dynamic range. This range is correlated with the threshold and spontaneous rate of the neurone; high spontaneous rates and low thresholds are associated with small dynamic ranges. For most neurones the dynamic range is between 20 and 50 dB, but a few neurones do not show complete saturation; instead the firing rate continues to increase gradually with increasing sound level even at high sound levels. This has been called 'sloping saturation' (Sachs and Abbas 1974) and it occurs particularly for neurones with low spontaneous rates and high thresholds.

The shapes of rate versus level functions can be understood in terms of two functions (Yates 1990; Patuzzi 1992). This is illustrated in Figure 1.12. The first function is the input–output function on the BM, illustrated schematically in the top-right panel. The second is the function relating BM displacement or velocity to the rate of spike generation for the particular neurone under consideration. This second function is similar in form for different neurones, showing saturation when the BM amplitude is a certain factor above the value required for threshold, but it varies in the amplitude required for threshold. This is illustrated in the top-left panel of Figure 1.12.

The variation across neurones probably depends mainly on the type of synapse, as discussed earlier. Neurones with low thresholds have large sensitive synapses. They start to respond at very low sound levels, where the input–output function

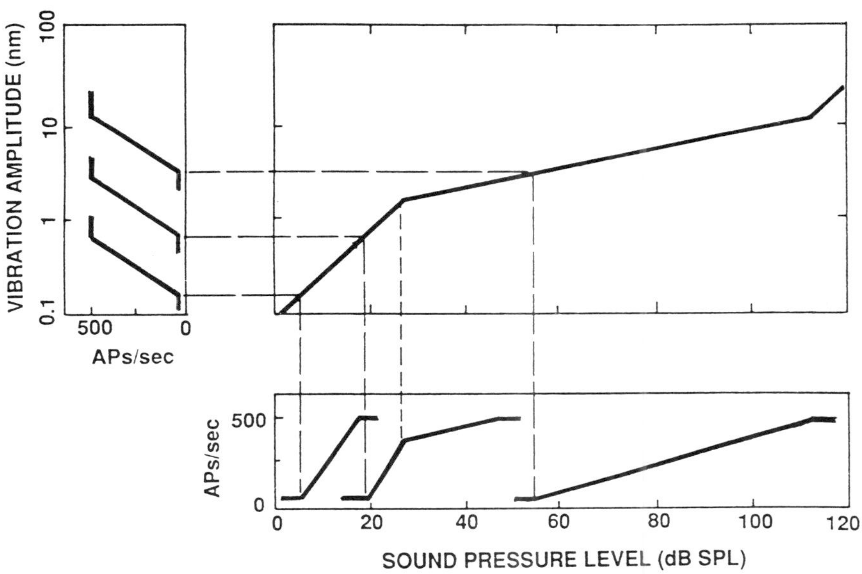

Fig. 1.12. Schematic illustration of how the shapes of rate-versus-level functions can be accounted for in terms of the BM input–output function (top-right panel), and the functions relating neural firing rate (APs/sec) to amplitude on vibration on the BM (top-left panel). Three such functions are shown, corresponding to synapses with different sensitivities. The resulting three rate-versus-level functions are shown in the bottom panel. Adapted from Patuzzi (1992).

on the BM is nearly linear. As the sound level increases, the BM displacement increases in a linear manner, and the neurone saturates relatively early, giving a small dynamic range, as shown by the left-most curve in the lower panel. Neurones with higher thresholds have less sensitive synapses. They respond over the range of sound levels where the BM input-output function shows a strong compressive nonlinearity. Hence a large increase in sound level is needed to increase the BM displacement to the point where the neurone saturates, and the neurone has a wide dynamic range, as shown by the right-most curve in the lower panel.

Phase locking

In response to a pure tone with a frequency below about 5 kHz, the nerve firings tend to be phase locked or synchronized to the stimulating waveform. A given nerve fibre does not necessarily fire on every cycle of the stimulus but, when firings do occur, they occur at roughly the same phase of the waveform each time. Thus the time intervals between firings are (approximately) integer multiples of the period of the stimulating waveform. For example, a 500-Hz tone has a period of 2 milliseconds (2 ms), so the intervals between nerve firings are approximately 2 ms, or 4 ms, or 6 ms, or 8 ms, etc. In general, a neurone does not fire in a completely regular manner, so that there are not exactly 500, or 250 or 125 spikes/s. However, information about the period of the stimulating waveform is

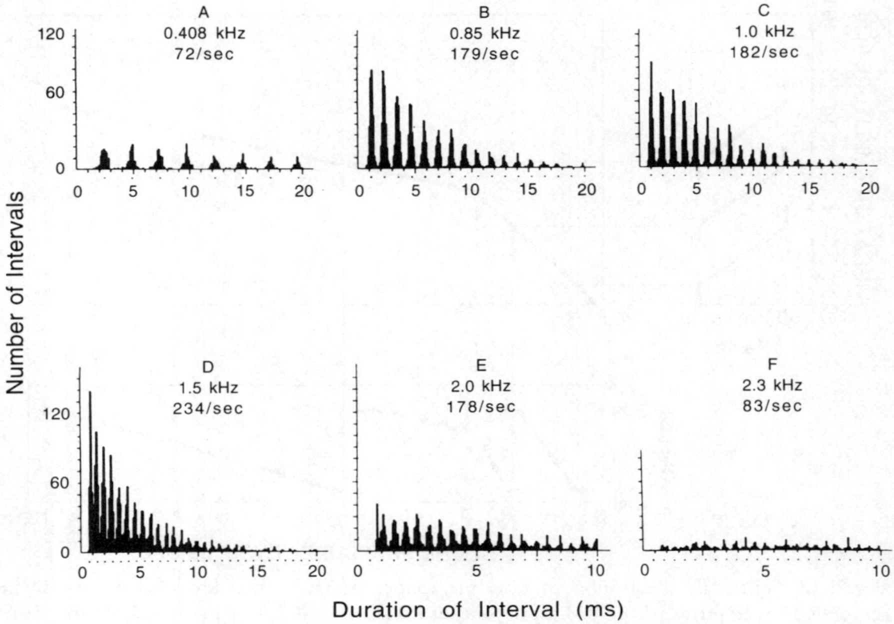

Fig. 1.13. Interspike interval histograms for a single auditory neurone (in the squirrel monkey) with a CF of 1.6 kHz. The frequency of the stimulating tone and the mean response rate in spikes per second are indicated above each histogram. All tones were at 80 dB SPL and of duration 1 s. Notice that the time scales in E and F differ from those in A to D. Redrawn from Rose *et al.* (1968).

carried unambiguously in the temporal pattern of firing of a single neurone. Phase locking is just what would be expected to occur as a result of the transduction process. Deflection of the stereocilia on the IHCs towards the outside of the cochlea, produced by movement of the BM towards the tectorial membrane, leads to neural excitation. No excitation occurs when the BM moves in the opposite direction. (This description is somewhat over-simplified; see, for example, Ruggero *et al.* 1986). Thus, nerve firings tend to occur on a deflection of the BM towards the tectorial membrane produced by the rarefaction phase of the signal.

One way to demonstrate phase locking in a single auditory nerve fibre is to plot a histogram of the time intervals between successive nerve firings. Several such interspike interval histograms are shown in Figure 1.13, for a neurone with a CF of 1.6 kHz. For each of the different stimulating frequencies (from 0.408 to 2.3 kHz in this case) the intervals between nerve spikes lie predominantly at integer multiples of the period of the stimulating tone. These intervals are indicated by dots below each abscissa. Thus, although the neurone does not fire on every cycle of the stimulus, the distribution of time intervals between nerve firings depends closely on the frequency of the stimulating waveform.

Phase locking does not occur over the whole range of audible frequencies. In most mammals it becomes progressively less precise for stimulus frequencies above

1 kHz, and it disappears completely at about 4–5 kHz (Rose *et al.* 1968), although the exact upper limit varies somewhat across species (Palmer and Russell 1986). Phase locking improves in precision with increasing sound level at low levels, and then stays roughly constant in precision over a very wide range of sound levels.

There is still considerable controversy over the extent to which information carried in the timing of neural impulses is actually used in perceptual processes. Most workers accept that the ability to localize sounds depends in part on a comparison of the temporal information from the two ears, but the relevance of temporal information in masking and in pitch perception is still hotly debated. These problems are discussed more fully in chapter 5.

Two-tone suppression

Auditory neurones show an effect that is exactly analogous to the two-tone suppression on the BM that was described earlier. Indeed, the neural effect was discovered long before the BM effect. The tone-driven activity of a single fibre in response to one tone can be suppressed by the presence of a second tone. This was originally called two-tone inhibition (Sachs and Kiang 1968), although the term 'two-tone suppression' is now generally preferred, since the effect does not appear to involve neural inhibition. Typically the phenomenon is investigated by presenting a tone at, or close to, the CF of a neurone. A second tone is then presented, its frequency and intensity are varied, and the effects of this on the response of the neurone are noted. When the frequency and intensity of the second tone fall within the excitatory area bounded by the tuning curve, this usually produces an increase in firing rate. However, when it falls just outside that area, the response

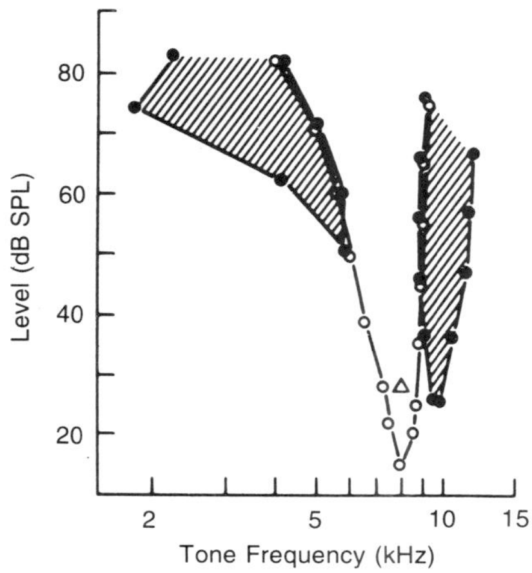

Fig. 1.14. Illustration of two-tone rate suppression. The open circles show the tuning curve (threshold versus frequency) of a single neurone with a CF at 8 kHz. The neurone was stimulated with a tone at CF, and just above threshold (indicated by the open triangle). A second tone was then added and its frequency and intensity varied. Any tone within the shaded areas bounded by the solid circles would reduce the response to the tone at CF by 20% or more. These are the suppression areas. Data from Arthur *et al.* (1971).

to the first tone is reduced or suppressed. The effect is usually greatest in two suppression regions at frequencies slightly above or below the area of the unit's excitatory response to a single tone, as illustrated in Figure 1.14. The suppression effect begins and ceases very rapidly, within a few milliseconds of the onset and termination of the second tone (Arthur *et al.* 1971), consistent with its likely origin as a mechanical effect on the BM.

Physiology and functional properties of the damaged cochlea

As reviewed above, there is strong evidence that the functioning of the normal cochlea depends upon the operation of an active mechanism that is especially dependent on the integrity of the OHCs. This mechanism may involve feedback of energy onto the BM, via the OHCs, and it plays an important role in producing the high sensitivity of the BM to weak sounds and the sharp tuning on the BM. The normal BM shows several nonlinearities, including compressive input–output functions, two-tone suppression, and combination-tone generation.

Cochlear hearing loss often involves damage to the OHCs and IHCs; the stereocilia may be distorted or destroyed, or entire hair cells may die. The OHCs are generally more vulnerable to damage than the IHCs. Some examples of OHC damage are shown in Figure 1.15 (more details are given below). When OHCs are damaged, the active mechanism tends to be reduced in effectiveness or lost altogether. As a result, several changes occur: the sensitivity to weak sounds is reduced, so sounds need to be more intense to produce a given magnitude of response on the BM; the tuning curves on the BM become much more broadly tuned; and all of the frequency-selective nonlinear effects disappear.

Neural responses

Some of the first evidence for a physiologically vulnerable active mechanism came from studies of the responses of single neurones in the auditory nerve. Robertson and Manley (1974) showed that the normal, sharp tuning seen in auditory neurones could be altered by reducing the oxygen supply to the animal. Slowing the rate of ventilation made the tuning curves less sharp, and at the same time decreased the sensitivity around the tip. These changes were reversible. Similar effects have been reported by Evans (1975), who also found that a reversible degradation in tuning could be produced by the ototoxic agents cyanide and frusemide. Evans and Harrison (1976) used the drug kanamycin to produce selective damage to the OHCs. They found that the threshold and tuning properties of auditory nerve fibres are dependent on the integrity of the OHCs.

BM responses

There have been a great many studies showing that the responses on the BM are highly physiologically vulnerable; some of these have been described earlier. The changes seen in responses of single neurones when the cochlea is damaged largely reflect the changes in BM responses. One example has already been given; see

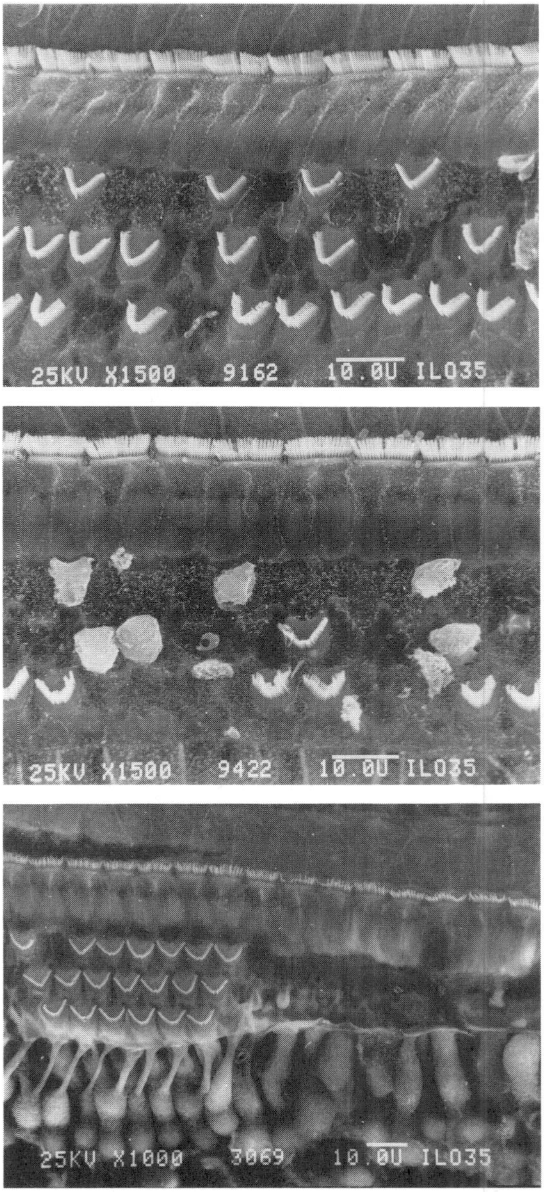

Fig. 1.15. Examples of patterns of damage to the OHCs. For the top two panels, the damage was caused by administration of aminoglycosides. For the bottom panel, the damage was of unknown origin. In the upper panel the stereocilia of some OHCs are missing. In the middle panel the stereocilia of the OHCs are mostly either missing or grossly deformed. In the bottom panel, the stereocilia of the OHCs are completely missing over a certain region. The bottom panel also shows expansion of the supporting cells to replace lost hair cells (compare Figure 1.4). The electronmicrographs were supplied by Dr. Andrew Forge of the Institute of Laryngology and Otology, University College London Medical School.

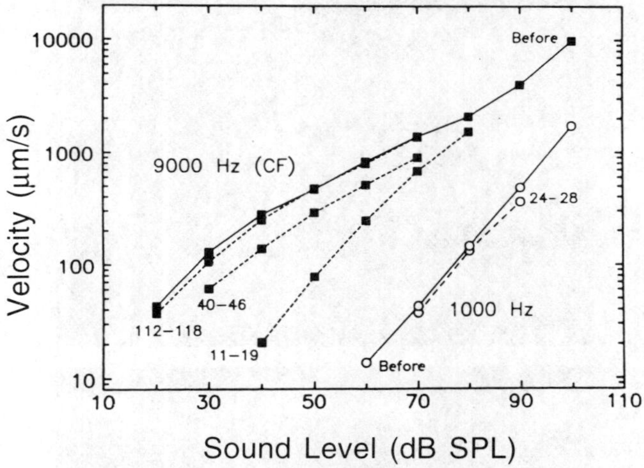

Fig. 1.16. Input-output functions on the BM immediately preceding (solid lines) and following (broken lines) an intravenous furosemide injection. See text for details. From Ruggero and Rich (1991).

Figure 1.6. In the great majority of studies, the changes in BM responses have been associated with some form of damage to the OHCs, either directly, or via some form of metabolic disturbance.

The effects of cochlear damage on the input–output functions of the BM of a chinchilla are illustrated in Figure 1.16 (Ruggero and Rich 1991). The solid curve with black squares, labelled 'Before', shows the input–output function obtained when the cochlea was in good condition; the stimulus was a CF tone at 9000 Hz. The curve shows a compressive nonlinearity for input sound levels between about 30 and 90 dB SPL. In contrast, the response to a tone with a frequency of 1000 Hz, well below the CF, is steeper and is almost linear (solid curve with open circles).

To manipulate the functioning of the cochlea, the animal was injected with furosemide, a diuretic that is known to disrupt hair cell potentials. The dashed curves in Figure 1.16 were obtained at various times after injection of the drug; the time is indicated by a range in minutes next to each curve. Shortly after the injection (11–19 minutes) the input-output function for the CF tone was markedly altered. The biggest alteration was at low sound levels. To produce a given response on the BM (say, 40 µm/s), the input level had to be increased by about 25 dB relative to the level measured before the injection. However, the response to a CF tone at a high level (80 dB SPL) was almost normal. This is consistent with the idea that the contribution of the active mechanism reduces progressively as the sound level is increased above about 40 dB. After a sufficiently long time (112–118 minutes), the input–output function returned to normal. Thus, in this case, the cochlear damage was reversible. Larger doses of the drug, or treatment with other drugs, can result in permanent cochlear damage.

It is noteworthy that injection of the drug did not change the input–output function for the 1000-Hz tone (see the curve with open symbols labelled 24–28). This is consistent with the idea that the active mechanism mainly influences responses around the peak of the response pattern evoked by a tone. Responses to tones with frequencies well away from the CF are linear, and remain so when the active mechanism is damaged.

Structure–function correlation

Liberman and his colleagues have conducted a series of studies in which they have produced cochlear damage and then measured the responses of neurones and compared them with structural changes in the cochlea (for a review, see Liberman *et al.* 1986). Using noise exposures or treatment with ototoxic drugs they have produced a variety of types of damage. In some cases, the IHCs have been damaged while the OHCs have remained nearly normal. In other cases, the OHCs were damaged and the IHCs were largely intact. After studying the properties of a given single neurone, the neurone was injected with horseradish peroxidase. This labelled the neurone so that it could be traced to the IHC with which it synapsed in the organ of Corti. In this way, the neural response properties could be directly compared with the structural changes in the IHC and the immediately surrounding structures in the organ of Corti.

Figure 1.17 shows the situation when there is partial loss of, or damage to, the OHCs, with intact IHCs. This pattern of damage is typical of that associated with ototoxic drugs, but is less typical of noise exposure. The left part of the figure schematically illustrates the pattern of structural damage. The view is looking down

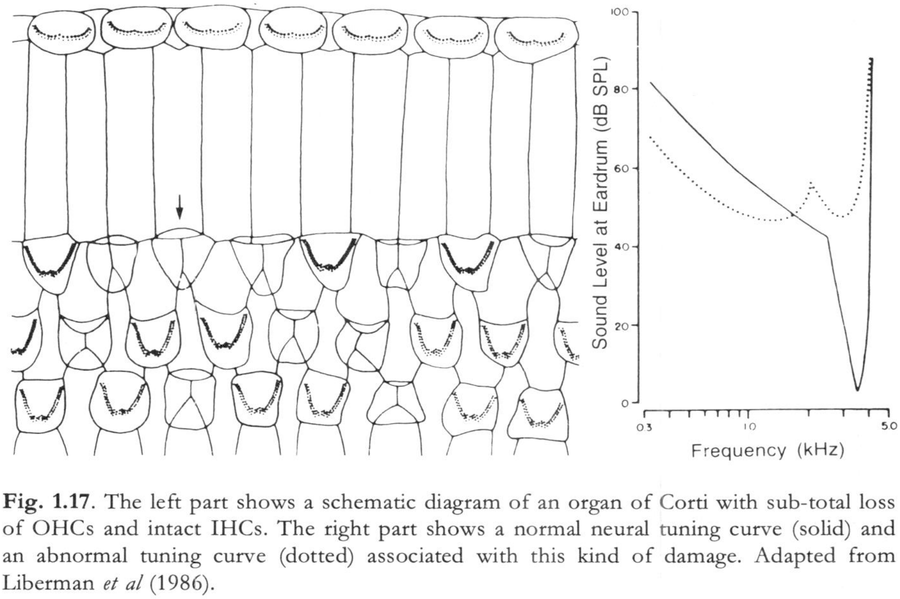

Fig. 1.17. The left part shows a schematic diagram of an organ of Corti with sub-total loss of OHCs and intact IHCs. The right part shows a normal neural tuning curve (solid) and an abnormal tuning curve (dotted) associated with this kind of damage. Adapted from Liberman *et al* (1986).

onto the tops of the hair cells, so each stereocilium appears as a small dot. The three rows of OHCs appear at the bottom. In the figure, some OHCs are missing or lack stereocilia (see arrow).

The right-hand part of Figure 1.17 shows a typical normal tuning curve (solid curve) and a tuning curve associated with this type of damage (dotted curve). The normal tuning curve shows a sharply tuned 'tip' and a broadly tuned 'tail'. The abnormal tuning curve also appears to have two sections, but the tip is elevated, and the tail is hypersensitive. The elevated tip may reflect the operation of the active mechanism at reduced effectiveness. The pattern of results suggests that the active mechanism is tuned to a frequency slightly above the resonance frequency of the passive mechanical BM at that place.

Figure 1.18 shows the situation when there is total loss of OHCs with intact IHCs. This pattern of damage is most easily produced with ototoxic drugs. The bowl-shaped abnormal tuning curve completely lacks the sharp tip, probably because the active mechanism is completely destroyed. The broad tuning of the curve probably depends largely on the passive mechanical properties of the BM.

Figure 1.19 shows the situation where there is severe damage to both the IHC and the OHC stereocilia. The damage to the OHCs is largely confined to the first row (the row closest to the IHCs). The damage to the OHCs is sufficient to eliminate completely the sharply tuned tip of the tuning curve, suggesting that the active mechanism is particularly dependent on the first row of OHCs. In addition the whole curve is shifted upwards, i.e. sensitivity is much less than normal. This overall loss of sensitivity (compare the tuning curves in Figures 1.18 and 1.19) can probably be attributed to the IHC damage. According to Liberman *et al.*, significant damage to the IHC stereocilia is always associated with reduced sensitivity on the tail of the tuning curve.

Liberman *et al.* did not find any cases of pure IHC damage, without OHC damage. It appears that the OHCs are generally more vulnerable to damage than

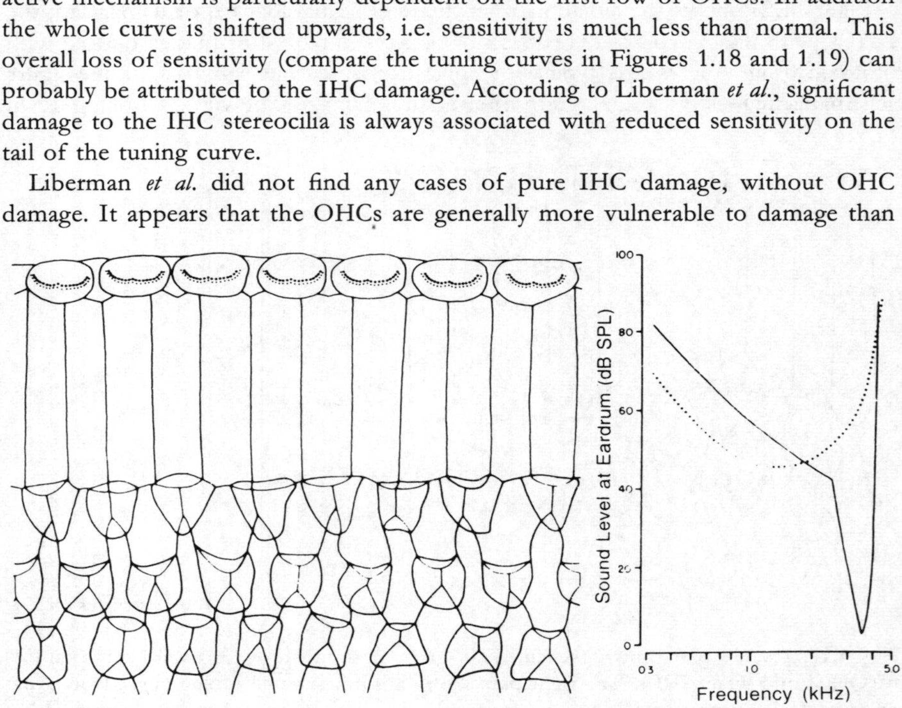

Fig. 1.18. As Figure 1.17, but for the situation with total loss of OHCs with intact IHCs.

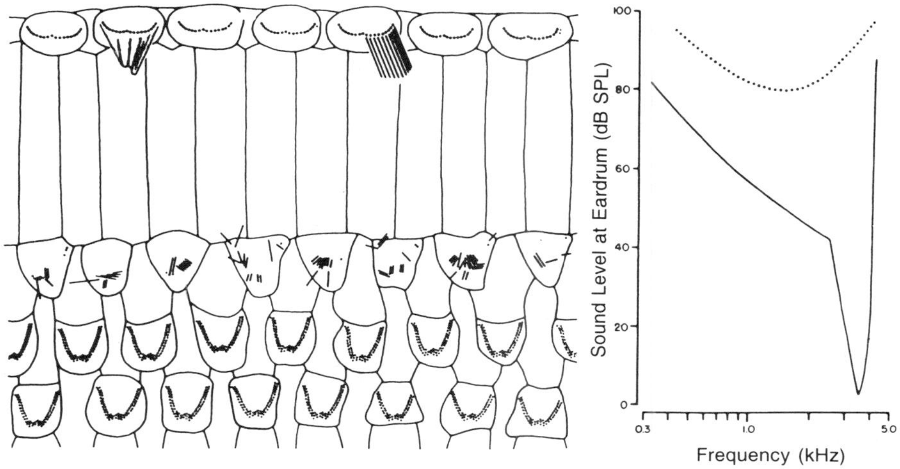

Fig. 1.19. As Figure 1.17, but for the situation with severe damage to both OHC and IHC stereocilia. Most of the damage to the OHC stereocilia is confined to the first row of cells.

the IHCs, and so damage to the IHCs is nearly always associated with damage to the OHCs. However, cases approximating pure IHC damage were sometimes found. Figure 1.20 shows the case of a neurone contacting an IHC missing the entire tall row of stereocilia (see arrow) in a region with only modest disarray of OHC stereocilia. The tuning curve shows a tip that is almost normal in shape, but the whole curve is shifted upwards by about 40 dB. It appears that the active

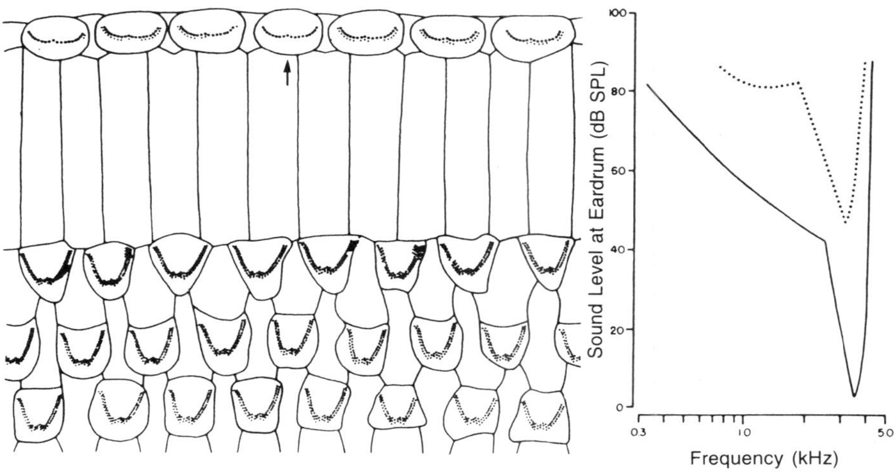

Fig. 1.20. As Figure 1.17, but for a situation with moderate damage to IHC stereocilia and minimal damage to OHC stereocilia.

mechanism was operating, but the transduction mechanism had greatly reduced sensitivity.

These findings can be summarised as follows. The OHCs appear to be responsible for the sharp tips of the tuning curves. When the OHCs are damaged the sharp tip becomes elevated, or may disappear altogether. This can cause a threshold elevation around the tip of the tuning curve of 40–50 dB. The condition of the OHCs determines the ratio of tip-to-tail thresholds. Damage to the IHCs causes an overall loss of sensitivity. This is apparent in the tail of the tuning curve, whether or not the OHCs are damaged. Pure OHC damage either leaves the tail unaffected or causes hypersensitivity (lower thresholds) in the tail. When both OHCs and IHCs are damaged, thresholds are usually greatly elevated, by 80 dB or more, and the tuning curve is broad, without any sign of a sharp tip.

Liberman *et al.* found that they could 'account for' most of the threshold shift in the auditory nerve by evaluating the presence or absence of OHCs and IHCs and the condition of their stereocilia. Furthermore, behavioural thresholds after noise exposure have been found to be correlated with patterns of damage in hair cell stereocilia (Slepecky *et al.* 1982). It seems likely that, for many types of cochlear hearing loss, the primary cause of the loss is damage to the OHCs and/or IHCs. For moderate losses, where thresholds are elevated by less than 50 dB, it may often be the case that the main cause of the loss is damage to the OHCs, with consequent loss or impairment of the active mechanism. For more severe losses, it is likely that both OHCs and IHCs are damaged.

Phase locking

The effect of cochlear damage on phase locking is not entirely clear. Harrison and Evans (1979) used the ototoxic drug kanamycin to produce hair cell damage (mainly to OHCs) in the guinea pig, and found that phase locking was not affected. However, Woolf *et al.* (1981) carried out a similar experiment using the chinchilla and found that phase locking was adversely affected by damage to the OHCs. For neurones with CFs corresponding to frequencies where the behavioural thresholds were elevated by 40 dB or more compared to normal, phase locking was significantly reduced. There was a reduction in the highest frequency at which phase locking could be observed, and the precision of phase locking over the range 0.4 to 3 kHz was reduced.

The reason for the discrepancy between studies is unclear. It could be related to a species difference. Another possibility is that the data of Harrison and Evans are atypical. Woolf *et al.* pointed out that the upper limit of phase locking reported by Harrison and Evans (5–7 kHz) is higher than usually observed in the guinea pig. The reason why phase locking should deteriorate as a consequence of cochlear damage is also unclear. Woolf *et al.* suggested that it could be connected with mechanical coupling between the tallest stereocilia of the OHCs and the tectorial membrane. Whatever the reason, it seems clear that phase locking can be affected by cochlear damage, and this may have important perceptual consequences.

Conclusions

The functioning of the normal cochlea is strongly dependent on an active mechanism that is physiologically vulnerable. This mechanism appears to depend upon the integrity of the OHCs, and particularly their stereocilia. The active mechanism is responsible for the high sensitivity and sharp tuning of the BM. It is also responsible for a variety of nonlinear effects that can be observed in BM responses and neural responses. These effects include: the nonlinear input–output functions on the BM; the reduction in sharpness of tuning with increasing sound level; two-tone suppression; and combination-tone generation. Finally the active mechanism is probably responsible for the generation of evoked and spontaneous otoacoustic emissions. The active mechanism strongly influences responses on the BM at low and medium sound levels, but its contribution progressively reduces as the sound level increases.

The OHCs are easily damaged by noise exposure, ototoxic chemicals, infection, and metabolic disturbances. When they are damaged, the active mechanism is reduced in effectiveness or destroyed completely. This has several important consequences: (1) Sensitivity is reduced, so that the tips of tuning curves are elevated by up to 40–50 dB; (2) The sharpness of tuning on the BM is greatly reduced. The tip of the tuning curve may be elevated or may disappear altogether, leaving only the broad tuning of the passive BM; (3) The nonlinearities are reduced or disappear altogether; (4) Evoked and spontaneous otoacoustic emissions usually disappear, at least in the frequency range corresponding to the damaged place.

The IHCs are the transducers of the cochlea. They are less susceptible to damage than the OHCs. When they are damaged, sensitivity is reduced. Damage primarily to the IHCs, with intact OHCs, is rare. When it does occur, sharp tuning may be preserved, but the whole tuning curve is elevated (less sensitive). More commonly, damage occurs both to the OHCs and IHCs. In this case the whole tuning curve is elevated, with a greater elevation around the tip than around the tail.

Damage to the IHCs can also result in a reduction in phase locking; the precision with which neural impulses are synchronised to the cochlear-filtered stimulating waveform is reduced. The reason why this occurs is unclear, but it may have important perceptual consequences.

2 Absolute thresholds and frequency selectivity in normal and impaired hearing

Introduction

The most obvious result of cochlear damage is reduced sensitivity to weak sounds; sounds below a certain level simply cannot be heard. While this is of major importance in creating hearing difficulty in everyday life, it is not the only factor involved. Cochlear damage produces a variety of changes in the perception of sounds that are well above the threshold for detection. The main emphasis in this book is on these suprathreshold perceptual changes. This chapter is mainly concerned with one specific aspect, namely frequency selectivity. However, it is helpful to consider first the loss of sensitivity.

Absolute threshold in normal and hearing-impaired subjects

The absolute threshold of a sound is the minimum detectable level of that sound in the absence of any other external sounds. It is important to define the way in which the physical intensity of the threshold stimulus is measured, and two methods have been in common use. One method requires the measurement of the sound pressure at some point close to the entrance of the ear canal or inside the ear canal, using a small 'probe' microphone. Ideally, the measurement is made very close to the eardrum. In all cases it is necessary to specify the exact position of the probe, since small changes in position can markedly affect the results at high frequencies. The threshold so determined is called the minimum audible pressure (MAP). The sounds are usually, but not always, delivered by headphone.

The other method uses tones delivered by loudspeaker, usually in a large anechoic chamber (a room whose walls are highly sound absorbing). The measurement of sound level is made after the listener is removed from the sound field, at the point which had been occupied by the centre of the listener's head. The threshold determined in this way is called the minimum audible field (MAF). The two methods give somewhat different results since the head, the pinna and the meatus do have an influence on the sound field.

The general shape of the curve relating threshold to frequency for normally hearing people (often called the audibility curve) is now well established. Figure 2.1 shows the MAF as a function of frequency; the curve is the result of averaging measurements from many young subjects with no history of any hearing disorder. Thresholds are lowest for frequencies in the range 1000–5000 Hz, and they

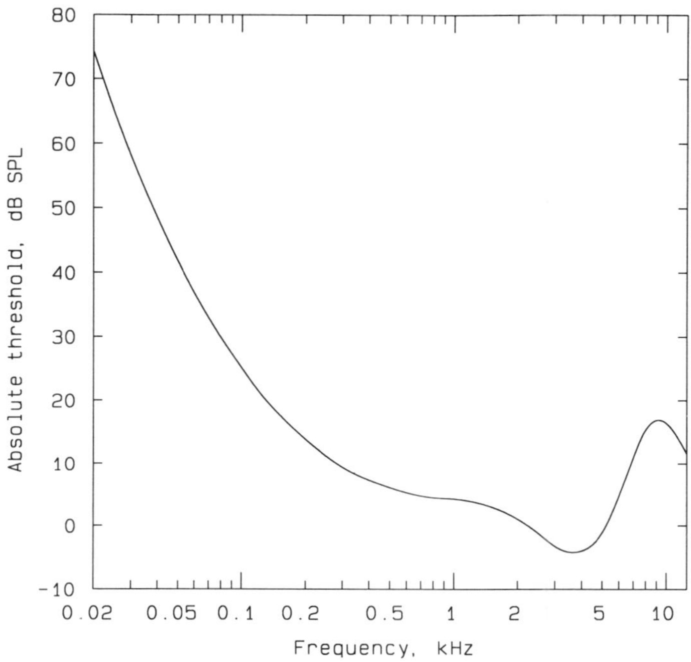

Fig. 2.1. The absolute threshold (Minimum Audible Field, MAF) plotted as a function of frequency for young normally hearing subjects. Data from Robinson and Dadson (1956).

increase at very high and very low frequencies. At least part of the sensitivity to middle frequencies derives from a broad resonance introduced by the pinna and ear canal. The outer ear enhances the sound pressure at the eardrum for frequencies in the range 1–9 kHz, with a maximum enhancement at 3 kHz of 10–15 dB. Another factor which contributes to the shape of the audibility curve is the transmission characteristic of the middle ear. Transmission is most efficient for midrange frequencies and drops off markedly for very low and very high frequencies. This can partly account for the rise in threshold at the low- and high-frequency ends of the audibility curve.

The highest audible frequency varies considerably with age. Young children can often hear tones with frequencies as high as 20 kHz, but for most adults threshold rises rapidly above about 15 kHz. The loss of sensitivity with increasing age (presbyacusis) is much greater at high frequencies than at low, and the variability between different people is also greater at high frequencies.

In audiology, thresholds are usually specified relative to the average threshold at each frequency for young, healthy listeners with 'normal' hearing. Thresholds specified in this way have units dB HL (hearing level) in Europe or dB HTL (hearing threshold level) in the USA. Thus, for example, a threshold of 40 dB HL at 1 kHz would mean that the patient had a threshold which was 40 dB higher than 'normal' at that frequency. In psychoacoustic work thresholds are normally plotted with threshold increasing upwards, as in Figure 2.1. However, in audiology, threshold elevations are shown as hearing losses, plotted downwards. The average 'normal' threshold is represented as a horizontal line at the top of the plot, and the degree of hearing loss is indicated by how much the threshold falls below this line. This type of plot is called an 'audiogram'.

When a sound is presented at a specified level above the absolute threshold of the subject for that sound, the level is referred to as a Sensation Level, abbreviated SL. For example, if the absolute threshold is 23 dB SPL, and the sound is presented at 33 dB SPL, then its level is 10 dB SL.

The most obvious sign of cochlear damage is a reduced sensitivity to weak sounds; the threshold for detecting sounds is higher than normal. This, in itself, is a major factor leading to difficulty in everyday life. The measurement of absolute thresholds provides the easiest way of detecting and measuring damage to the auditory system. A common way of quantifying hearing loss is in terms of the absolute threshold for sinusoids, expressed in dB HL, and averaged over the frequencies 500, 1000 and 2000 Hz; this is often known as the pure-tone average (PTA) hearing loss. Goodman (1965) proposed the following classification:

PTA −10 to 26 dB	Normal limits
PTA 27 to 40 dB	Mild hearing loss
PTA 41 to 55 dB	Moderate hearing loss
PTA 56 to 70 dB	Moderately severe hearing loss
PTA 71 to 90 dB	Severe hearing loss
PTA over 90 dB	Profound hearing loss

A similar classification is still used, although nowadays the boundary between normal hearing and mild hearing loss is usually put at a PTA of 16 dB. Generally, the categories are indicative of the problems that are likely to be experienced in everyday life; greater losses are associated with more difficulty. However, individuals with similar absolute thresholds may vary considerably in this respect.

Frequency selectivity

Frequency selectivity refers to the ability of the auditory system to separate or resolve (to a limited extent) the components in a complex sound. For example, if two tuning forks, each tuned to a different frequency, are struck simultaneously, two different tones can usually be heard, one corresponding to each frequency. This ability is also known as frequency analysis and frequency resolution; these terms will be used interchangeably in this book.

It seems likely that frequency selectivity depends to a large extent on the filtering that takes place in the cochlea (see chapter 1). Thus, any complex sound, such as a note produced by a musical instrument, or a vowel sound produced by the human voice, undergoes such an analysis at an early stage of auditory processing; the sinusoidal components of the sound are separated, and coded independently in the auditory nerve, provided that their frequency separation is sufficiently large. Furthermore, this stage of analysis cannot be by-passed; all sounds are subject to frequency analysis within the cochlea. Hence, the percept of such sounds as a coherent whole depends upon the representations of the individual components being 'reassembled' at some later stage in the auditory system.

It was shown in chapter 1 that damage to the cochlea leads to reduced sharpness of tuning on the basilar membrane and in single neurones of the auditory nerve. Hence, it would be expected that frequency selectivity as measured behaviourally would be poorer than normal in people with cochlear hearing loss. The present chapter shows that this is, indeed, the case, and it demonstrates how the changes in frequency selectivity can be measured.

Frequency selectivity is most often quantified by studying masking. Masking may be regarded as reflecting the limits of frequency selectivity. If a sound of a given frequency is masked by another sound with a different frequency, then the auditory system has failed to resolve the two sounds. Hence, by measuring when one sound is just masked by another, it is possible to characterize the frequency analysis capabilities of the auditory system.

The power spectrum model and the concept of the critical band

Many of the concepts used to explain and model masking effects derive from the early work of Fletcher (1940). He measured the threshold for detecting a sinusoidal signal as a function of the bandwidth of a bandpass noise masker. The noise was always centred at the signal frequency, and the noise power density was held

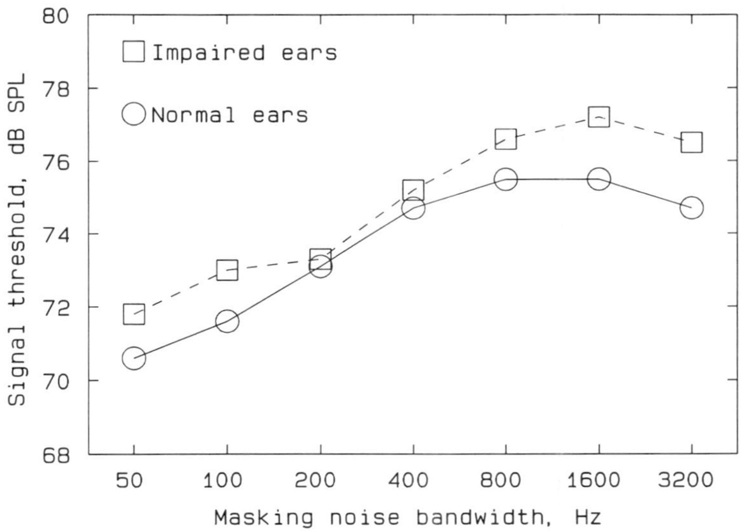

Fig. 2.2. The threshold of a 2-kHz sinusoidal signal plotted as a function of the bandwidth of a noise masker centred at 2 kHz. Results are averaged for the normal ears (circles) and impaired ears (squares) of three subjects with moderate unilateral cochlear hearing loss.

constant. Thus, the total noise power increased as the bandwidth increased. This experiment has been repeated several times since then, with similar results (Hamilton 1957; Greenwood 1961a; Spiegel 1981; Schooneveldt and Moore 1989; Bernstein and Raab 1990; Moore *et al.* 1993c). An example of the results, taken from Moore *et al.* (1993c), is given in Figure 2.2. The solid line with circles shows mean results from the normal ears of three subjects with a unilateral cochlear hearing loss. The threshold of the 2000-Hz signal increases at first as the noise bandwidth increases, but then flattens off; the threshold is roughly constant for bandwidths of 400 Hz and above. The dashed line with squares shows mean results from the impaired ears of the same three subjects. The pattern of results is broadly similar, but performance overall is worse, and the thresholds increase up to a somewhat greater bandwidth of about 800 Hz.

Fletcher (1940) suggested that the peripheral auditory system behaves as if it contained a bank of bandpass filters, with overlapping passbands. These filters are now called the 'auditory filters'. He suggested further that the signal was detected by using the output of the auditory filter centred on the signal frequency. Increases in noise bandwidth result in more noise passing through that filter, provided the noise bandwidth is less than the filter bandwidth. However, once the noise bandwidth exceeds the filter bandwidth, further increases in noise bandwidth do not increase the noise passing through the filter. Fletcher called the bandwidth at which the signal threshold ceased to increase the 'critical bandwidth' (CB). It is usually assumed that this bandwidth is closely related to the bandwidth of the auditory filter at the same centre frequency. The results in Figure 2.2 suggest that the CB is greater for the impaired ears than for the normal ears.

Fletcher's band-widening experiment does not provide a precise way of estimating the bandwidth of the auditory filter (Patterson and Moore 1986). It is obvious from Figure 2.2 that there is no distinct bandwidth at which thresholds cease to increase. Also, although the results of other experiments (described below) suggest that auditory filter bandwidths were considerably different for the normal and impaired ears of the subjects used to produce the data in Figure 2.2, the two curves in Figure 2.2 are not strikingly different in shape; the differences that are apparent could easily have arisen from errors of measurement. Nevertheless, the experiment is important for the concepts to which it gave rise.

Fletcher's experiment led to a model of masking known as the power-spectrum model, which is based on the following assumptions:

(1) The peripheral auditory system contains an array of linear overlapping bandpass filters.
(2) When trying to detect a signal in a noise background, the listener is assumed to make use of just one filter with a centre frequency close to that of the signal. Usually, it is assumed that the filter used is the one that has the highest signal-to-masker ratio at its output.
(3) Only the components in the noise which pass through the filter have any effect in masking the signal.

(4) The threshold for detecting the signal is determined by the amount of noise passing through the auditory filter; specifically, threshold is assumed to correspond to a certain signal-to-noise ratio, K, at the output of the filter. The stimuli are represented by their long-term power spectra, i.e. the relative phases of the components and the short-term fluctuations in the masker are ignored.

We now know that none of these assumptions is strictly correct: the filters are not linear, but are level-dependent (Moore and Glasberg 1987); listeners can combine information from more than one filter to enhance signal detection (Spiegel 1981; Buus *et al.* 1986); noise falling outside the passband of the auditory filter centred at the signal frequency can affect the detection of that signal (Hall *et al.* 1984a); and fluctuations in the masker can play a strong role (Patterson and Henning 1977; Kohlrausch 1988; Moore 1988).

These failures of the model do not mean that the basic concept of the auditory filter is wrong. Indeed, the concept is widely accepted and will be used extensively in the rest of this book. Nevertheless, it should be remembered that simplifying assumptions are often made in attempts to characterize and model the auditory filter.

Estimating the shape of the auditory filter

Most methods for estimating the shape of the auditory filter at a given centre frequency are based on the assumptions of the power-spectrum model of masking. If the masker is represented by its long-term power spectrum, N(f), and the weighting function or shape of the auditory filter is W(f), then the power-spectrum model is expressed by:

$$P_S = K \int_0^\infty W(f)N(f)df, \qquad \text{Eq. 2.1}$$

where P_s is the power of the signal at threshold and K is the signal-to-masker ratio at the output of the filter when the signal is at threshold. For a given subject and signal frequency, K is assumed to be constant. It is assumed that the filter in question is the one that gives the highest signal-to-masker ratio at its output. By manipulating the masker spectrum, N(f), and measuring the corresponding changes in P_s, it is possible to derive the filter shape, W(f).

The masker chosen to measure the auditory filter shape should be such that the assumptions of the power-spectrum model are not strongly violated. The factors affecting this choice have been reviewed elsewhere (Moore 1995). Generally, it appears that the assumptions are best satisfied using reasonably broad-band noise maskers. A second important consideration in choosing maskers for measuring auditory filter shapes is that the filter giving the highest signal-to-masker ratio is not necessarily centred at the signal frequency. For example, if the signal has a frequency of 1 kHz, and the masker spectrum consists entirely of frequencies above 1 kHz, the highest signal-to-masker ratio may occur for a filter centred below 1 kHz. The process of detecting the signal through a filter which is not centred at the signal frequency is called 'off-frequency listening'. In this context, it is the centre frequency of the filter that is 'off frequency'. If the masker is such that off-frequency listening might be substantial (i.e. the filter giving the highest signal-to-masker ratio may be centred far from the signal frequency), this makes the analysis of the results difficult, especially if the extent of off-frequency listening varies as the masker spectrum is altered. Ideally, the masker should be chosen to limit the degree to which off-frequency listening can occur.

Psychophysical tuning curves

The measurement of psychophysical (or psychoacoustical) tuning curves (PTCs) involves a procedure which is analogous in many ways to the determination of a neural tuning curve (Chistovich 1957; Small 1959); see chapter 1. The signal is fixed in level, usually at a very low level, say, 10 dB Sensation Level (SL). The masker can be either a sinusoid or a narrow band of noise.

For each of several masker centre frequencies, the level of the masker needed just to mask the signal is determined. Because the signal is at a low level it is assumed that it will produce activity primarily in one auditory filter. It is assumed further that, at threshold, the masker produces a constant output from that filter, in order to mask the fixed signal. Thus the PTC indicates the masker level required

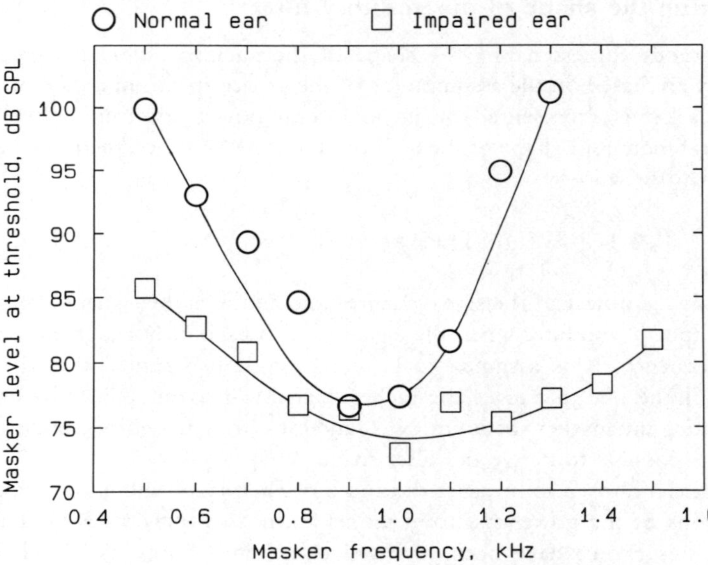

Fig. 2.3. Psychophysical tuning curves (PTCs) determined in simultaneous masking for the normal ear (circles) and the impaired ear (squares) of a subject with a unilateral cochlear hearing loss. The signal frequency was 1 kHz. The variable masker was a narrowband noise. A fixed notched noise was gated with the variable masker, to restrict off-frequency listening. The signal was presented at a level 10 dB above its masked threshold in the notched noise alone.

to produce a fixed output from the auditory filter as a function of frequency. Normally, a filter characteristic is determined by plotting the output from the filter for an input varying in frequency and fixed in level. However, if the filter is linear the same result can be obtained by plotting the input required to give a fixed output. Thus, if linearity is assumed, the shape of the auditory filter can be obtained simply by inverting the PTC. Two PTCs are shown in Figure 2.3; the data are taken from Moore and Glasberg (1986b). The circles show results from the normal ear of a subject with a unilateral cochlear hearing loss. The squares show results from the impaired ear of the same subject. It is obvious that the PTC is broader for the impaired ear.

There is good evidence that off-frequency listening can influence PTCs. When the masker frequency is above the signal frequency, the highest signal-to-masker ratio occurs for a filter centred below the signal frequency. Conversely, when the masker frequency is below the signal frequency, the highest signal-to-masker ratio occurs for a filter centred above the signal frequency. In both these cases, the masker level required for threshold is higher than would be the case if off-frequency listening did not occur. When the masker frequency equals the signal frequency, the signal-to-masker ratio is similar for all auditory filters that are excited, and off-frequency listening is not advantageous. The overall effect is that the PTC has a sharper tip than would be obtained if only one auditory filter were involved (Johnson-Davies and Patterson 1979; O'Loughlin and Moore 1981a,b).

One way to limit off-frequency listening is to add to the masker a fixed noise with a spectral notch centred at the signal frequency (O'Loughlin and Moore 1981a; Moore *et al.* 1984a; Patterson and Moore 1986). Such a masker should make it disadvantageous to use an auditory filter whose centre frequency is shifted much from the signal frequency, although it will not eliminate off-frequency listening entirely. A noise of this type was used when gathering the data shown in Figure 2.3.

A final difficulty in using PTCs as a measure of frequency selectivity is connected with the nonlinearity of the auditory filter. Evidence will be presented later indicating that the auditory filter is not strictly linear, but changes its shape with level. The shape seems to depend more on the level at the input to the filter than on the level at the output (although this is still a matter of some debate). However, in determining a PTC the input is varied while the output is held (roughly) constant. Thus, effectively, the underlying filter shape changes as the masker frequency is altered. This can give a misleading impression of the shape of the auditory filter; in particular it leads to an underestimation of the slope of the lower skirt of the filter, and an overestimation of the slope of the upper skirt (Verschuure 1981a,b; Moore and O'Loughlin 1986).

The notched-noise method

To satisfy the assumptions of the power-spectrum model, it is necessary to use a masker which limits the amount by which the centre frequency of the auditory filter can be shifted (off-frequency listening), and which limits the range of filter

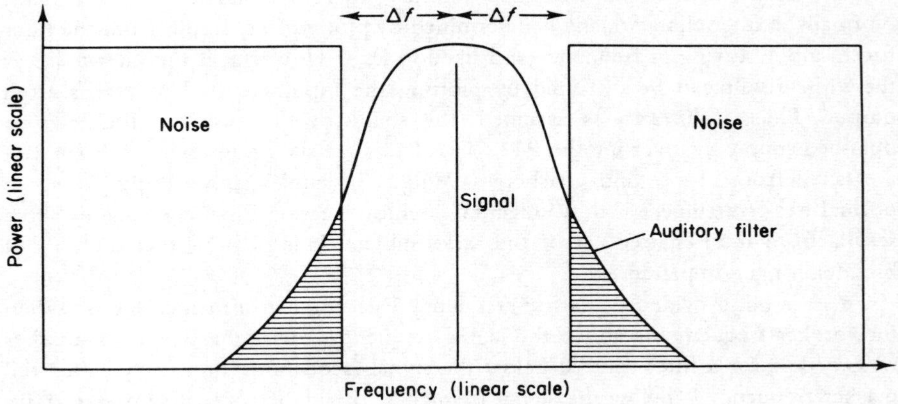

Fig. 2.4. Schematic illustration of the technique used by Patterson (1976) to determine the shape of the auditory filter. The threshold of the sinusoidal signal is measured as a function of the width of a spectral notch in the noise masker. The amount of noise passing through the auditory filter centred at the signal frequency is proportional to the shaded areas.

centre frequencies over which the signal-to-masker ratio is sufficiently high to be useful. This can be achieved using a noise masker with a spectral notch around the signal frequency. For such a masker, the highest signal-to-masker ratio occurs for a filter which is centred reasonably close to the signal frequency, and performance is not improved (or is improved very little) by combining information over filters covering a range of centre frequencies (Patterson 1976; Patterson and Moore 1986; Moore *et al.*1992a). The filter shape can then be estimated by measuring signal threshold as a function of the width of the notch.

For moderate noise levels, the auditory filter is almost symmetrical on a linear frequency scale (Patterson 1974, 1976; Patterson and Nimmo-Smith 1980; Moore and Glasberg 1987). Hence the auditory filter shape can be estimated using a notched-noise masker with the notch placed symmetrically about the signal frequency. The method is illustrated in Figure 2.4. For a masker with a notch width of $2\Delta f$, and centre frequency f_c Eq. 2.1 becomes

$$P_S = KN_0 \int_0^{f_c-\Delta f} W(f)df + KN_0 \int_{fc+\Delta f}^{\infty} W(f)df, \qquad \text{Eq. 2.2.}$$

where N_0 is the power spectral density of the noise in its passbands. The two integrals on the right-hand side of Eq. 2.2 represent the respective shaded areas in Figure 2.4 where the lower and upper noise bands overlap the filter. Since both the filter and the masker are symmetrical about the signal frequency, these two areas are equal. Thus, the function relating Ps to the width of the notch provides a measure of the integral of the auditory filter. Hence, the value of W(f) at a given deviation Δf from the centre frequency is given by the slope of the threshold function at a notch width of $2\Delta f$.

When the auditory filter is asymmetric, as it is at high masker levels (see later), then the filter shape can still be measured using a notched-noise masker if some reasonable assumptions are made, and if the range of measurements is extended to include conditions where the notch is placed asymmetrically about the signal frequency. It is necessary first to assume that the auditory filter shape can be approximated by a simple mathematical expression with a small number of free parameters. Patterson *et al.* (1982) suggested a family of such expressions, all having the form of an exponential with a rounded top, called 'roex' for brevity. The simplest of these expressions was called the roex(p) filter shape. It is convenient to measure frequency in terms of the absolute value of the deviation from the centre frequency of the filter, f_c, and to normalize this frequency variable by dividing by the centre frequency of the filter. The new frequency variable, g, is:

$$g = |f - f_c| / f_c \qquad \text{Eq. 2.3}$$

The roex(p) filter shape is then given by:

$$W(g) = (1 + pg)\exp(-pg) \qquad \text{Eq. 2.4}$$

where p is a parameter which determines both the bandwidth and the slope of the skirts of the auditory filter. The higher the value of p, the more sharply tuned is the filter. The equivalent rectangular bandwidth (ERB) is equal to $4f_c/p$. The ERB is about 11% greater than the half-power (−3 dB) bandwidth. When the filter is assumed to be asymmetric, then p is allowed to have different values on the two sides of the filter: p_l for the lower branch and p_u for the upper branch. The ERB in this case is $2f_c/p_l + 2f_c/p_u$. The values of p_l and p_u that give the best fit to the data define the filter shape; for details see Patterson and Moore (1986).

The roex(p) filter shape is usually quite successful in predicting the data from notched-noise experiments, except when the thresholds cover a wide range of levels or when the masked thresholds approach absolute threshold. In such cases there is a decrease in the slope of the function relating threshold to notch width, a decrease which is not predicted by the roex(p) filter shape. One way of dealing with this is to limit the dynamic range of the filter, using a second parameter, r. This gives the roex(p,r) filter shape of Patterson *et al.* (1982):

$$W(g) = (1 - r)(1 + pg)\exp(-pg) + r. \qquad \text{Eq. 2.5}$$

As before, p can have different values for the upper and lower branches of the filter. However, the data can generally be well predicted using the same value of r for the two sides of the filter (Tyler *et al.* 1984; Glasberg and Moore 1986).

One limitation of the notched-noise method occurs when the auditory filter is markedly asymmetric, as it is in some hearing-impaired people. In such cases, the method does not define the sharper side of the filter very well. As a rule of thumb, when the value of p for one side of the filter is more than twice that for the other, the slope of the steeper side is very poorly determined.

The rippled-noise method

Several researchers have estimated auditory filter shapes using rippled noise, sometimes also called comb filtered noise, as a masker. This is produced by adding white noise to a copy of itself which has been delayed by T seconds. The resulting spectrum has peaks spaced at 1/T Hz, with minima in between. When the delayed version of the noise is added to the original in phase, the first peak in the spectrum of the noise occurs at 0 Hz; this noise is referred to as cosine+. When the polarity of the delayed noise is reversed, the first peak is at 0.5/T Hz; this is referred to as cosine−. The signal is usually a sinusoid that is fixed in frequency, and the values of T are chosen so that the signal falls at either a maximum or minimum in the masker spectrum; the signal threshold is measured for both cosine+ and cosine− noise for various ripple densities (different values of T).

The auditory filter shape can be derived from the data either by approximating the auditory filter as a Fourier series (Houtgast 1977; Pick 1980) or by a method similar to that described for the notched-noise method (Glasberg *et al.* 1984; Patterson and Moore 1986). The filter shapes obtained in this way are generally similar to those obtained using the notched-noise method, although they tend to have a slightly broader and flatter top (Glasberg *et al.* 1984). The method seems to be quite good for defining the shape of the tip of the auditory filter, but it does not allow the auditory filter shape to be measured over a wide dynamic range.

Allowing for the transfer function of the outer and middle ear

The transfer function of the outer and middle ear varies markedly with frequency, particularly at very low and high frequencies. Clearly this can have a significant influence on measures of frequency selectivity. For example, if one of the bands of noise in a notched-noise experiment is very low or high in centre frequency, it will be strongly attenuated by the middle ear, and so will not do much masking. It is possible to conceive of the auditory filter shape as resulting from the overall response properties of the outer/middle ear and the cochlea. However, it is theoretically more appealing to conceive of the auditory filter as resulting from processes occurring after the outer/middle ear. The effect of the outer and middle ear can be thought of as a fixed spectral shaping applied to all stimuli before auditory filtering takes place. If this is the case, then the spectral shaping should be taken into account in the fitting procedure for deriving filter shapes. Glasberg and Moore (1990) have described how this can be done.

An example of measurement of the auditory filter shape

Figure 2.5 shows an example of data obtained using the notched-noise method, and of the filter shape obtained. The data are for a normally hearing subject and a signal frequency of 200 Hz. In the left panel, signal thresholds are plotted as a function of the width of the spectral notch in the noise masker. Asterisks indicate conditions where the spectral notch was placed symmetrically about the signal frequency; the notch width, Δ, is specified as the deviation of each edge of the

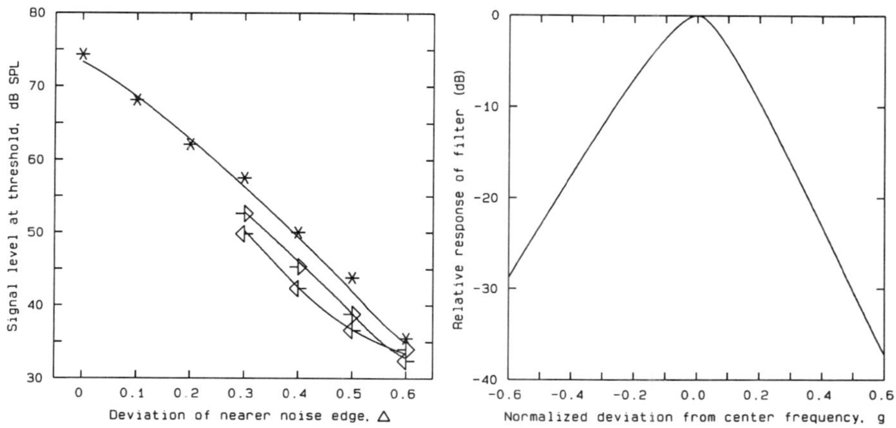

Fig. 2.5. The left panel shows thresholds for a 200-Hz signal as a function of the width of a notch in a noise masker. The value on the abscissa is the deviation of the nearer edge of the notch from the signal frequency, divided by the signal frequency, represented by the symbol Δ. Asterisks (*) indicate conditions where the notch was placed symmetrically about the signal frequency. Right-pointing arrows indicate conditions where the upper edge of the notch was 0.2 units farther away from the signal frequency than the lower edge. Left-pointing arrows indicate conditions where the lower edge of the notch was 0.2 units farther away than the upper edge. The fact that the left-pointing arrows are markedly below the right-pointing arrows indicates that the filter is asymmetric. The right panel shows the auditory filter shape derived from the data. From Moore *et al.* (1990).

notch from the signal frequency, divided by the signal frequency. The left-pointing arrows indicate conditions where the lower edge of the notch was 0.2 units farther from the signal frequency than the upper edge. The right-pointing arrows indicate conditions where the upper edge of the notch was 0.2 units farther from the signal frequency than the lower edge. Moving the lower edge of the notch farther from the signal frequency has a greater effect than moving the upper edge farther from the signal frequency.

The lines in the left panel are the fitted values derived from the roex(p,r) model, after allowing for the transfer function of the outer and middle ear, as described by Glasberg and Moore (1990). The model fits the data well. The derived filter shape is shown in the right panel. The filter is somewhat asymmetric, with a shallower lower branch. The ERB is 48 Hz, which is typical at this centre frequency.

Summary of the characteristics of the auditory filter in normally hearing subjects

Variation with centre frequency

Moore and Glasberg (1983c) presented a summary of experiments measuring auditory filter shapes using symmetric notched-noise maskers and rippled-noise

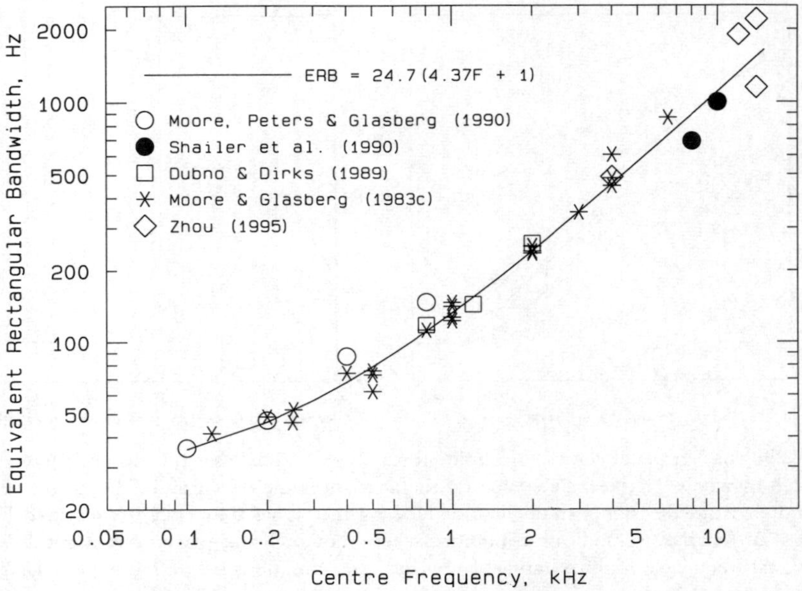

Fig. 2.6. Estimates of the auditory filter bandwidth from a variety of experiments, plotted as a function of centre frequency. The solid line represents the equation suggested by Glasberg and Moore (1990; Eq. 2.6). Two points are shown for a centre frequency of 14 kHz, since filter bandwidths were estimated for two different noise spectrum levels, 40 and 50 dB; the ERB was greater at the higher level.

maskers. All of the data were obtained at moderate noise levels and were analyzed using the roex(p,r) filter shape. Glasberg and Moore (1990) updated that summary, including results that extend the frequency range of the measurements, and including data from experiments using asymmetric notches. Figure 2.6 shows the ERBs of the filters obtained in the various studies, including a recent study by Zhou (1995). The solid line in Figure 2.6 provides a good fit to the ERB values over the whole frequency range tested. It is described by the following equation:

$$\text{ERB} = 24.7(4.37\text{F} + 1) \qquad \text{Eq. 2.6}$$

where the ERB is in Hertz and F is centre frequency in kHz. This equation is a modification of one originally suggested by Greenwood (1961b) to describe the variation of the CB with centre frequency. He based it on the assumption that each CB corresponds to a constant distance along the basilar membrane. Although the constants in Eq. 2.6 differ from those given by Greenwood, the form of the equation is the same as his. Each ERB corresponds to a distance of about 0.89 mm on the BM.

Auditory filter shapes for young normally hearing subjects vary relatively little across subjects; the standard deviation of the ERB is typically about 10% of its mean value (Moore 1987b; Moore *et al.* 1990). However, the variability tends to increase at very low frequencies (Moore *et al.* 1990) and at very high frequencies (Patterson *et al.* 1982; Shailer *et al.* 1990).

Sometimes it is useful to plot psychoacoustical data on a frequency scale related to the ERB. Essentially, the ERB is used as the unit of frequency. For example, the value of the ERB for a centre frequency of 1 kHz is about 130 Hz, so an increase in frequency from 935 to 1065 Hz represents a step of one ERB. A formula relating number of ERBs to frequency can be derived from Eq. 2.6 (Glasberg and Moore 1990):

$$\text{Number of ERBS} = 21.4\log_{10}(4.37F + 1) \qquad \text{Eq. 2.7}$$

where F is frequency in kHz. This scale is conceptually similar to the tonalness scale or Bark scale proposed by Zwicker and co-workers (Zwicker and Terhardt 1980), although it differs somewhat in numerical values.

The variation of the auditory filter shape with level

If the auditory filter were linear, then its shape would not vary with the level of the noise used to measure it. Unfortunately, this is not the case. Moore and Glasberg (1987) presented a summary of measurements of the auditory filter shape using maskers with notches placed both symmetrically and asymmetrically about the signal frequency. They concluded that the lower skirt of the filter becomes less sharp with increasing level, while the higher skirt becomes slightly steeper. Glasberg and Moore (1990) re-analysed the data from the studies summarised in that paper, but using a modified fitting procedure including 'corrections' for the transfer function of the middle ear. They also examined the data presented in Moore *et al.* (1990) and Shailer *et al.* (1990). The re-analysis led to the following conclusions:

(1) The auditory filter for a centre frequency of 1 kHz is roughly symmetric on a linear frequency scale when the level of the noise is approximately 51 dB/ERB. This corresponds to a noise spectrum level of about 30 dB. The auditory filters at other centre frequencies are approximately symmetric when the effective input levels to the filters are equivalent to the level of 51 dB/ERB at 1 kHz (after making allowance for changes in relative level produced by passage of the sound through the outer and middle ear).
(2) The low-frequency skirt of the auditory filter becomes less sharp with increasing level.
(3) Changes in slope of the high-frequency skirt of the filter with level are less consistent. At medium centre frequencies (1–4 kHz) there is a trend for the slope to increase with increasing level, but at low centre frequencies there is no clear trend with level, and the filters at high centre frequencies show a slight decrease in slope with increasing level.

The statements above are based on the assumption that, although the auditory filter is not linear, it may be considered as approximately linear at any given noise

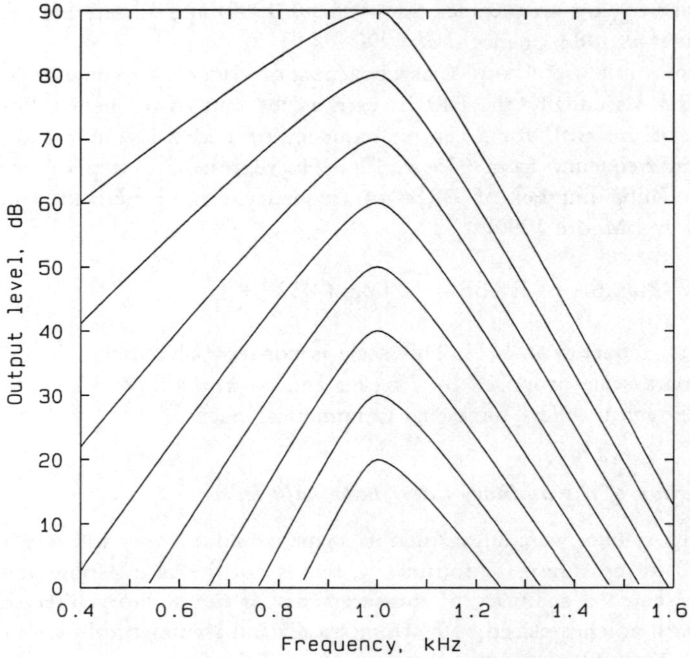

Fig. 2.7. The shape of the auditory filter centred at 1 kHz, plotted for input sound levels ranging from 20 to 90 dB SPL/ERB in 10-dB steps. The output of the filter is plotted as a function of frequency. On the low-frequency side, the filter becomes progressively less sharply tuned with increasing sound level. On the high-frequency side, the sharpness of tuning increases slightly with increasing sound level. At moderate sound levels the filter is approximately symmetric on the linear frequency scale used.

level. Furthermore, the sharpness of the filter is assumed to depend on the input level to the filter, not the output level (Moore and Glasberg 1987). Figure 2.7 illustrates how the shape of the auditory filter varies with input level for a centre frequency of 1 kHz.

As mentioned earlier, the notched-noise method does not give a precise estimate of the slope of the steeper side of the filter when the filter is markedly asymmetric. This is a particular problem at high sound levels, where the lower branch becomes very shallow. Thus, at high levels, there may well be significant errors in the estimates of the sharpness of the high-frequency side of the filter.

Masking patterns and excitation patterns

In the masking experiments described so far, the frequency of the signal was held constant, while the masker was varied. These experiments are most appropriate for estimating the shape of the auditory filter at a given centre frequency. However, many experiments on masking do the opposite; the signal frequency is varied while the masker is held constant.

Wegel and Lane (1924) published the first systematic investigation of the masking of one pure tone by another. They determined the threshold of a signal with adjustable frequency in the presence of a masker with fixed frequency and intensity. The function relating masked threshold to the signal frequency is known as a masking pattern, or sometimes as a masked audiogram. The results of Wegel and Lane were complicated by the occurrence of beats (amplitude fluctuations) when the signal and masker were close together in frequency. To avoid this problem, later experimenters (Egan and Hake 1950; Fastl 1976a) have used a narrow band of noise as either the signal or the masker.

The masking patterns obtained in these experiments show steep slopes on the low-frequency side, of between 80 and 240 dB/octave for pure-tone masking and 55–190 dB/octave for narrowband noise masking. The slopes on the high-frequency side are less steep and depend on the level of the masker. A typical set of results is shown in Figure 2.8; the data are taken from Egan and Hake (1950). Notice that on the high-frequency side the slopes of the curves tend to become shallower at high levels. Thus, if the level of a low-frequency masker is increased by, say, 10 dB, the masked threshold of a high-frequency signal is elevated by more than 10 dB; the amount of masking grows non-linearly on the high-frequency side. This has been called the 'upward spread of masking'.

The masking patterns do not reflect the use of a single auditory filter. Rather, for each signal frequency the listener uses a filter centred close to the signal frequency. Thus the auditory filter is shifted as the signal frequency is altered. One way of interpreting the masking pattern is as a crude indicator of the excitation

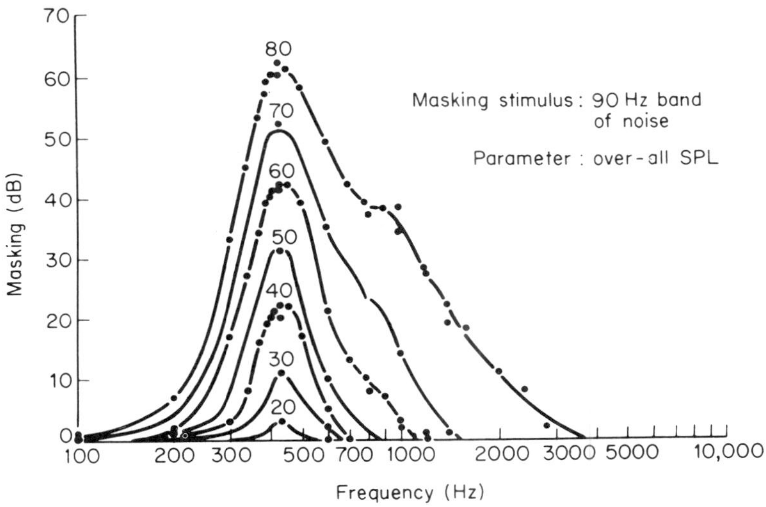

Fig. 2.8. Masking patterns (masked audiograms) for a narrow band of noise centred at 410 Hz. Each curve shows the elevation in threshold of a sinusoidal signal as a function of signal frequency. The overall noise level for each curve is indicated in the figure. Data from Egan and Hake (1950).

pattern of the masker. The excitation pattern of a sound is a representation of the activity or excitation evoked by that sound as a function of characteristic frequency or 'place' in the auditory system (Zwicker 1970). In the case of a masking pattern, one might assume that the signal is detected when the excitation it produces is some constant proportion of the excitation produced by the masker in the frequency region of the signal. Thus the threshold of the signal as a function of frequency is proportional to the masker's excitation level. The masking pattern should be parallel to the excitation pattern of the masker, but shifted vertically by a small amount. In practice, the situation is not so straightforward, since the shape of the masking pattern is influenced by factors such as off-frequency listening and the detection of combination tones produced by the interaction of the signal and the masker (Greenwood 1971).

Relationship of the auditory filter to the excitation pattern

Moore and Glasberg (1983c) have described a way of deriving the shapes of excitation patterns using the concept of the auditory filter. They suggested that the excitation pattern of a given sound can be thought of as the output of the auditory

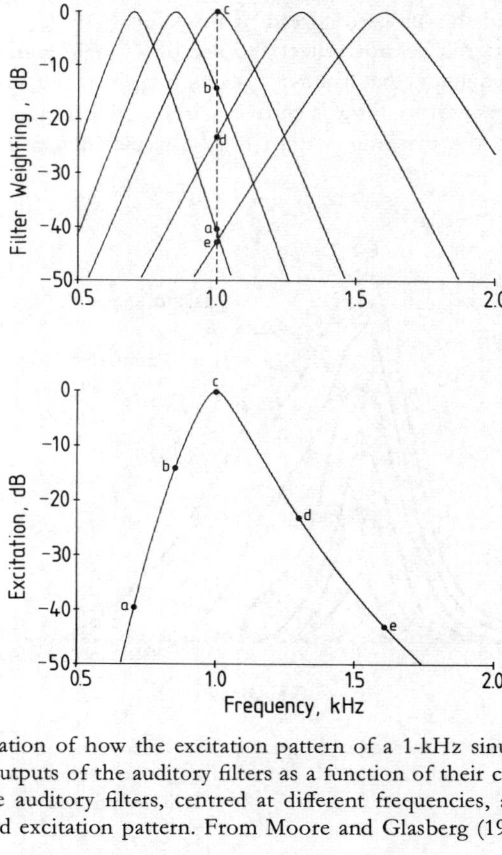

Fig. 2.9. An illustration of how the excitation pattern of a 1-kHz sinusoid can be derived by calculating the outputs of the auditory filters as a function of their centre frequency. The top half shows five auditory filters, centred at different frequencies, and the bottom half shows the calculated excitation pattern. From Moore and Glasberg (1983c).

filters as a function of their centre frequency. This idea is illustrated in Figure. 2.9. The upper portion of the figure shows auditory filter shapes for five centre frequencies. Each filter is symmetrical on the linear frequency scale used, but the bandwidths of the filters increase with increasing centre frequency. The dashed line represents a 1-kHz sinusoidal signal whose excitation pattern is to be derived. The lower panel shows the output from each filter in response to the 1 kHz signal, plotted as a function of the centre frequency of each filter; this is the desired excitation pattern.

To see how this pattern is derived, consider the output from the filter with the lowest centre frequency. This has a relative output in response to the 1 kHz tone of about −40 dB, as indicated by point 'a' in the upper panel. In the lower panel, this gives rise to the point 'a' on the excitation pattern; the point has an ordinate value of −40 dB and is positioned on the abscissa at a frequency corresponding to the centre frequency of the lowest filter illustrated. The relative outputs of the other filters are indicated, in order of increasing centre frequency, by points 'b' to 'e', and each leads to a corresponding point on the excitation pattern. The complete excitation pattern was actually derived by calculating the filter outputs for filters spaced at 10-Hz intervals. In deriving the excitation pattern, excitation levels were expressed relative to the level at the tip of the pattern, which was arbitrarily labelled as 0 dB. To calculate the excitation pattern for a 1-kHz tone with a level of, say, 60 dB, the level at the tip would be labelled as 60 dB, and all other excitation levels would correspondingly be increased by 60 dB.

Note that, although the auditory filters were assumed to be symmetric on a linear frequency scale, the derived excitation pattern is asymmetric. This happens because the bandwidth of the auditory filter increases with increasing centre frequency. Note also that the excitation pattern has the same general form as the masking patterns shown in Figure. 2.8.

Changes in excitation patterns with level

In the normal auditory system, auditory filters broaden on the low-frequency side with increasing sound level (Figure 2.7). Correspondingly, the excitation patterns evoked by narrowband sounds broaden on the high-frequency side. This is illustrated in Figure 2.10, which shows excitation patterns for a 1-kHz sinusoid at levels from 20 to 90 dB, calculated in a manner similar to that described above.

Non-simultaneous masking

'Simultaneous masking' describes situations where the masker is present for the whole time that the signal occurs. Masking can also occur when a brief signal is presented just before or after the masker; this is called non-simultaneous masking. Non-simultaneous masking is introduced here since it can be used as a tool to measure a nonlinear effect known as suppression, which has a significant influence on the internal representation of sounds in the normal auditory system, but which has reduced effects in people with cochlear hearing loss.

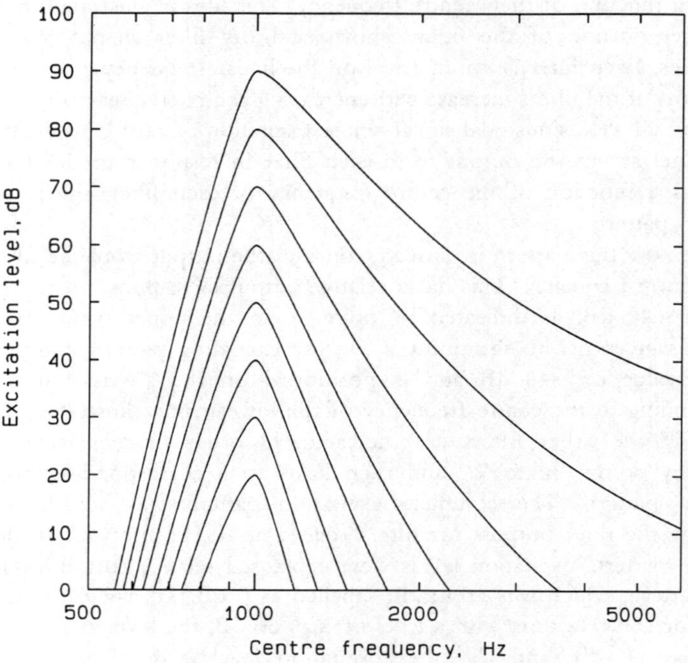

Fig. 2.10. Excitation patterns calculated according to the procedure described in the text for 1-kHz sinusoids ranging in level from 20 to 90 dB SPL in 10-dB steps.

Two basic types of non-simultaneous masking can be distinguished: (1) backward masking, in which the signal precedes the masker (also known as pre-stimulatory masking); and (2) forward masking, in which the signal follows the masker (also known as post-stimulatory masking). I will concentrate on forward masking, since it is generally the greater of the two types of masking, at least in well-trained subjects, and since it is better understood than backward masking.

The main properties of forward masking are as follows:

(1) Forward masking is greater the nearer in time to the masker that the signal occurs. This is illustrated in the left panel of Figure 2.11. When the delay D of the signal after the end of the masker is plotted on a logarithmic scale, the data fall roughly on a straight line. In other words, the amount of forward masking, in dB, is a linear function of log(D).
(2) The rate of recovery from forward masking is greater for higher masker levels. Thus, regardless of the initial amount of forward masking, the masking decays to zero after 100–200 ms.
(3) Increments in masker level do not produce equal increments in amount of forward masking. For example, if the masker level is increased by 10 dB, the masked threshold may only increase by 3 dB. This contrasts with simultaneous masking, where, at least for wideband maskers, threshold usually corresponds to a constant signal-to-masker

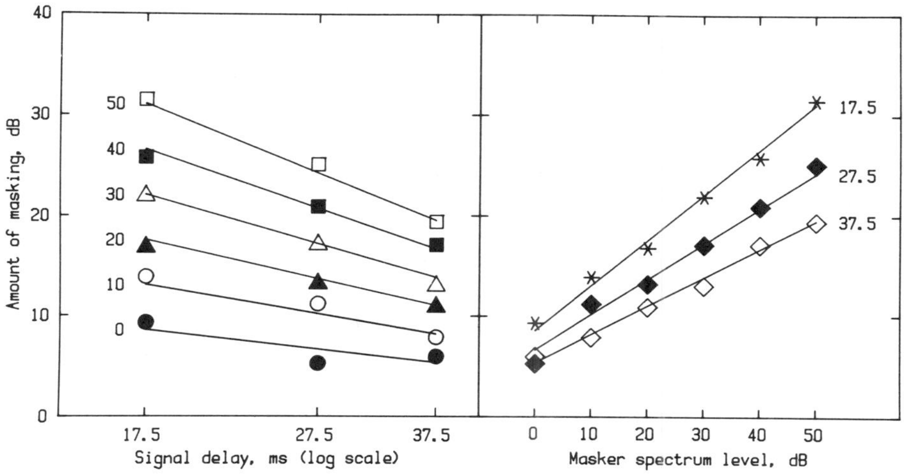

Fig. 2.11. The left panel shows the amount of forward masking of a brief 2-kHz signal, plotted as a function of the time delay of the signal after the end of the noise masker. Each curve shows results for a different noise spectrum level (10–50 dB). The results for each spectrum level fall on a straight line when the signal delay is plotted on a logarithmic scale, as here. The right panel shows the same thresholds plotted as a function of masker spectrum level. Each curve shows results for a different signal delay time (17.5, 27.5 or 37.5 ms). Note that the slopes of these growth of masking functions decrease with increasing signal delay. Adapted from Moore and Glasberg (1983a).

ratio. This effect can be quantified by plotting the signal threshold as a function of masker level. The resulting function is called a growth of masking function. Several such functions are shown in the right panel of Figure 2.11. In simultaneous masking such functions would have slopes close to one. In forward masking the slopes are less than one, and the slopes decrease as the value of D increases.

(4) The amount of forward masking increases with increasing masker duration for durations up to at least 20 ms. The results for greater masker durations vary somewhat across studies. Some studies show an effect of masker duration for durations up to 200 ms (Kidd and Feth 1982), while others show little effect for durations beyond 50 ms (Fastl 1976b).

The mechanisms underlying forward masking are not clear. It could be explained in terms of a reduction in sensitivity of recently stimulated neurones, or in terms of a persistence in the pattern of neural activity evoked by the masker. Both points of view can be found in the literature. In addition, the response of the basilar membrane to the masker takes a certain time to decay, and for small intervals between the signal and the masker this may result in forward masking (Duifhuis 1973).

Evidence for lateral suppression from non-simultaneous masking

Measurements of BM motion (Ruggero 1992), or in single neurones (Arthur *et al.* 1971), show that the response to a tone of a given frequency can sometimes be suppressed by a tone with a different frequency, a phenomenon known as two-tone suppression; see chapter 1. For other complex signals, similar phenomena occur and are given the general name lateral suppression or suppression. This can be characterized in the following way. Strong activity at a given characteristic frequency (CF) can suppress weaker activity at adjacent CFs. In this way, peaks in the excitation pattern are enhanced relative to adjacent dips.

The question now arises as to what are the perceptual consequences of suppression, and how its effects can be measured. Houtgast (1972) has argued that simultaneous masking is not an appropriate tool for detecting the effects of suppression. In simultaneous masking, the masking stimulus and the signal are processed simultaneously in the same frequency-selective channel. Thus any suppression in that channel will affect the neural activity caused by both the signal and the masker. In other words, the signal-to-masker ratio in a given frequency region will be unaffected by suppression, and thus the threshold of the signal will remain unaltered.

Houtgast suggested that this difficulty could be overcome by presenting the masker and the signal successively, for example, by using forward masking. If suppression does occur, then its effects will be seen in forward masking provided: (1) in the chain of levels of neural processing, the level at which the suppression occurs is not later than the level at which most of the forward masking effect arises; (2) the suppression built up by the masker has decayed by the time that the signal is presented (otherwise the problems described for simultaneous masking will be encountered).

Following the pioneering work of Houtgast (1972, 1973, 1974) many workers have reported that there are systematic differences between the results obtained using simultaneous and non-simultaneous masking techniques. An extensive review is provided by Moore and O'Loughlin (1986). One major difference is that non-simultaneous masking reveals effects that can be directly attributed to suppression. A good demonstration of this involves a psychophysical analogue of neural two-tone suppression. Houtgast (1973, 1974) measured the threshold for a 1-kHz signal and a 1-kHz non-simultaneous masker. He then added a second tone to the masker and measured the threshold again. He found that sometimes the addition of this second tone produced a reduction in the threshold, an effect that has been called 'two-tone unmasking'. He attributed this to a suppression of the 1-kHz component in the masker by the second component. If the 1-kHz component is suppressed, then there will be less activity in the frequency region around 1 kHz, producing a drop in the threshold for detecting the signal. The second tone was most effective as a 'suppressor' when it was somewhat more intense than the 1-kHz component, and above it in frequency. Similar results have been obtained by Shannon (1976).

Under some circumstances, the reduction in threshold (unmasking) produced by adding one or more extra components to a masker can be partly explained in terms of additional cues provided by the added components, rather than in terms of suppression. Specifically, in forward masking the added components may reduce 'confusion' of the signal with the masker by indicating exactly when the masker ends and the signal begins (Moore 1980, 1981; Moore and Glasberg 1982, 1985; Neff 1985; Moore and O'Loughlin 1986). This may have led some researchers to over-estimate the magnitude of suppression as indicated in non-simultaneous masking experiments. However, it seems clear that not all unmasking can be explained in this way.

The enhancement of frequency selectivity revealed in non-simultaneous masking

A second major difference between simultaneous and non-simultaneous masking is that the frequency selectivity revealed in non-simultaneous masking is greater than that revealed in simultaneous masking. A well-studied example of this is the psychophysical tuning curve (PTC). PTCs determined in forward masking, are typically sharper than those obtained in simultaneous masking (Moore 1978). Some examples are given in Figure 2.12. A low-level notched-noise masker was gated with the main narrowband noise masker to restrict off-frequency listening and to provide a consistent detection cue in forward masking. The differences between the PTCs for simultaneous and forward masking are particularly marked on the high-frequency side. According to Houtgast (1974) this difference arises because the internal representation of the masker (its excitation pattern), is sharpened by a

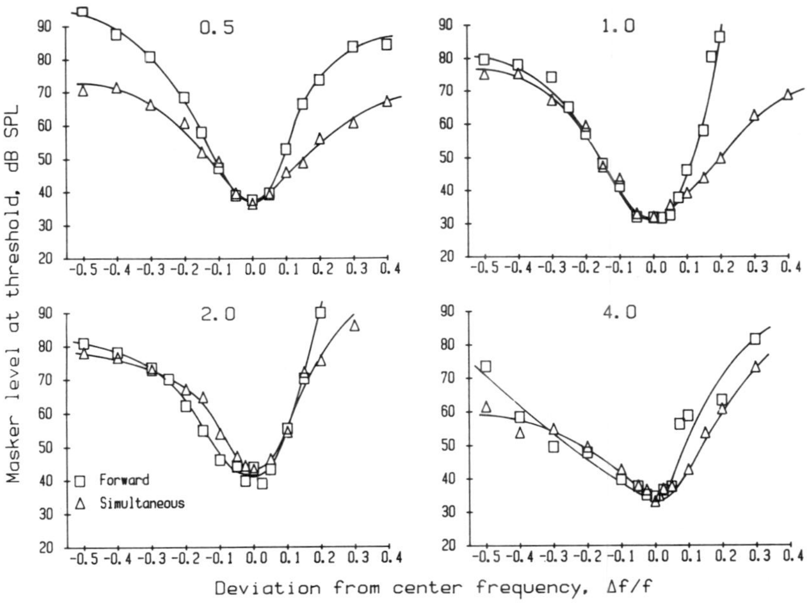

Fig. 2.12. Comparison of psychophysical tuning curves (PTCs) determined in simultaneous masking (triangles) and forward masking (squares). The masker frequency is plotted as deviation from the centre frequency divided by the centre frequency (Δf/f). The centre frequency is indicated in kHz in each panel. A low-level notched noise was gated with the masker to provide a consistent detection cue in forward masking and to restrict off-frequency listening. From Moore *et al.* (1984a).

suppression process, with the greatest sharpening occurring on the low-frequency side. In simultaneous masking, the effects of suppression are not seen, since any reduction of the masker activity in the frequency region of the signal is accompanied by a similar reduction in signal-evoked activity. In other words, the signal-to-masker ratio in the frequency region of the signal is unaffected by the suppression. In forward masking, on the other hand, the suppression does not affect the signal. For maskers with frequencies above that of the signal, the effect of suppression is to sharpen the excitation pattern of the masker, resulting in an increase of the masker level required to mask the signal. Thus the suppression is revealed as an increase in the slopes of the PTC.

An alternative explanation is that, in simultaneous masking, the low-level signal may be suppressed by the masker, so that it falls below absolute threshold. The neural data indicate that tones falling outside of the region bounded by the neural tuning curve can produce suppression. Thus the PTC in simultaneous masking might map out the boundaries of the more broadly tuned suppression region (Moore *et al.* 1987; Delgutte 1988, 1990).

Several other methods of estimating frequency selectivity have indicated sharper tuning in non-simultaneous masking than in simultaneous masking. For example, auditory filter shapes estimated in forward masking using a notched-noise masker, have smaller bandwidths and greater slopes than those estimated in simultaneous masking (Moore and Glasberg 1981). This encourages the belief that a general consequence of suppression is an enhancement of frequency selectivity.

Frequency selectivity in simultaneous masking for subjects with cochlear hearing loss

Comparisons of frequency selectivity in normal and hearing-impaired subjects are complicated by several factors. One factor is the sound level of the stimuli used. As mentioned above, the auditory filters of normally hearing subjects broaden on the low-frequency side with increasing level. This effect probably depends on the active mechanism in the cochlea. At low sound levels, this mechanism probably strongly enhances the tuning on the low-frequency side of the auditory filter. However, as the sound level increases, the contribution of the active mechanism is progressively reduced, and the low-frequency side of the auditory filter broadens.

It seems likely that the active mechanism is usually damaged or completely non-functioning in ears with cochlear damage. Hence, changes in frequency selectivity with level are absent or much less pronounced (Moore *et al.* 1985c; Stelmachowicz *et al.* 1987). As a result, the differences between normal and hearing-impaired subjects tend to decrease at high sound levels. Also, it may be inappropriate to compare frequency selectivity measured using a low sound level in normal subjects with that measured at a high sound level in hearing-impaired subjects.

A second complicating factor is off-frequency listening. Some measures of frequency selectivity, especially PTCs, can be strongly influenced by off-frequency listening. More importantly, the role of off-frequency listening may vary markedly depending on the sensation level of the stimuli and the frequency selectivity of the subject. For example, if PTCs are measured for a normally hearing subject using a signal at 70 dB SPL, there is a strong potential for off-frequency listening in some conditions. On the other hand, if a hearing-impaired subject with an absolute threshold of 60 dB SPL is tested with a 70 dB SPL signal, the potential for off-frequency listening is much reduced. Although these problems can be reduced by gating a notched noise with the variable masker, as described earlier, this has not usually been done in studies with hearing-impaired subjects. Hence, in what follows, studies of PTCs will be described only briefly, while measures controlling off-frequency listening will be described in more detail. For a more detailed review of the results of PTC measurements, see Tyler (1986).

Psychophysical tuning curves

There have been several studies comparing PTCs in normal subjects and subjects with cochlear hearing loss (Leshowitz *et al.* 1975; Hoekstra and Ritsma 1977; Zwicker and Schorn 1978; Bonding 1979b; Florentine *et al.* 1980; Tyler *et al.* 1982b; Carney and Nelson 1983; Festen and Plomp 1983; Stelmachowicz *et al.* 1985; Nelson 1991). Although the studies differ in detail, their results are in general agreement that PTCs are broader than normal in the impaired subjects. However, it is difficult to quantify the differences from normal, owing to the problems discussed above. Most studies have found that the sharpness of tuning of the PTCs decreases with increasing absolute threshold, although the correlation between the two varies markedly across studies. No systematic differences in PTCs have been reported between cochlear losses of different origin, such as noise-induced, Ménière's, aging, and hereditary losses. In some cases, PTCs have been found that are W-shaped rather than V-shaped (Hoekstra and Ritsma 1977). These may be a psychoacoustical analogue of the W-shaped neural tuning curves that are sometimes found in animals with cochlear damage (see Figure 1.14).

In rare cases, PTCs have been found whose tips are shifted well away from the signal frequency (Thornton and Abbas 1980; Florentine and Houtsma 1983; Turner *et al.* 1983). This can happen when cochlear damage is restricted to low-frequency regions of the cochlea and there are no functioning IHCs with CFs corresponding to the frequency region of the loss. The detection of low-frequency tones is then mediated by neurones with high CFs. If the signal to be detected has a frequency corresponding to the region of the hearing loss, the tip of the tuning curve lies well above the signal frequency. In other words, a masker centred well above the signal in frequency is more effective than a masker centred close to the signal frequency. This happens because the higher-frequency masker lies closer to the CFs of the neurones mediating detection of the signal.

Auditory filter shapes measured using rippled noise

Pick *et al.* (1977) estimated auditory filter bandwidths using a rippled-noise masker, for both normal subjects and subjects with cochlear hearing loss. The overall noise level was either 90 or 100 dB SPL. Test frequencies of 0.5, 1, 2 and 4 kHz were used. When the absolute thresholds of the hearing-impaired subjects were less than about 20 dB HL at the test frequency, the filter bandwidths were generally within the normal range. With increasing hearing loss above 20 dB, the filter bandwidths generally increased. On average, bandwidths reached about twice the normal values for absolute thresholds in the range 40–50 dB HL, although considerable scatter was evident in the data. For example, some subjects with thresholds of about 50 dB HL had almost normal bandwidths, while others had bandwidths four to five

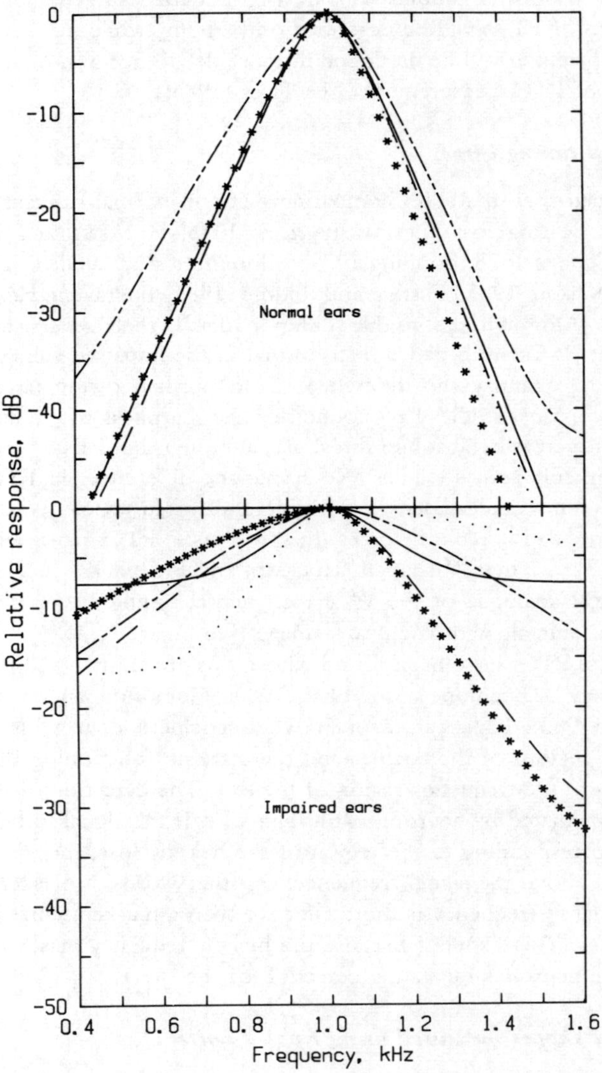

Fig. 2.13. Auditory filter shapes at a centre frequency of 1 kHz for the normal (top) and impaired (bottom) ears of six subjects with unilateral cochlear impairments.

times greater than normal. Broadly comparable results were obtained by Hoekstra (1979) and by Festen and Plomp (1983).

Auditory filter shapes measured with notched noise

Auditory filter shapes of subjects with cochlear impairments have been estimated in several studies using notched-noise maskers (Tyler *et al.* 1984; Glasberg and Moore 1986; Dubno and Dirks 1989; Laroche *et al.* 1992; Peters and Moore 1992; Stone *et al.* 1992; Leek and Summers 1993; Sommers and Humes 1993; Leeuw and Dreschler 1994). The results generally agree in showing that auditory filters are broader than normal in hearing-impaired subjects and that, on average, the degree of broadening increases with increasing hearing loss.

As an example, we will describe the study of Glasberg and Moore (1986). They measured auditory filter shapes in subjects with unilateral and bilateral cochlear impairments; in the former case differences between the normal and impaired ears cannot be attributed to extraneous factors such as age or ability to concentrate. The same noise spectrum level (50 dB, corresponding to an overall level of 79 dB SPL) was used for the normal and impaired ears. Results for six subjects at a centre frequency of 1 kHz are shown in Figure 2.13. The filter shapes for the normal ears (top panel) are similar to one another, and all show a high degree of frequency selectivity. The filter shapes for the impaired ears vary greatly in shape across subjects, but they are all broader than those for the normal ears on at least one side. The most common feature is a marked broadening on the low-frequency side. This indicates a marked susceptibility to masking by low-frequency sounds, such as car noise and air-conditioning noise.

Figure 2.14 summarizes values of the ERB of the auditory filter obtained from subjects with cochlear hearing loss in my laboratory and in the laboratory of Robert Peters. The summary was prepared by Michael Stone. The upper panel shows ERB values plotted relative to the value for young normally hearing subjects at moderate sound levels, as given by Eq. 2.6. The lower panel shows ERB values plotted relative to the value for young normal subjects tested at the same sound pressure level as the impaired subjects, assuming that the ERB for normal subjects varies with level as described by Glasberg and Moore (1990); see Figure 2.7. In both cases, the ERB values are plotted as a function of the absolute threshold (dB HL) at the test frequency. There is a clear trend for the ERB to increase with increasing absolute threshold. The increase is less in the lower panel, since the auditory filters for normal subjects broaden with increasing level of the test stimuli. However, the trend is still quite clear. There is also considerable scatter in the data, indicating that the ERB of the auditory filter cannot be predicted reliably from the absolute threshold.

Figure 2.15 shows the asymmetry of the auditory filter, expressed as the ratio p_l/p_u, plotted relative to the asymmetry for normally hearing subjects tested at the same sound level. The scatter in the results increases considerably as the absolute threshold increases. The majority of subjects show a positive asymmetry, indicating a broad lower skirt to the auditory filter and an increased susceptibility to the

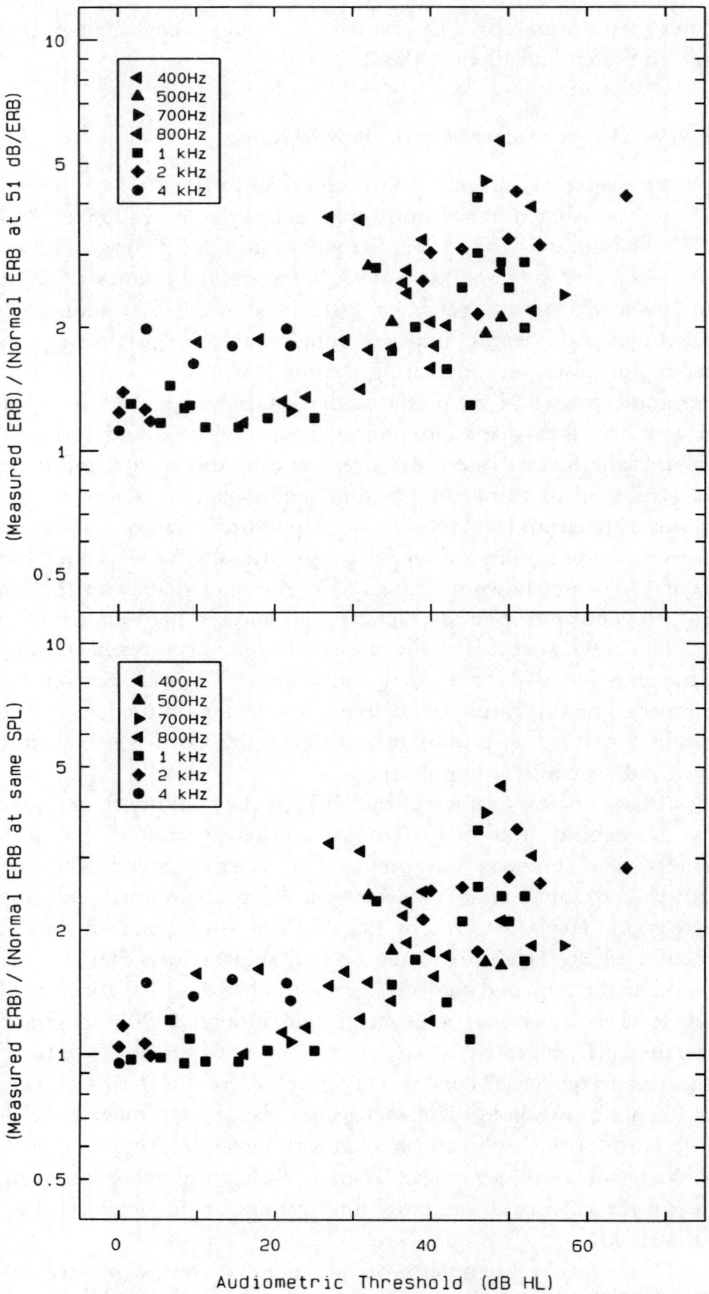

Fig. 2.14. Values of the ERB of the auditory filter for subjects with cochlear hearing loss, plotted as a function of absolute threshold (dB HL) at the test frequency. The ERB values are plotted either relative to the values given by Eq. 2.6, or relative to the ERBs for young normal subjects tested at the same sound level.

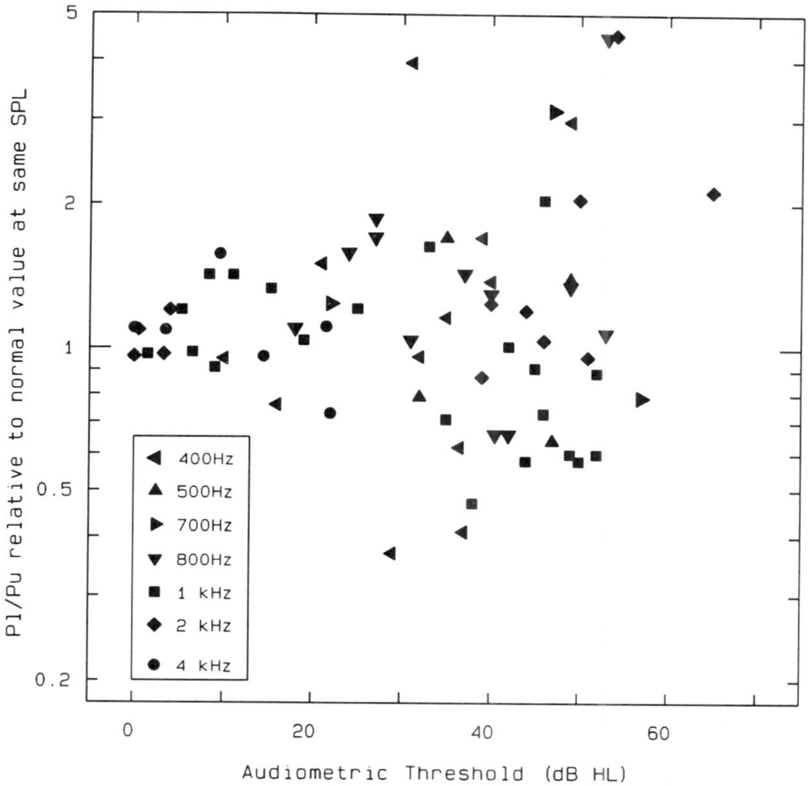

Fig. 2.15. As figure 2.14, but showing the asymmetry of the auditory filters, relative to the asymmetry for normal subjects tested at the same sound level.

upward spread of masking from low frequencies. However, some subjects show the opposite asymmetry, indicating an increased susceptibility to the downward spread of masking from high frequencies.

The scatter in the data shown in Figures 2.14 and 2.15 may reflect different ways in which cochlear damage can occur, as described in chapter 1 (Liberman and Dodds 1984; Liberman *et al.* 1986). In one common case, the damage is primarily to the outer hair cells (OHCs) and the inner hair cells (IHCs) are intact. This results in reduced effectiveness of the active mechanism, but a relatively normal mechanism for transducing basilar-membrane movement into neural responses. In this case, the degree of auditory-filter broadening is correlated with the loss of sensitivity (elevated absolute threshold), and the broadening of the auditory filter can occur on both sides or mainly on the low-frequency side. Sometimes the filter response shows two peaks rather than one (the tuning curve is W-shaped).

In a second case, both the OHCs and IHCs are damaged. Both the active mechanism and the transducer mechanism are adversely affected. This results in a considerable elevation of absolute threshold and the filter is normally broadened on both sides. In a final (rare) case, the damage is mainly to the IHCs, with minimal damage to the OHCs. The transducer mechanism is severely affected in this case, but the active mechanism still functions, albeit with reduced effectiveness because of the high sound level needed to evoke a neural response. In this case, the absolute threshold is elevated, but the sharpness of tuning is only slightly worse than normal.

In summary, all methods of estimating frequency selectivity suggest that it decreases with increasing hearing loss. However, for a given elevation in absolute threshold, there can be considerable scatter both in the degree of broadening and in the asymmetry of the auditory filter. This large variability may arise from different patterns of damage within the cochlea.

Forward masking and suppression in subjects with cochlear hearing loss

Several workers have compared results from simultaneous and forward masking in an attempt to measure suppression effects in hearing-impaired subjects. To avoid problems associated with the nonlinear growth and decay of forward masking, as described earlier, the signal level has usually been fixed, and the masker has been varied to determine a masked threshold. Essentially, it is assumed that threshold is reached when the masker produces a fixed output from the auditory filter centred at the signal frequency.

Wightman *et al.* (1977) compared PTCs in simultaneous and forward masking for subjects with high-frequency hearing losses. They found that, when both the signal and the masker were in regions of normal sensitivity, the PTCs obtained in forward masking were sharper than those found in simultaneous masking. However, when the signal was in the frequency region of reduced sensitivity, or just below it, the differences were much reduced. They also attempted to measure suppression more directly, using the two-tone unmasking paradigm described earlier. Unmasking was observed when the 'suppressor' tone fell in frequency regions of normal sensitivity, but not when it fell in the region of the hearing loss. Wightman *et al.* concluded that the suppression mechanism was rendered ineffective by the hearing loss. They took their results to support the hypothesis that, in normally hearing subjects, suppression is responsible for the differences between PTCs in simultaneous and forward masking. Penner (1980b) and Mills and Schmeidt (1983) studied two-tone unmasking in subjects with noise-induced hearing loss, and obtained similar results to those of Wightman *et al.*

Moore and Glasberg (1986b) measured PTCs in simultaneous and forward masking separately for each ear of subjects with unilateral moderate cochlear losses. A notched noise was gated with the narrowband variable masker to restrict off-frequency listening, to provide a consistent detection cue in forward masking, and to equate the levels of the PTCs around their tips for the normal and impaired ears. For the normal ears, they found, as expected, that the PTCs were usually sharper in forward masking than in simultaneous masking. For the impaired ears, the PTCs were broader, and the differences between simultaneous and forward

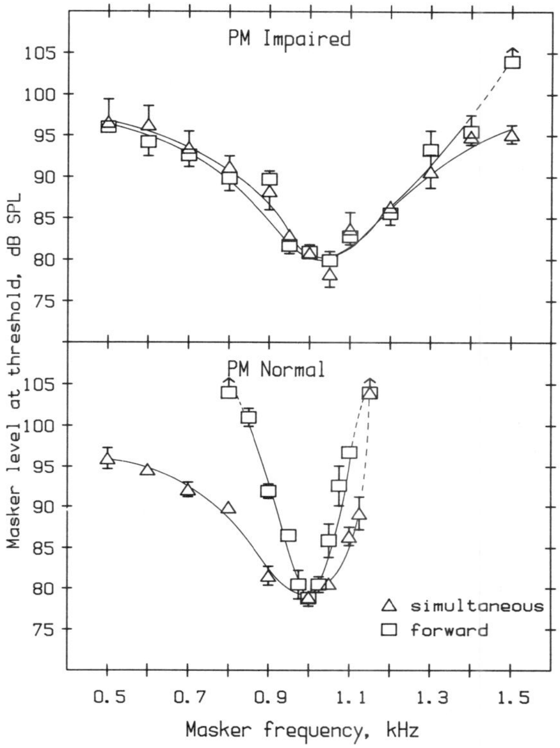

Fig. 2.16. PTCs determined for the normal (bottom) and impaired (top) ears of a subject with a unilateral cochlear impairment, for simultaneous masking (triangles) and forward masking (squares). Up-pointing arrows indicate that the masker level required for threshold was greater than 105 dB SPL. Data from Moore and Glasberg (1986b).

masking were reduced or absent. An example of their results is given in Figure 2.16. These results are consistent with the idea that suppression is reduced or absent in people with cochlear hearing loss.

In another experiment using five subjects with unilateral cochlear impairments, Moore and Glasberg (1986b) used notched noise as a simultaneous and a forward masker. The signal level was fixed and the masker level was varied to determine threshold for each notch width used. For the normal ears, the rate of change of masker level at threshold with notch width was greater in forward masking than in simultaneous masking, indicating a higher effective degree of frequency selectivity in forward masking. For the impaired ears, the differences between simultaneous and forward masking were smaller, although they were completely absent for only one subject. These results suggest that the suppression mechanism was reduced in effectiveness in the impaired ears, but was not completely inoperative, except in one case.

Festen and Plomp (1983) compared simultaneous and forward masking for a rippled-noise masker, again keeping the level of the signal fixed (at about 15 dB

SL) and varying the level of the masker to determine threshold. The differences between thresholds in simultaneous and forward masking were much smaller for impaired than for normal subjects, which they interpreted as indicating that suppression was greatly reduced in effectiveness in the hearing-impaired subjects.

In summary, the results of the various experiments are in agreement in showing that:

(1) Two-tone unmasking in forward masking is small or absent when the stimuli fall in a frequency region where there is cochlear hearing loss.
(2) Differences in frequency selectivity between simultaneous and forward masking are much smaller than normal in hearing-impaired subjects.

Taken together, these findings strongly support the idea that lateral suppression is reduced or absent in people with cochlear hearing loss.

Perceptual consequences of reduced frequency selectivity

Frequency selectivity plays an important role in many aspects of auditory perception. Hence, when frequency selectivity is reduced in persons with cochlear hearing loss, these aspects of perception can be expected to alter. Some of these aspects, specifically, loudness perception, frequency discrimination, pitch perception and speech perception, are discussed in more detail in later chapters of this book. This section will consider some of the other aspects of perception that are affected by reduced frequency selectivity.

Susceptibility to masking

It is obvious from the studies discussed earlier that masking effects are often more pronounced in hearing-impaired than in normal subjects. However, the size of the difference depends greatly on the spectral characteristics of the signal and masker. When the signal and masker overlap spectrally (for example, when the signal is a sinusoid and the masker is a broadband noise without distinct spectral peaks), masked thresholds are usually only slightly greater for hearing-impaired than for normal listeners. However, when the signal and masker differ in spectrum, masking may be considerably greater in the hearing-impaired. There are two obvious situations where this might apply. One is when the average spectrum of a masking sound differs from that of a signal. For example, the signal may be a high-frequency warning siren, and the masker may be primarily low-frequency noise from air-conditioning or machinery. The second is when the signal and the masker differ in their short-term spectra. For example, the signal might be a vowel sound from an attended talker and the masker might be a different vowel sound from an interfering talker. A hearing-impaired person with reduced frequency selectivity will be less able than normal to take advantage of the spectral differences betweeen the two vowels. This issue is examined in more detail in chapter 7.

Timbre perception

Timbre is often defined as 'that attribute of auditory sensation in terms of which a listener can judge that two sounds having the same loudness and pitch are dissimilar'. Differences in timbre allow us to distinguish between the same note played on, say, the piano or the flute. Timbre depends on both spectral and temporal aspects of sounds. Changing either the long term spectral shape of a sound or its temporal envelope may lead to a change in perceived timbre (see Handel 1995, for a review).

The aspects of timbre perception that are affected by spectral shape almost certainly depend on the frequency selectivity of the ear. The spectral shape of a sound is represented in the excitation pattern evoked by the sound, and the timbre is related to the shape of the excitation pattern (Plomp 1976). In an ear with cochlear damage, frequency selectivity is usually reduced. Hence, the excitation pattern contains less detail about the spectrum than would be the case for a normal ear. This would be expected to lead to a reduced ability to distinguish sounds on the basis of their spectral shape.

For many sounds, such as different musical instruments (e.g. xylophone versus harpsichord) the differences in spectral shape are so large that even very poor frequency selectivity allows their discrimination. However, it may be more difficult for a person with reduced frequency selectivity to distinguish sounds that differ in spectrum in more subtle ways. There has been little study of the ability of hearing-impaired people to distinguish musical instruments. However, different steady-state vowels are primarily distinguished by their spectral shapes, and studies of vowel perception suggest that reduced frequency selectivity can, indeed, lead to difficulties in the discrimination and identification of vowels. These studies are reviewed in chapter 7.

3 Loudness perception and intensity resolution in people with normal and impaired hearing

Introduction

Loudness is defined as that attribute of auditory sensation in terms of which sounds can be ordered on a scale extending from quiet to loud. A problem which arises in studying the loudness of sounds, particularly when these are complex or of a transient nature, is that loudness is a subjective quantity, and as such cannot be measured directly. This chapter starts by describing some of the ways in which loudness perception has been studied in normally hearing people. It then goes on to consider changes in loudness perception associated with cochlear damage.

Loudness perception in normally hearing people

Equal-loudness contours and loudness level

It is often useful to be able to compare the loudness of sounds with that of a standard, reference sound. The most common reference sound is a 1000-Hz sinusoid. The loudness level of a sound is defined as the level of a 1000-Hz sinusoid that is equal in loudness to the sound. To determine the loudness level of a given sound, the subject is asked to adjust the level of a 1000-Hz sinusoid until it appears to have the same loudness as the test sound. The 1000-Hz sinusoid and the test sound are presented alternately rather than simultaneously. The unit of loudness level is the phon. Thus, the loudness level of any sound in phons is the level (in dB SPL) of the 1000-Hz sinusoid to which it sounds equal in loudness.

In a variation of this procedure, the 1000-Hz sinusoid is fixed in level, and the test sound adjusted to give a loudness match. If this is repeated for various different frequencies of a sinusoidal test sound, an equal-loudness contour is generated (Fletcher and Munson 1933). Some typical results are shown in Figure 3.1 (Robinson and Dadson 1956). This figure shows equal-loudness contours for loudness levels from 20 phons to 120 phons, and it also includes the absolute threshold (MAF) curve. The equal-loudness contours are of similar shape to the threshold curve, but tend to become flatter at high loudness levels. This means that the rate of growth of loudness differs for tones of different frequency. For example,

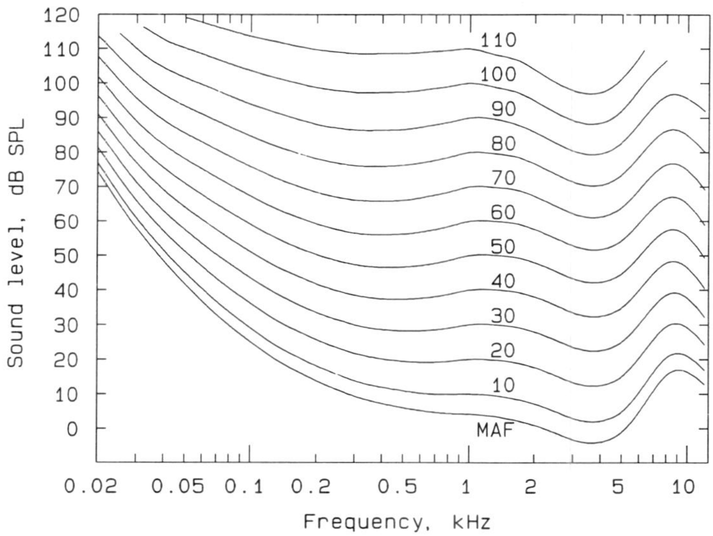

Fig. 3.1. Equal-loudness contours for various loudness levels. The lowest curve is the absolute threshold (MAF) curve. Data from Robinson and Dadson (1956).

the absolute threshold for a 100-Hz tone is about 20 dB above that for a 1000-Hz tone (thresholds at 23 and 3 dB SPL). But for the 100-phon contour, the intensities are nearly the same at 100 and 1000 Hz (102 and 100 dB SPL). For the same range of loudness level, from threshold to 100 phons, the level of the 1000-Hz tone must be increased by 97 dB, while that of the 100-Hz tone must be increased by only 79 dB. Thus the rate of growth of loudness with increasing intensity is greater for low frequencies (and to some extent for very high frequencies) than for middle frequencies.

The scaling of loudness

Several methods have been developed that attempt to measure 'directly' the relationship between the physical magnitude of sound and perceived loudness. The development of scales of loudness and of other sensory dimensions was pioneered by S. S. Stevens, and the reader is referred to his work for further details (Stevens 1957). Two methods have been commonly used to derive scales of loudness. In one, called magnitude estimation, sounds with various different levels are presented, and the subject is asked to assign a number to each one according to its perceived loudness. In a second method, called magnitude production, the subject is asked to adjust the level of a sound until it has a loudness corresponding to a specified number.

On the basis of results from experiments of this type, Stevens suggested that loudness, L, was a power function of physical intensity, I:

$$L = kI^{0.3} \qquad \text{Eq. 3.1}$$

where k is a constant depending on the subject and the units used. In other words, the loudness of a given sound is proportional to its intensity raised to the power 0.3. A simple approximation to this is that a two-fold change in loudness is produced by a 10 dB step in level. Stevens proposed the 'sone' as the unit of loudness. One sone is defined arbitrarily as the loudness of a 1000-Hz sinusoid at 40 dB SPL. A 1000-Hz sinsuoid with a level of 50 dB SPL is usually judged as about twice as loud as a 40-dB sinusoid, and has a loudness of 2 sones.

Another method of relating loudness sensations to physical intensity involves categorical judgements of loudness. This method has been used mainly with hearing-impaired people, and it will be described later in this chapter.

The detection of intensity changes

The normal auditory system is remarkable both in terms of its absolute sensitivity and in terms of the range of sound intensities to which it can respond. The most intense sound that can be heard without damaging the ears has a level about 120 dB above that of the faintest sound that can be detected. This corresponds to a ratio of intensities of 1,000,000,000,000:1. Over this whole range, relatively small changes in sound intensity can be detected.

The smallest detectable change in intensity has been measured for many different types of stimuli by a variety of methods. The three main methods are:

(1) Modulation detection. The stimulus is amplitude modulated (i.e. made to vary in amplitude) at a slow regular rate and the subject is required to detect the modulation.
(2) Increment detection. A continuous background stimulus is presented, and the subject is required to detect an increment in the level of the background.
(3) Intensity discrimination of gated or pulsed stimuli. Two separate pulses of sound are presented successively, one being more intense than the other, and the subject is required to indicate which was the more intense.

Although there are some minor discrepancies in the experimental results for the different types of method, the general trend is similar. Thresholds for detecting intensity changes are usually specified in decibels, i.e. as the change in level at threshold. For wideband noise, or for bandpass filtered noise, the smallest detectable intensity change is approximately a constant fraction of the intensity of the stimulus. If I is the intensity of a noise band, and ΔI the smallest detectable change in intensity, then ΔI is roughly constant. This is an example of Weber's Law, which states that the smallest detectable change in a stimulus is proportional to the magnitude of that stimulus. The value of $\Delta I/I$ is called the Weber fraction. If the smallest detectable change is expressed in decibels, i.e. as $10\log[(I + \Delta I/ I]$then this, too, is constant. Thus the just-detectable change in level, ΔL, is constant, regardless of the absolute level, and for wideband noise has a value of about 0.5–1 dB. This holds from about 20 dB above threshold to 100 dB above threshold (Miller 1947). The value of ΔL increases for sounds which are close to the absolute threshold.

For sinusoids the situation is somewhat different. Riesz's (1928) data for modulated tones, and data from a number of other workers using pulsed tones, show that Weber's Law does not hold (Harris 1963; Viemeister 1972; Jesteadt *et al.* 1977b). Instead it is found that if ΔI (in dB) is plotted against I (also in dB), a straight line is obtained with a slope of about 0.9; Weber's law would give a slope of 1.0. Thus discrimination, as measured by the Weber fraction, improves at high levels. This has been called the 'near miss' to Weber's Law. The data of Riesz for modulation detection show a value of ΔL of 1.5 dB at 20 dB SL, 0.7 dB at 40 dB SL, and 0.3 dB at 80 dB SL (all at 1000 Hz). The change in ΔL with level is somewhat less for pulsed tones than for modulated tones.

Loudness recruitment and reduced dynamic range in people with cochlear damage

Most, if not all, people with cochlear damage show a phenomenon referred to as loudness recruitment (Fowler 1936; Steinberg and Gardner 1937). The phenomenon may be described as follows. The absolute threshold is higher than normal. However, when a sound is increased in level above the absolute threshold, the rate of growth of loudness with increasing sound level is greater than normal. When the level is sufficiently high, usually around 90 to 100 dB SPL, the loudness reaches its 'normal' value; the sound appears as loud to the person with impaired hearing as it would to a normally hearing person. With further increases in sound level above 90–100 dB SPL, the loudness grows in an almost normal manner.

A complementary way of describing the same effect is in terms of dynamic range. This refers to the range of sound levels over which sounds are both audible and comfortable. The lower end of the dynamic range is determined by the absolute threshold for detecting sounds. The upper end is determined by the level at which sounds start to become uncomfortably loud. Typically, in people with cochlear hearing loss, the absolute threshold is elevated, but the level at which sounds become uncomfortably loud is about the same as normal. Hence the dynamic range is reduced compared to normal. Sometimes, especially in cases of severe hearing loss, the loudness does not reach its 'normal' value at high sound levels, but remains somewhat below that which would occur in normal hearing. This is called 'under recruitment' or 'partial recruitment'. The opposite case also sometimes occurs, where high-level sounds appear louder to a hearing-impaired person than to a normally hearing person. This is called 'over recruitment'. However, the commonest pattern is that of complete recruitment, where for sounds at high levels the loudness is about the same for normally hearing and hearing-impaired persons.

Loudness recruitment is most easily demonstrated in people who have a cochlear hearing impairment in one ear only. It is then possible to obtain loudness matches between the two ears. Figure 3.2 shows the mean results of measurements of this type obtained by Moore *et al.* (1985a) for five subjects with unilateral cochlear hearing loss. The subjects were chosen to have relatively 'flat' losses across frequency, and their absolute thresholds at the test frequency (either 1.0 or 1.5

kHz) were in the range 45–60 dB HL. Sinusoidal tone bursts of 500 ms duration were presented in alternation to the normal and impaired ears, with an interval of 500 ms between the tones. The tone in the impaired ear was fixed in level, and the tone in the normal ear was varied under computer control in a Békésy tracking procedure. The starting level of the variable tone was determined randomly for each trial. The loudness match was estimated as the mean level at the last eight 'turnpoints', and three such estimates were obtained for each subject. The mean level of the loudness match in the normal ear is plotted as a function of the level in the impaired ear. For comparison, the mean results from three subjects with normal hearing in both ears are also shown (dashed line).

For the normal ears, as expected, the loudness in the two ears is matched when the tones are approximately equal in level at the two ears; the line has a slope close to one (in fact, there is a bias for the level of the matching tone to be slightly below the level of the fixed tone, for the higher levels used, since subjects tend to avoid very high sound levels). In contrast, for the impaired ears, the slope is greater than one. A level of 60 dB SPL in the impaired ears is matched by a level of about 27 dB in the normal ears, reflecting the elevation in absolute threshold in the impaired ears. However, at high sound levels, the discrepancy between the normal and impaired ears is much reduced. A level of 90 dB SPL in the impaired ears is

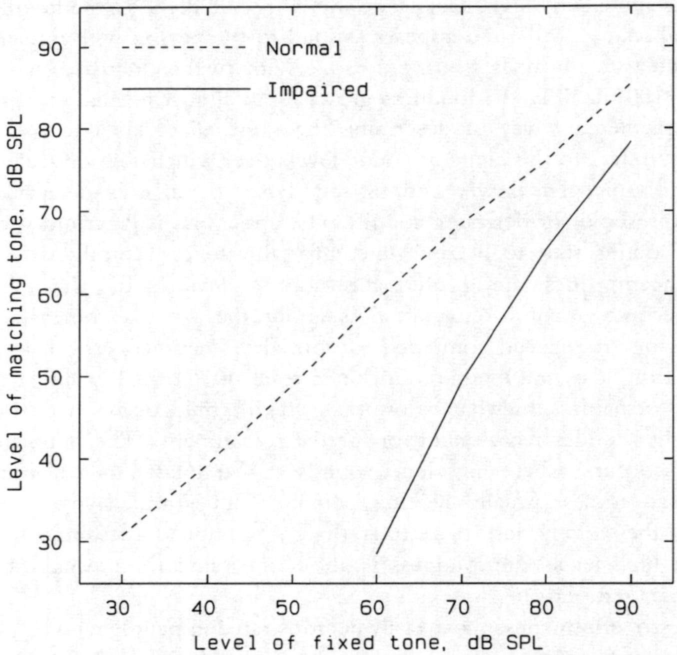

Fig. 3.2. Results of loudness matches between sinusoidal tone bursts presented alternately to the two ears for normally hearing subjects (dashed line) and subjects with unilateral cochlear hearing loss (continuous line). The tone was fixed at a series of levels in one ear (the impaired ear of the subjects with unilateral impairment) and the level in the other ear was varied to determine the point corresponding to equal loudness.

matched by a level of about 80 dB SPL in the normal ears. If higher levels had been used, the loudness in the impaired ears would probably have 'caught up' completely with that in the normal ears. However, for these subjects, the sounds started to become uncomfortably loud at levels above 90 dB SPL.

Loudness recruitment can also be demonstrated in people with cochlear damage in both ears. One method of doing this involves the use of a categorical loudness scaling procedure. The subject is presented with a test sound, and is asked to judge its loudness by using one of several verbal categories (Pascoe 1978; Hellbrück and Moser 1985; Kiessling *et al.* 1993). An example is the Loudness Growth in half-Octave Bands (LGOB) test described by Allen and Jeng (1990) and adapted by Pluvinage (1989) and by Moore *et al.* (1992b). The stimuli are half-octave wide bands of noise centred at 500, 1000, 2000 and 4000 Hz. In an initial phase of the test, each centre frequency is tested separately. On each trial, the noise band is presented as a series of three bursts, and the subject is required to indicate the loudness of the bursts by pressing one of seven buttons labelled 'cannot hear', 'very soft', 'soft', 'comfortable', 'loud', 'very loud', and 'too loud'. The sound level is varied randomly from trial to trial over the range from 30 to 110 dB SPL.

In the second phase, all stimuli consistently eliciting responses of 'can't hear' or 'too loud' are eliminated, and a series of trials is presented in which both the centre frequency and level of the noise bands are randomized. The step size in level is determined on the basis of the subject's dynamic range, varying from 8 dB for a normal dynamic range to 4 dB for a narrow one (<50 dB). The results of the second phase are used to construct functions relating perceived loudness to level at each centre frequency. These curves give a quantitative measure of loudness recruitment; the steeper the slope, the greater the recruitment. The test is applied separately for each ear.

Some examples of growth-of-loudness curves are given in Figure 3.3 (data from Moore *et al.* 1992b). The numbers 1–5 correspond to the five categories of loudness from 'very soft' to 'very loud'. In each panel, the dashed line indicates typical results for subjects with normal hearing. The four panels at the top show results for a subject with marked loudness recruitment; all of the curves have steep slopes, and at high levels the loudness reaches or even exceeds that which would occur in a normal ear. The bottom four panels show results for a subject with little or no loudness recruitment. The curves are shifted down vertically relative to those for normally hearing subjects, but the slopes are almost normal. This pattern of results is common in cases of conductive hearing loss, but rare in cases of cochlear damage. Most subjects with cochlear impairments give results between these two extremes, a typical example being shown in the middle four panels.

A third way of measuring loudness recruitment is to use magnitude estimation (ME) or magnitude production (MP), as described earlier for normally hearing subjects (Stevens 1957). These techniques give a similar pattern of results to the categorical loudness scaling procedures; almost all subjects with cochlear damage show some degree of loudness recruitment, as indicated by the fact that the rate of growth of loudness with increasing sound level is greater than normal (Hellman and Meiselman 1990, 1993).

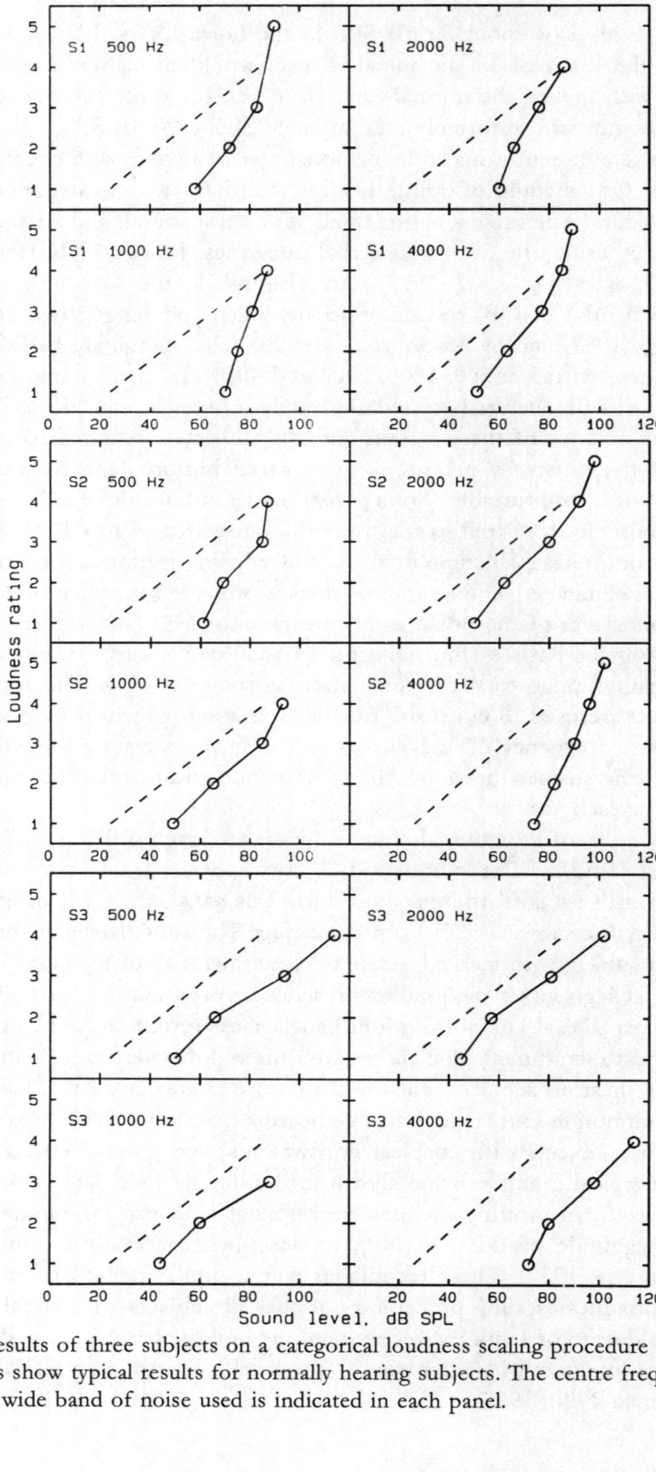

Fig. 3.3. Results of three subjects on a categorical loudness scaling procedure (circles). The dashed lines show typical results for normally hearing subjects. The centre frequency of the half-octave wide band of noise used is indicated in each panel.

Although there can be considerable individual differences using all three techniques for measuring recruitment, on average the steepness of the loudness growth curves increases with increasing absolute threshold at the test frequency (Miskolczy-Fodor 1960; Glasberg and Moore 1989; Hellman and Meiselman 1990, 1993; Kiessling *et al.* 1993). This is consistent with the idea that threshold elevation and loudness recruitment are both linked to the loss of the active mechanism in the cochlea. When the absolute threshold is high, the dynamic range can be very small indeed. For example, for subject S2 in Figure 3.3, a 75-dB tone at 4000 Hz was judged 'very soft', while a 100-dB tone was judged 'very loud', indicating a dynamic range of only about 25 dB. In some cases, the dynamic range can be as small as 10 dB.

Models of loudness perception

The mechanisms underlying the perception of loudness are not fully understood. A common assumption is that loudness is somehow related to the total neural activity evoked by a sound. If this is the case, then the loudness of a sinusoidal tone is determined not only by activity in neurones with CFs close to the frequency of the tone, but also by the spread of activity to neurones with adjacent CFs. Put another way, loudness may depend upon a summation of neural activity across different frequency channels.

Models incorporating these basic concepts have been proposed by Fletcher and Munson (1933, 1937), Zwicker (1958), and Zwicker and Scharf (1965). The first stage of Zwicker's model is a fixed filter to account for the transmission of sound through the outer and middle ear. The next stage is the calculation of an excitation pattern for the sound under consideration; the concept of the excitation pattern was described in chapter 2. This pattern can be thought of as representing the distribution of excitation at different points along the BM. Zwicker's model uses as a starting point the masking patterns for narrowband noises (Zwicker 1958). He assumed that the excitation patterns evoked by such noises were similar in shape to the masking patterns, but shifted by a few dB, the exact amount of shift depending on frequency. However, it is also possible to calculate excitation patterns from auditory filter shapes, as described in chapter 2. This is done in a revised version of Zwicker's loudness model described by Moore and Glasberg (1995).

The next stage is the transformation of the frequency scale of the excitation pattern to a scale more closely related to how the sound is represented in the auditory system. In Zwicker's model, this scale was referred to as 'tonalness' or the 'Bark' scale. An alternative is the ERB scale described in chapter 2.

The next stage in Zwicker's model is the transformation from excitation level to specific loudness, N', which is the loudness per critical band. This transformation involves a compressive nonlinearity. Although Zwicker's model is based on psychoacoustical data, this transformation can be thought of as representing the way that physical excitation is transformed into neural activity; the specific loudness is probably related to the amount of neural activity at the corresponding

CF. The overall loudness of a given sound, in sones, is assumed to be proportional to the total area under the specific loudness pattern plotted as N′ versus Bark. One might think of this area as approximately proportional to the total neural activity evoked by a sound.

Zwicker described the relationship between excitation and N′ in terms of excitation in power units, E, rather than excitation level in dB, L_E:

$$L_E = 10\log_{10}(E/E_0) \qquad \text{Eq. 3.2}$$

where E_0 is the excitation corresponding to a sound at 0 dB SPL. The specific loudness is related to the excitation at a given CF by the following equation:

$$N' = C(E_{THRQ})^{\alpha}\ [(0.5E_{SIG}/E_{THRQ} + 0.5)^{\alpha} - 1\ ] \quad \text{for } E_{SIG} > E_{THRQ}$$

$$N' = 0 \text{ for } E_{SIG} < E_{THRQ} \qquad \text{Eq. 3.3}$$

where E_{SIG} is the excitation produced by the stimulus, E_{THRQ} is the excitation at absolute threshold at that CF, and C and α are constants. The value of α is less than one ($\alpha \approx 0.23$), so Eq. 3.3 defines a compressive relationship between excitation and specific loudness. However, the function becomes steeper when E_{SIG} approaches E_{THRQ}. Moore and Glasberg (1995) have proposed a slightly different equation relating specific loudness to excitation, but, again, it involves a compressive nonlinearity:

$$N' = C[(E_{SIG}/E_0)^{\alpha} - (E_{THRQ}/E_0)^{\alpha}] \quad \text{for } E_{SIG} \geq E_{THRQ} \qquad \text{Eq. 3.4}$$

$$N' = 0 \quad \text{for } E_{SIG} < E_{THRQ}$$

Just as in Zwicker's model, the function is highly compressive when the signal excitation is well above the threshold excitation, but becomes steeper when E_{SIG} approaches E_{THRQ}. The compressive nonlinearity in the models can be thought of as representing the overall effects of the transformation from the physical stimulus to neural activity. At least two nonlinearities contribute to this overall effect: the compressive nonlinearity of the BM input–output function, as described in chapter 1; and the nonlinear transformation from BM velocity or amplitude to neural activity.

The function defined by Eq. 3.4 is plotted in Figure 3.4 for a series of values of the excitation level at absolute threshold, E_{THRQ}. The value of N′ is plotted on a log scale as a function of excitation level in decibels (also a log scale). At high excitation levels, the curves show an asymptotic slope corresponding to the value of the constant α. However, the steepness of the initial part of the curves depends on the value of E_{THRQ}; the higher E_{THRQ}, the steeper the curve. Thus the functions show a recruitment-like effect. Higher thresholds automatically are associated with steeper functions. This resembles the way that higher thresholds on the BM are associated with steeper input–output functions, and higher behavioural absolute thresholds lead to steeper loudness growth curves.

The mechanisms underlying loudness recruitment

Theoretical considerations

Consider now the changes that occur in an ear with cochlear damage, and how these might affect the perception of loudness. The first such change is an elevation in absolute threshold, or, equivalently, a reduced sensitivity to weak sounds. Accompanying this is a reduction in or loss of the compressive nonlinearity in the input-output function of the BM; this is usually associated with damage to the OHCs. In an ear where the damage is confined largely to the OHCs, with IHCs intact, the transformation from BM velocity or amplitude to neural activity probably remains largely normal. However, in an ear with damage to the IHCs as well, this nonlinearity may also be affected.

If the input–output function on the BM is steeper (less compressive) than normal in an ear with cochlear damage, this would be expected to lead to an increased rate of growth of loudness with increasing sound level. However, at high sound levels, around 90–100 dB SPL, the input–output function becomes almost linear in both normal and impaired ears. The magnitude of the BM response at high sound levels is roughly the same in a normal and an impaired ear (see, for example, Figure 1.13). This could explain why the loudness in an impaired ear usually 'catches up' with that in a normal ear at sound levels around 90–100 dB SPL.

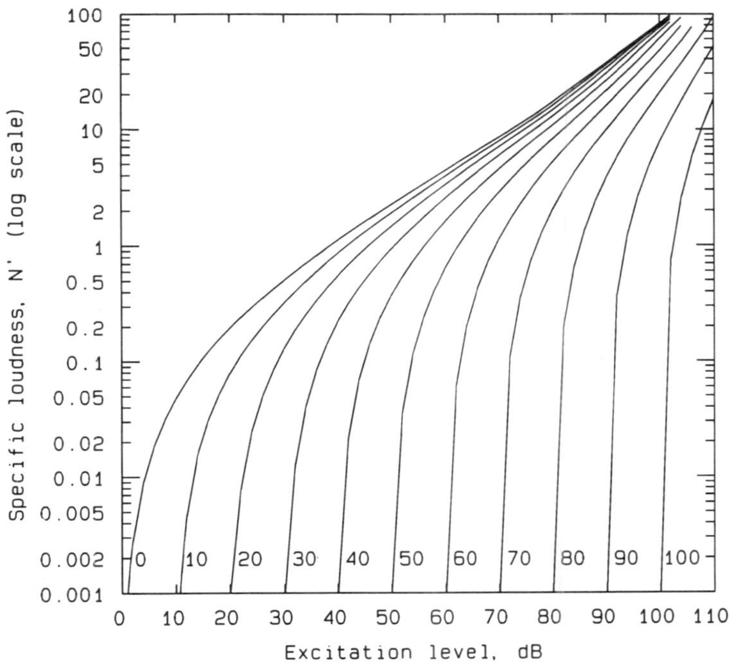

Fig. 3.4. Functions relating specific loudness, N′, to excitation level in dB, as defined by Eq. 3.4. The parameter is the excitation level at threshold for the CF under consideration.

In terms of the loudness model outlined above, the fact that the absolute threshold is higher than normal (E_{THRQ} in Eqs. 3.3 and 3.4) automatically leads to a steeper function relating specific loudness to excitation, as illustrated in Figure 3.4; this mimics the effect seen on the BM. To assess whether this is sufficient on its own to account for loudness recruitment, the predictions of the model have been compared with data from Miskolczy-Fodor (1960). Figure 3.5 shows loudness-matching data for subjects with unilateral hearing losses; subjects were selected to have absolute thresholds about 50 dB higher than normal or 80 dB higher than normal, and results are shown for many different subjects. The solid curves show the predictions of the loudness model of Moore and Glasberg (1995). The parameters in the model were exactly the same as would apply to loudness predictions for normally hearing subjects, except that the values of E_{THRQ} were increased by 50 dB (left curve) or 80 dB (right curve). The curves fit the data rather well, suggesting that loudness recruitment can be largely accounted for by the

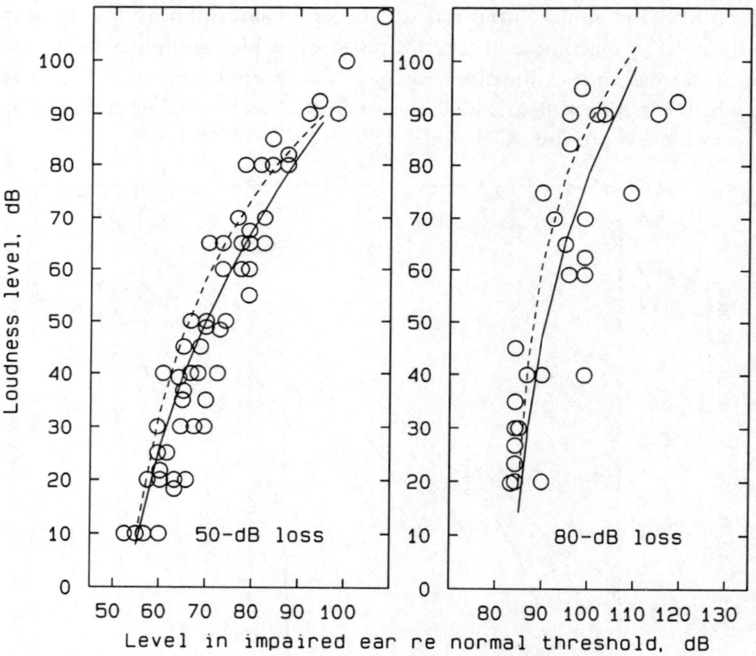

Fig. 3.5. The circles show loudness matching data presented by Miskolczy-Fodor (1960) for subjects with unilateral hearing loss of 50 dB (left panel) or 80 dB (right panel). The level in the impaired ear is expressed relative to the normal absolute threshold at the test frequency. The matching level in the normal ear is expressed as loudness level in dB, equivalent to the SPL of an equally-loud 1-kHz sinusoid. The continuous lines show the predictions of the loudness model of Moore and Glasberg (1995) when frequency selectivity was assumed to be normal but absolute thresholds were elevated. The dashed lines show the predictions when the auditory filters were assumed to be broader than normal.

elevated absolute threshold and the associated steeper growth of specific loudness with increasing excitation level. Note, however, that the data show a large scatter; the model accounts for the mean data quite well, but it does not account for the individual differences.

Another change that occurs in cases of cochlear damage is a reduction in frequency selectivity, as reviewed in chapters 1 and 2. For a sinusoidal stimulus, this leads to an excitation pattern which is broader (spreads over a greater range of CFs) in an impaired than in a normal ear. Kiang *et al.* (1970) and Evans (1975) suggested that this might be the main factor contributing to loudness recruitment. They suggested that, once the level of a sound exceeds threshold, the excitation in an ear with cochlear damage spreads more rapidly than normal across the array of neurones, and this leads to the abnormally rapid growth of loudness with increasing level.

The theoretical importance of reduced frequency selectivity can be assessed by modifying the loudness model described above by introducing broader-than-normal auditory filters. This has been done to model the data shown in Figure 3.5. For the subjects with absolute thresholds about 50 dB higher than normal, it was assumed that the auditory filters were twice as broad as normal at levels just above threshold and increased slightly in bandwidth with increasing level. For the subjects with absolute thresholds about 80 dB higher than normal, it was assumed that the auditory filters were four times as broad as normal, but were invariant with level. The predictions obtained using these assumptions are shown as the dashed lines in Figure 3.5.

The assumed broadening of the auditory filters has the effect of increasing the predicted loudness in the impaired ears. However, this effect occurs over almost the whole range of levels covered, with little effect on the slopes of the curves. Thus, while reduced frequency selectivity is predicted to influence perceived loudness to some extent, it is not predicted to play a major role in producing the steep slopes of the loudness growth curves obtained from subjects with loudness recruitment.

Experimental tests of the role of frequency selectivity in loudness recruitment

Moore *et al.* (1985a) carried out an experimental test of whether abnormal spread of excitation could account for loudness recruitment, using subjects with unilateral cochlear hearing loss. The subjects were those whose loudness-matching data are shown in Figure 3.2. They carried out a loudness-matching experiment similar to that described earlier, except that the fixed tone presented to the impaired ear had a noise gated on and off with it. The noise was filtered so as to have a spectral notch extending from 0.6 to 1.4 times the signal frequency. The ratio of the level of the tone to the spectrum level of the noise within its passbands was either 20, 30 or 40 dB.

The idea of this experiment was as follows. Provided that the subjects have some degree of frequency selectivity, the background noise should mask neural activity evoked by the tone at CFs far from the signal frequency, but should not mask activity at CFs close to the signal frequency, owing to the presence of the spectral notch. The frequency selectivity of the subjects was measured with the notched-noise method described in chapter 2, to confirm that the subjects had reduced frequency selectivity in their impaired ears, but that frequency selectivity was not completely absent. This turned out to be the case for all subjects. As the level of the noise relative to the tone was increased, the noise would have masked more and more of the activity at CFs remote from the signal frequency. If the activity at these remote CFs were responsible for the loudness recruitment, then the noise should have greatly reduced the loudness of the tone, especially at high tone levels.

The mean results are shown in Figure 3.6. It is obvious that the noise had only a small effect on the loudness of the tone in the impaired ear. The noise did result in a slightly lower level for the matching tone, but not by very much. Further, the noise had almost no effect on the slope of the curves. The loudness was not reduced more at high tone levels than at low tone levels, as would be expected if abnormal spread of excitation were responsible for loudness recruitment.

These results suggest that abnormal spread of excitation is not the main cause of loudness recruitment. This is consistent with the theoretical analysis based on

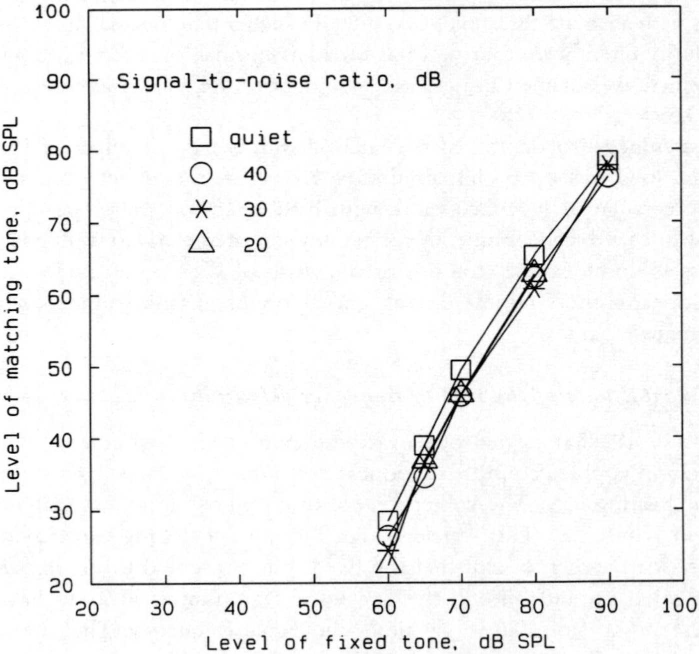

Fig. 3.6. Mean results of loudness matches between sinusoidal tone bursts presented alternately to the two ears for subjects with unilateral cochlear hearing loss. The tone in the impaired ear was presented either in quiet (squares) or in a notched noise designed to mask tone-evoked neural activity at CFs away from the frequency of the tone. The ratio of the signal level to the noise spectrum level in its passbands is indicated in the figure.

the loudness model. A similar conclusion has been reached by others who have studied the role of spread of excitation in loudness (Hellman 1978; Hellman and Meiselman 1986; Zeng and Turner 1991). Although spread of excitation may play a small role, the loss of compressive nonlinearity on the BM seems to be a more dominant factor.

In some cases of cochlear damage, it appears that a reduction in effective spread of excitation can reduce the rate of growth of loudness with increasing intensity at frequencies where hearing is normal. Hellman (1994) studied loudness growth in 21 subjects with normal hearing at low frequencies and hearing loss at high frequencies (above about 2 kHz), using the methods of magnitude estimation and magnitude production. Subjects were divided into two groups according to the rate of increase of threshold with increasing frequency in the region of hearing loss; group I had rates of 30–49 dB/octave and group II had rates of 51–71 dB/octave. For group I, the slopes of the loudness growth functions were similar for a sinusoidal signal at the upper edge of the frequency region of normal hearing and for a signal well within the region of normal hearing. However, for group II, the slopes of the loudness growth functions were shallower, at medium to high levels (40–80 dB SL), when the signal was at the upper edge of the frequency region of normal hearing than when it was well within the region of normal hearing. This can be explained by assuming that, in subjects with losses that increase rapidly with frequency, the excitation produced by a tone with a frequency close to the region of the loss does not spread effectively to high CFs. The reduced spread of excitation leads to reduced loudness growth.

Loudness summation in impaired subjects

In normally hearing subjects, if the bandwidth of a sound is varied keeping the overall intensity fixed, the loudness remains constant as long as the bandwidth is less than a certain value (called the critical bandwidth, CB, for loudness). If the bandwidth is increased beyond the CB, the loudness increases (Zwicker *et al.* 1957). The reason that loudness remains constant for sub-critical bandwidths can be understood by considering how the specific loudness patterns change with bandwidth. With increasing bandwidth up to the CB, the specific loudness patterns become lower at their tips, but broader; the decrease in area around the tip is almost exactly cancelled by the increase on the skirts, so that the total area remains almost constant (Moore and Glasberg 1986d; Moore and Glasberg 1995). This is illustrated in Figure 3.7. When the bandwidth is increased beyond the CB, the increase on the skirts is greater than the decrease around the tip, and the total area, and hence the predicted loudness, increases. Since the increase depends on the summation of specific loudness at different CFs, the increase in loudness is often described as 'loudness summation'.

Several studies have shown that loudness summation is reduced in people with cochlear hearing loss; the increase in loudness with increasing bandwidth is less than occurs in normally hearing people (Scharf and Hellman 1966; Bonding 1979a; Florentine and Zwicker 1979; Bonding and Elberling 1980). Florentine and

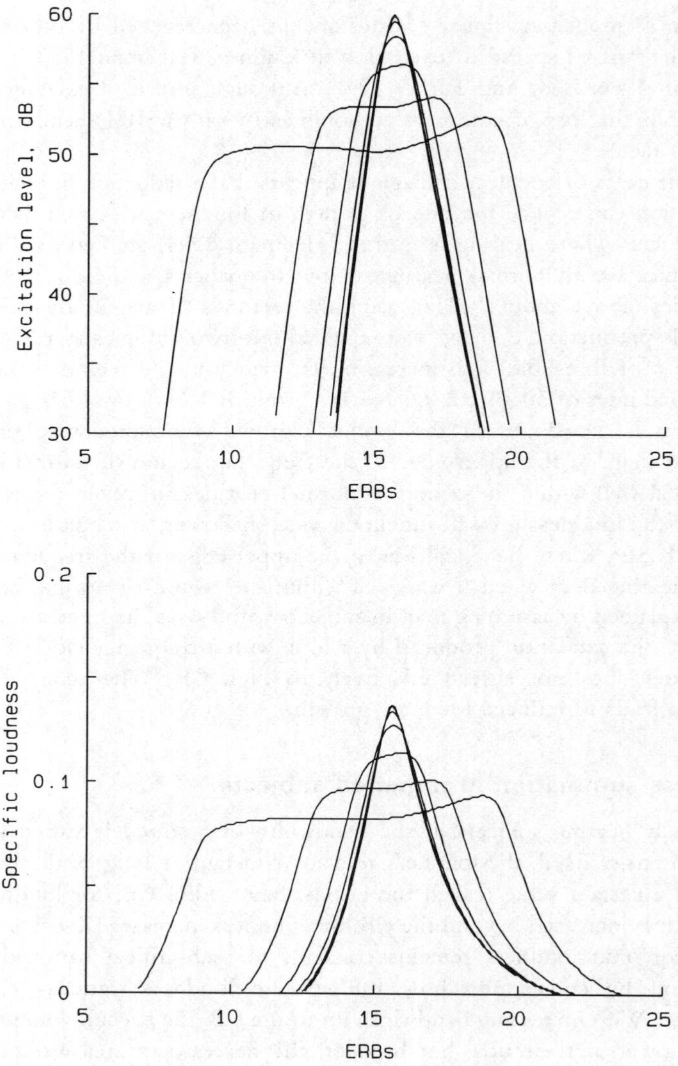

Fig. 3.7. Excitation patterns (top) and specific loudness patterns (bottom) for bands of noise with constant overall level and centre frequency, but varying bandwidth. The patterns were calculated using the model of Moore and Glasberg (1995). The frequency scale has been transformed to an ERB scale, which corresponds reasonably well to distance along the BM; see chapter 2 for details. It is assumed that the loudness of a given sound corresponds to the total area under its specific loudness pattern.

Zwicker (1979) measured the level difference needed for equal loudness between a 709-Hz wide noise and a 5909-Hz wide noise, both geometrically centred at 4000 Hz, using subjects with noise-induced hearing loss. The absolute thresholds of the subjects were about 45 dB higher than normal at 4000 Hz. Their results are shown by the open circles in Figure 3.8. The difference in level between the two noise bands required for equal loudness is plotted as a function of the level of the narrower band of noise, L_{NBN}. The difference varies somewhat with level, but is generally smaller than they obtained with normally hearing subjects.

Florentine and Zwicker (1979) considered whether their data could be accounted for by Zwicker's loudness model, based on various modifications to the model to take account of the hearing impairment. They found that if the only modification was to the value of E_{THRQ}, the excitation at absolute threshold at each CF, then the model predicted more loudness summation (a greater level difference) than was obtained. Recall that increasing E_{THRQ} has the effect of increasing the slope of the function relating specific loudness to excitation level, so the change in E_{THRQ} effectively incorporates the main factor influencing loudness recruitment. From this they concluded that loudness recruitment alone does not account for the reduced loudness summation. If they took into account reduced frequency selectivity, then the predicted level differences were closer to the obtained differences, although still somewhat larger. A similar analysis is presented here

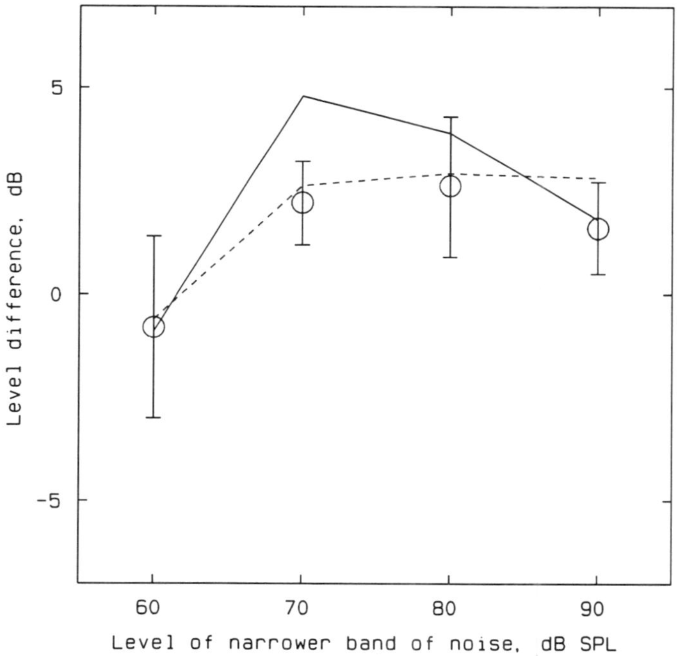

Fig. 3.8. The circles show the level difference needed for equal loudness between a 709-Hz wide noise and a 5909-Hz wide noise, both geometrically centred at 4000 Hz, using subjects with noise-induced hearing loss (data from Florentine and Zwicker, 1979). Error bars indicate inter-quartile ranges. The continuous line shows the predictions of the loudness model of Moore and Glasberg (1995) when frequency selectivity was assumed to be normal but absolute thresholds were elevated. The dashed line shows the predictions when the auditory filters were assumed to be broader than normal.

using the modified version of Zwicker's loudness model described by Moore and Glasberg (1995).

The solid line in Figure 3.8 shows the predictions of the model when the value of E_{THRQ} was increased by 45 dB relative to the value for normally hearing subjects, but frequency selectivity was assumed to be normal. The model correctly predicts that the level difference is slightly negative for L_{NBN} = 60 dB, and is slightly positive at higher levels. The decrease in loudness with increasing bandwidth at L_{NBN} = 60 dB occurs for the same reason that, for normally hearing subjects, loudness decreases with increasing bandwidth at very low overall sound levels. The reason is as follows. At low SLs, specific loudness increases very rapidly with increasing excitation level (see Figure 3.4). As the bandwidth is increased, keeping overall intensity constant, the excitation spreads over a wider range of CFs, but the excitation in the central part of the excitation pattern decreases. This leads to a large decrease in specific loudness. The decrease in the central part of the specific loudness pattern more than offsets the increase at the edges, so overall loudness decreases.

At high sound levels, the predicted level differences are positive, as are the obtained values. However, for L_{NBN} = 70 and 80 dB the differences are somewhat larger than the obtained values. The dashed line shows the predictions of the model when E_{THRQ} was set to a value 45 dB higher than normal, and the auditory filters were assumed to be twice as broad as normal, but invariant with level. The predicted and obtained values are very close. It seems reasonable to conclude that the reduced loudness summation observed in subjects with cochlear hearing loss depends both on loss of the compressive nonlinearity on the BM (which is the main cause of loudness recruitment) and on reduced frequency selectivity.

Intensity resolution in cases of cochlear damage

The ability to detect changes in intensity, or to compare the intensity of two separate sounds, is usually assumed to be based on the loudness sensations evoked by the sounds. In persons with cochlear damage, a given change in intensity usually results in a larger-than-normal change in loudness. Hence, it might be expected that intensity discrimination would be *better* than normal. However, this expectation is based on the assumption that the just-detectable change in loudness is unaffected by the cochlear damage, and this assumption may not be valid.

Following early evidence that loudness recruitment was specific to cochlear damage (Dix *et al.* 1948), there were many studies exploring the possibility that better-than-normal intensity discrimination could be used as an indirect measure of loudness recruitment, and hence as an indicator of cochlear damage (Lüscher and Zwislocki 1949). These studies led to the Short Increment Sensitivity Index (SISI) test (Jerger *et al.* 1959; Jerger 1962), reviewed by Buus *et al.* (1982a,b). In this test, a continuous tone is presented at 20 dB above the absolute threshold (20 dB SL). The level is increased by 1 dB every 5 seconds, with a rise/fall time of 50 ms, and a steady-state duration of 200 ms. Larger, 5-dB increments are used to familiarise the patient with the task, and 'catch' trials may be presented to control for false positives and eliminate rhythmic responding. The subject is asked to press a button whenever a small jump in loudness is heard and 20 test increments are presented. The number of increments to which a patient responds multiplied by five gives the SISI score in percent. Normally hearing people, and patients with conductive or retrocochlear losses, typically score below 20%, whereas patients with cochlear losses typically score more than 60%. In other words, for this specific test, cochlear damage leads to an improvement in the ability to detect changes in intensity.

Although the SISI test does appear to be useful as a clinical indicator of cochlear damage, this should not be taken to indicate that, more generally, intensity resolution is better than normal in persons with cochlear damage. It turns out that the results depend on the nature of the task used, on the level of testing and on the pattern of hearing loss of the subject.

Detection of amplitude modulation

The SISI test involves detection of changes in level of an ongoing sound. A related task is that of detecting amplitude modulation at a low rate. In a review, Buus *et al.* (1982b) concluded that subjects with cochlear impairment show higher SISI scores, and lower difference limens (DLs) for detecting amplitude modulation when compared to normal listeners at equal Sensation Level (SL), i.e. equal amounts above absolute threshold. However, when compared at equal SPL, the performance of subjects with cochlear damage is not better than normal, and may be worse than normal.

This conclusion is generally supported by more recent data (Glasberg and Moore 1989; Turner *et al.* 1989). As an example, some data from Glasberg and Moore (1989) are presented here. They tested nine subjects with unilateral cochlear impairments and six subjects with bilateral cochlear impairments. Most of the subjects had relatively 'flat' moderate losses. Subjects were presented with two successive tone pulses, one of which had a constant amplitude, and the other of which was sinusoidally amplitude modulated at a 4-Hz rate. Subjects were required to detect which tone was modulated. The level of the unmodulated tone presented to the impaired ears was 80 dB SPL. The normal ears were tested both at the same SPL and at the same SL (determined separately for each subject). Each tone lasted 1020 ms, including the 10-ms raised-cosine onset and offset ramps.

The threshold for detecting the amplitude modulation was measured using an adaptive procedure and is specified as the peak-to-valley ratio in dB required for 71% correct. The threshold value will be denoted by the term AMDL (amplitude modulation difference limen). Tests were conducted both in quiet and in the presence of a continuous one-octave wide noise; this noise was designed to mask the upper side of the excitation pattern of the tone, to assess the influence of nonlinearities on the high-frequency side of the excitation pattern; see chapter 2 and below for more details. The lower cutoff frequency of the noise (−3 dB point) was twice the signal frequency, slopes were 96 dB/oct, and the overall level of the noise was 77 dB SPL.

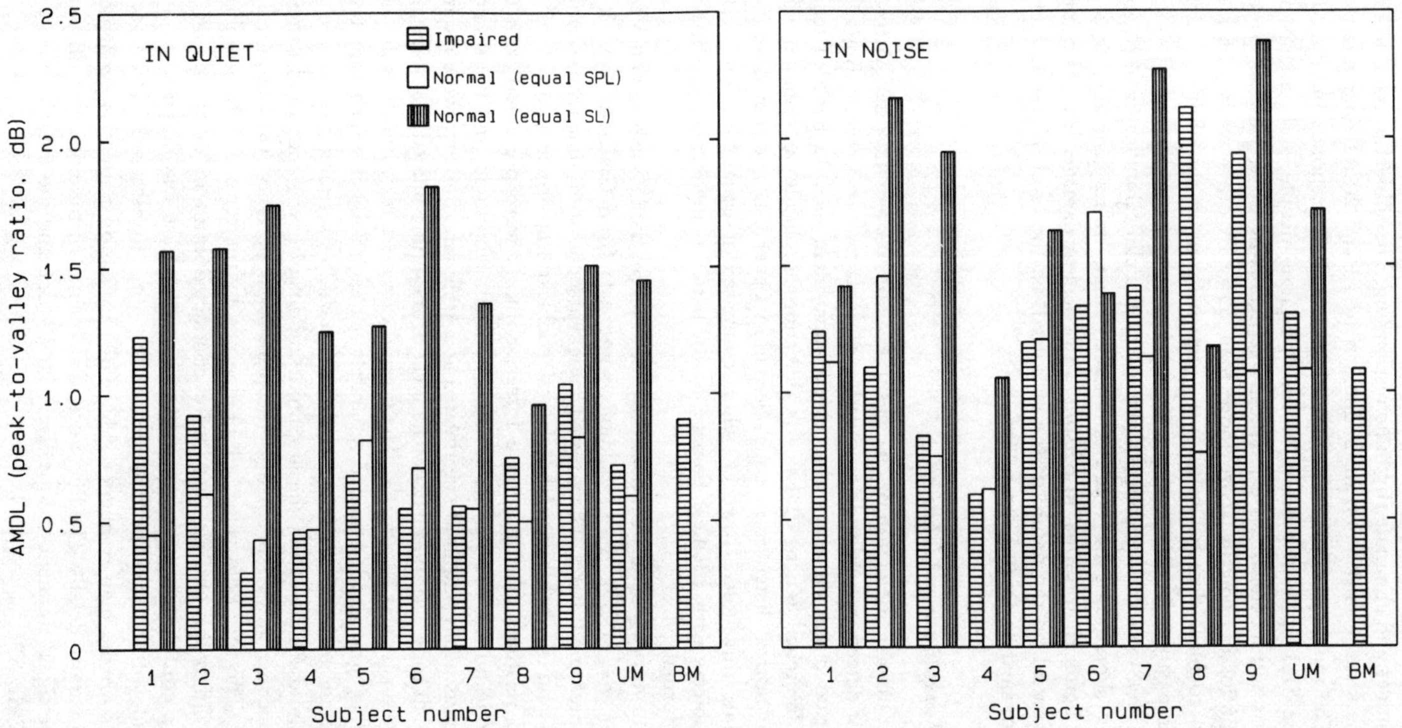

Fig. 3.9. Thresholds for detecting amplitude modulation, AMDLs, averaged for the frequencies 0.5, 1.0 and 2.0 kHz. Individual results are shown for nine subjects with unilateral cochlear hearing loss. Mean results are also shown for those nine subjects (UM) and for six subjects with bilateral cochlear hearing loss (BM). Stimuli were presented either in quiet (left panel) or in noise designed to mask part of the high-frequency side of the excitation pattern (right panel).

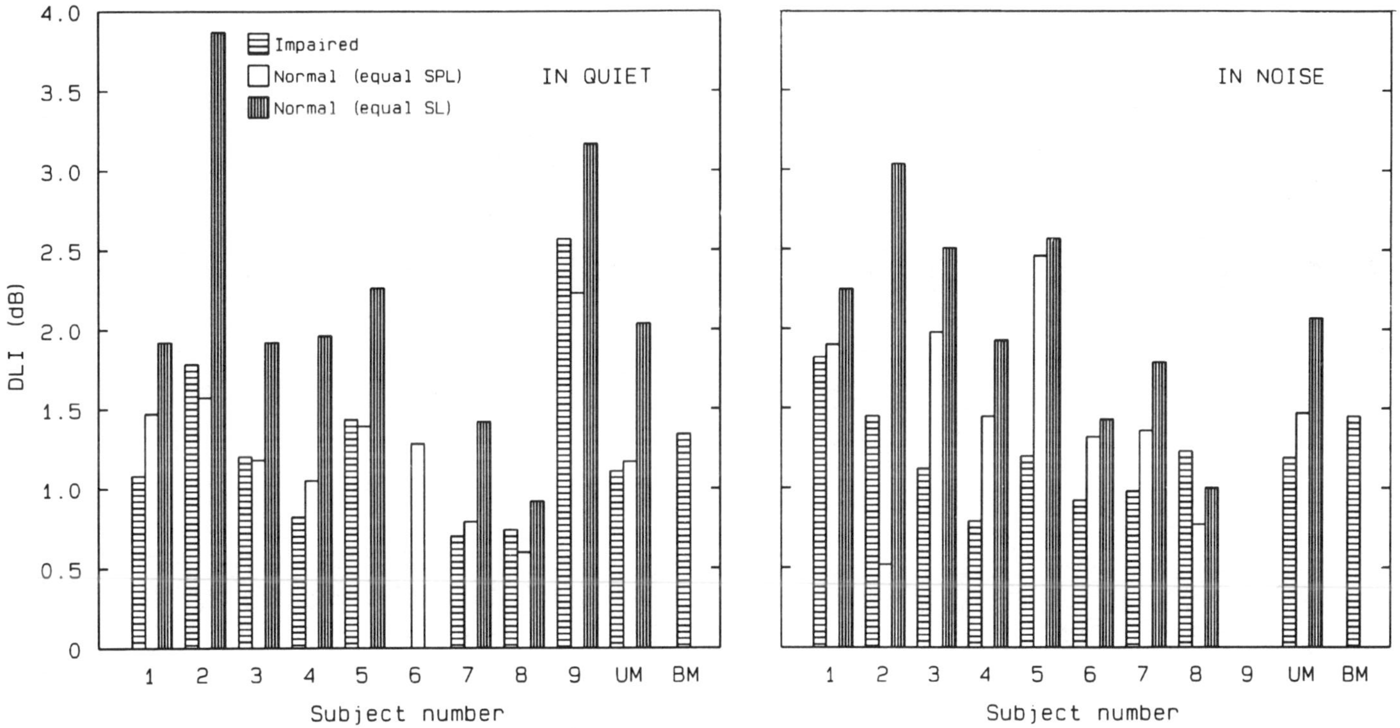

Fig. 3.10. As Figure 3.9 but showing thresholds for detecting an intensity difference between two tone pulses, DLIs.

Figure 3.9 shows the AMDLs, in quiet (left panel) and in high-pass noise (right panel). Individual results are shown for the nine unilaterally impaired subjects, but only mean results are shown for the bilaterally impaired subjects. At equal SPL, thresholds are sometimes larger for the impaired ear than the normal ear (e.g. subjects 1 and 8), and are sometimes smaller (e.g. subject 6). At equal SL, thresholds are consistently smaller for the impaired ear in quiet, and are usually so in noise. The subjects with bilateral impairments show similar thresholds to those of the impaired ears of the unilaterally impaired subjects. The high-pass noise resulted in increased AMDLs for both the normal and impaired ears, consistent with the idea that information from the high-frequency side of the excitation pattern is important for the detection of amplitude modulation.

Intensity discrimination of tone pulses

A different measure of intensity resolution requires subjects to detect differences of intensity between two separate tone pulses. This task is sometimes described as a gated-pedestal paradigm, in contrast to the continuous-pedestal paradigm used in the SISI test. The threshold change in level, in dB, will be denoted by DLI (difference limen for intensity). Except when the signals are very short in duration, thresholds measured with gated pedestals are larger than when a continuous pedestal is used (Turner *et al.* 1989). However, at least in some studies, the differences between normally hearing subjects and subjects with cochlear damage are similar to those obtained with continuous pedestals. Specifically, at equal SLs, subjects with cochlear damage have smaller values of DLI than normal, whereas at equal SPLs, they usually have DLI values that are similar to normal (Glasberg and Moore 1989; Turner *et al.* 1989; Schroder *et al.* 1994).

As an example, some data from Glasberg and Moore (1989) are presented here for the same nine subjects with unilateral cochlear impairments and six subjects with bilateral cochlear impairments as described earlier. Subjects were required to identify which of two tone pulses was more intense. For the impaired ears, the level of the less intense tone pulse was 80 dB SPL. The normal ear was tested both at equal SL and at equal SPL. Each tone pulse had a 200-ms steady state portion and 10-ms raised-cosine onset and offset ramps. As with the AMDLs, thresholds were measured both in quiet and in the presence of noise, which was identical to that described for amplitude modulation detection.

Figure 3.10 shows thresholds for the intensity discrimination of pulsed tones in quiet (left panel) and in high-pass noise (right panel). At equal SPL there is no consistent effect of hearing impairment, while at equal SL the thresholds tend to be smaller for the impaired ears than for the normal ears. The high-pass noise has only a small effect on the thresholds, suggesting that information from the high-frequency side of the excitation pattern is less important for DLIs than it is for AMDLs.

The relation of intensity discrimination to loudness

Zwislocki and Jordan (1986) presented evidence suggesting that AMDLs for detecting trapezoidal-shaped amplitude modulation were related to loudness rather than to the slope of the function relating loudness to sound level. They compared AMDLs for normally hearing subjects and for subjects with hearing loss accompanied by loudness recruitment and found that the AMDLs for the two groups were roughly equal when the loudnesses were equal. They argued that this result could be accounted for if the variability of the loudness sensation from one stimulus to the next depended both on the loudness and on the derivative (the slope) of the function relating loudness to sound level. Essentially, the variability was assumed to increase in proportion to the slope of the loudness growth function. A steeper loudness growth function in an ear with recruitment leads to a larger change in average loudness for a given change in intensity, but this does not lead to improved intensity discrimination because the variability of the loudness sensation increases by the same factor.

While some other studies have lent support to the hypothesis of Zwislocki and Jordan (Hellman *et al.* 1987; Schlauch and Wier 1987; Stillman *et al.* 1993), others have questioned its generality. Rankovic *et al.* (1988) measured intensity discrimination of normally hearing subjects using both continuous and gated pedestals, in quiet and in the presence of a broadband background noise with a spectrum level of 40 dB. They also obtained loudness matches between the tones in quiet and the tones in noise. They found that equally loud tones did not yield equal intensity discrimination thresholds for mid-range levels of the gated pedestals and over a wide range of levels of the continuous pedestals. Schlauch (1994) carried out a similar experiment, but using high-pass noise instead of broadband noise. He found that intensity discrimination thresholds were generally higher in the presence of the high-pass noise than in quiet, even for tones judged equally loud. Florentine *et al.* (1993) have reported cases of subjects with loudness recruitment for whom equal loudness did not lead to equal DLIs, for tones presented in quiet.

Overall, it appears that the hypothesis of Zwislocki and Jordan (1986), that equal loudness leads to equal intensity discrimination thresholds, is not always applicable, although it appears to work reasonably well on average for tones in quiet. It does seem plausible that the steep loudness growth functions of subjects with loudness recruitment are associated with greater variability in the loudness sensation, giving little or no advantage in intensity discrimination.

The role of spread of excitation in intensity discrimination

Several of the studies referred to above have shown that noise can have an adverse effect on intensity discrimination, both for normal and for hearing-impaired subjects. Noise designed to mask the upper side of the excitation pattern evoked by the signal appears to have particularly deleterious effects. Information from the high-frequency side of the excitation pattern may be important for two reasons. Firstly, in normally hearing subjects, the excitation pattern grows with increasing level in a nonlinear manner on the high-frequency side (Zwicker 1970); see Figure 2.10. For example, a one-decibel change in stimulus level may lead to a change in excitation level as large as two or three decibels on the high-frequency side of the pattern. In an intensity discrimination task, it would be advantageous to use information from the part of the pattern that changes most (Zwicker 1956). Secondly, at medium to high levels the excitation pattern is asymmetric, spreading more towards CFs above the signal frequency than below the signal frequency. If subjects combine information across different CFs, more information will be gained from the high side of the pattern than from the low side (Florentine and Buus 1981; Moore and Sek 1994).

In subjects with cochlear damage, the nonlinearity on the high-frequency side of the pattern tends to be reduced or absent, as discussed in chapter two. This would be expected to impair intensity discrimination. On the other hand, cochlear damage is often associated with an unusually large spread of excitation on the high-frequency side of the pattern. This might lead to improved intensity discrimination, and it would certainly increase the relative importance of information from the high-frequency side of the pattern.

The role of spread of excitation in intensity discrimination has been studied by Florentine *et al.* (1993). They measured intensity discrimination for 1-kHz pulsed tones in hearing-impaired subjects with various configurations of hearing loss. Subjects with increasing hearing loss above 1 kHz generally showed larger than normal DLIs when compared at equal SPL and at equal loudness, but not when compared at equal SL. Subjects with decreasing hearing loss above 1 kHz showed DLIs close to normal when compared at equal SPL and equal loudness, and showed smaller than normal DLIs when compared at equal SL. These results are consistent with the idea that information on the high-frequency side of the excitation pattern is important for intensity discrimination. When the coding of intensity on the high-frequency side of the pattern is disrupted, by increasing hearing loss at high frequencies, this leads to impaired intensity discrimination.

A role for the spread of excitation in intensity discrimination is also indicated by a recent study of Schroder *et al.* (1994). They measured DLIs in three subjects with normal hearing, two subjects with moderate-to-severe flat cochlear losses, and three subjects with near-normal hearing at low frequencies and severe losses at high frequencies. In frequency regions where there was a hearing loss, the DLIs were sometimes similar to those of the normally hearing subjects tested at the same SPL. In these cases, the DLIs at medium to high levels were markedly elevated by the addition of high-pass noise to mask the spread of excitation, suggesting that spread of excitation allowed the good performance without noise. In other cases, the DLIs were larger than normal, and the addition of high-pass noise had little effect on the DLIs, suggesting that these subjects were unable to use spread of excitation.

Perceptual consequences of altered loudness perception

Consequences of loudness recruitment and reduced dynamic range

The most prominent change in loudness perception associated with cochlear damage is loudness recruitment and reduced dynamic range. For sounds with inherent amplitude fluctuations, such as speech or music, this results in an exaggeration of the perceived dynamic qualities. The sound appears to fluctuate more in loudness than it would for a normally hearing person. When listening to music, the *forte* passages may be perceived at almost normal loudness, but the *piano* passages may be inaudible. One might regard the normal auditory system as containing a built in fast-acting automatic gain control system; this system is lacking or reduced in effectiveness in people with cochlear damage. The perception of exaggerated loudness changes can play a role in several other aspects of auditory perception. The role in temporal processing is reviewed in chapter 4, and the role in speech perception is reviewed in chapter 7.

The reduction in dynamic range has practical implications for the design and use of hearing aids. Many hearing aids act primarily as linear amplifiers, except that they have some form of output limiting or clipping to prevent the user from being exposed to excessively loud sounds (see chapter 8 for details). The limiting/clipping is usually associated with unpleasant sounding distortion, so in practice, users set the volume control so as to avoid limiting/clipping in most everyday situations. Thus, the aid acts as a linear amplifier most of the time; the amplification is independent of the input sound level.

When linear amplification is used, and the volume control is set so that the more intense sounds are at a comfortable loudness, then some weak sounds may be inaudible, owing to the reduced dynamic range. If the volume control is set to make the weak sounds audible, then intense sounds will be unpleasantly loud. In practice, the amount of amplification selected for use in everyday life is often rather small (Leijon 1989), meaning that many weak environmental and speech sounds would be inaudible. Hearing aid users probably select low gains for use in everyday life partly to be sure of avoiding unpleasantly loud sounds, and partly to avoid the distorted sound associated with limiting/clipping.

These problems can be largely overcome by the use of hearing aids incorporating automatic volume control or compression; such aids are described in more detail in chapter 8.

Perceptual consequences of reduced loudness summation

As described earlier, a narrowband sound and a broadband sound with the same intensity usually differ considerably in loudness for normally hearing people (the broadband sound being louder), but differ less or not at all in loudness for hearing-impaired people. This means that the relative loudness of complex sounds may differ for normally hearing and hearing-impaired people; sound A might be judged louder than sound B by a normally hearing person, but might be judged as less loud than sound B by a hearing-impaired person.

The difference in level required for equal loudness in an impaired ear and a normal ear is typically greater for a broadband sound than for a narrowband sound. Consider as an example a person with unilateral cochlear damage, and an absolute threshold in the damaged ear about 50 dB higher than normal. A sinusoidal signal with a level of 80 dB in the impaired ear might be matched in loudness by a signal with a level of about 65 dB in the normal ear (see Figure 3.2). In other words, the signal in the impaired ear has to be about 15 dB higher in level in the impaired ear to achieve equal loudness. However, if the sinusoidal signal is replaced by a broadband signal, the loudness will go up in the normal ear, but will change only slightly, if at all, in the impaired ear. For the broadband sound, a level of about 55 dB in the normal ear might be matched by a level of 80 dB in the impaired ear, a difference of 25 dB. Hence, to restore 'normal' loudness in an impaired ear for complex broadband sounds such as speech or music, more amplification may be required than suggested by measurements with narrowband sounds.

There are, however, some advantages of reduced loudness summation in hearing-impaired persons. One advantage is in the fitting of hearing aids. Such fitting often involves the determination of the most comfortable level (MCL), the highest comfortable level (HCL) and/or the uncomfortable loudness level (UCL or ULL). Nearly always, determination of the MCL, HCL or UCL is done using narrowband sounds, either sinusoids or narrow bands of noise. For normally hearing persons, the levels determined using narrowband sounds can be very different to MCLs, HCLs or UCLs for complex broadband sounds, such as speech. However, in people with cochlear damage, the loudness would not be as different for broadband and narrowband sounds. Exceptions to this occur when loudness is strongly influenced by changes with centre frequency, as tends to happen when the hearing loss varies markedly with frequency (Byrne 1986). However, for subjects with 'flat' losses, MCLs and HCLs determined using narrowband sounds can be used to predict, with reasonable accuracy, MCLs and HCLs for speech. Of course, the accuracy will not be perfect, since the loudness of speech is influenced by its fluctuations over time and by its exact spectral shape, as well as by its overall level.

Perceptual consequences of altered intensity discrimination

As reviewed above, intensity discrimination by people with cochlear hearing loss can be better than, worse than, or about the same as normal, depending on whether the comparison is made at equal SL, equal SPL or equal loudness, and also depending on the pattern of hearing loss as a function of frequency. In practice, hearing-impaired people often listen at lower SLs than normally hearing people, so their intensity discrimination can be worse than normal. However, this does not appear to lead to marked problems, since it is rare in everyday life for critical information to be carried by small changes in intensity. Although intensity contrasts can convey information in speech, the contrasts involve rather large changes in intensity, changes that are well above the threshold of detection for both normally hearing and hearing-impaired persons.

Potential problems can arise when hearing aids incorporating fast-acting compression are used; details are given in chapter 8. Such hearing aids reduce differences in level between sounds. If a large amount of compression is used, then information-bearing intensity contrasts may be reduced to the point where they are difficult for the hearing-impaired person to discriminate. This can lead to impaired speech perception (Plomp 1994). However, moderate amounts of compression do not seem to have such deleterious effects, and even have beneficial effects by restoring audibility of weak sounds. These issues are discussed further in chapter 8.

Conclusions

This chapter has described three main ways in which loudness perception is altered by cochlear damage. Firstly, the rate of growth of loudness with increasing intensity is greater than normal; the threshold for detecting sounds is elevated, but the level at which sounds become uncomfortably loud is similar to normal. This is called loudness recruitment. The effect can also be described as a reduced dynamic range; the range of levels over which sounds are both comfortable and audible is smaller than normal. Loudness models and experimental data suggest that loudness recruitment can be explained primarily in terms of steeper input–output functions on the BM, associated with loss of, or damage to, the active mechanism. Reduced frequency selectivity may also play a small role.

The second change in loudness perception produced by cochlear damage is reduced loudness summation; when the bandwidth of a sound is increased keeping the overall intensity constant, the loudness at medium to high intensities increases markedly for people with normal hearing, but increases only slightly, or not at all, in people with cochlear damage. Modelling of this effect suggests that it depends both on steeper input–output functions on the BM, and on reduced frequency selectivity.

The third change in loudness perception is in the ability to detect changes in intensity. Intensity discrimination by people with cochlear hearing loss can be better than, worse than, or about the same as normal, depending on whether the comparison is made at equal SL, equal SPL or equal loudness, and also depending on the pattern of hearing loss as a function of frequency. At equal low SLs, intensity discrimination is usually better than normal in persons with cochlear hearing loss, and this is exploited in the SISI test. However, in everyday life people with cochlear damage usually listen at lower SLs than normally hearing people, and in this situation their intensity discrimination may be either better or worse than normal.

At first sight it appears surprising that intensity discrimination is not consistently better than normal in people with cochlear damage, since the functions relating loudness to sound intensity are steeper than normal, and intensity discrimination is usually assumed to be based on loudness sensations. However, it seems likely that steeper loudness-growth functions are associated with greater variability in the loudness sensation; a sound of fixed level, presented repeatedly, evokes a loudness sensation that varies more across presentations. This increase in variability offsets any advantage that might be gained from the steeper-than-average loudness growth.

4 Effects of cochlear damage on temporal resolution and temporal integration

Introduction

Many studies have shown that temporal resolution can be adversely affected by cochlear damage. At first sight, it is not obvious why this should be the case. Neurophysiological data obtained from animals with noise-induced or drug-induced cochlear damage indicate that the temporal patterns of suprathreshold stimuli are accurately represented in the responses of primary auditory neurones. Furthermore, as described in chapter 2, the auditory filters in subjects with cochlear damage are typically broader than normal, which might be expected to lead to better-than-normal temporal resolution, since broad filters respond more quickly to changes in their input than narrow filters. Nevertheless, psychoacoustic data indicate that temporal processing for certain types of stimuli is strongly affected by cochlear damage, with temporal resolution usually being worse than normal. To understand the reasons for these effects, it is helpful to use a model of temporal processing in the normal auditory system and to consider how the different stages of the model may be altered by cochlear pathology.

In characterizing temporal resolution in the auditory system, it is essential to take account of the filtering that takes place in the peripheral auditory system. Temporal resolution depends on two main processes: analysis of the time pattern occurring within each frequency channel; and comparison of the time patterns across channels. This chapter concentrates mainly on within-channel processes, since there have been few studies of across-channel processing in hearing-impaired subjects.

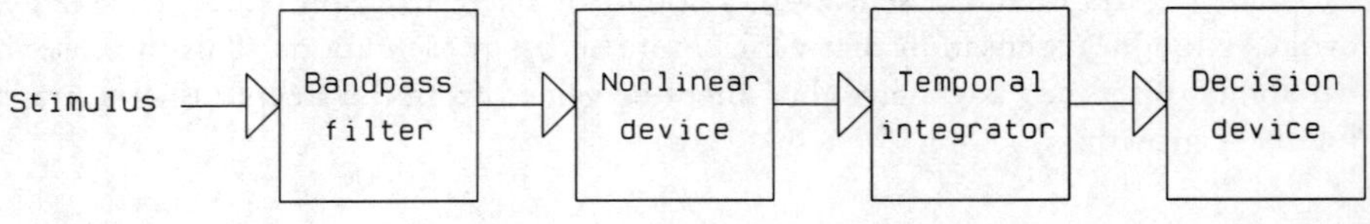

Fig. 4.1. A block diagram showing the stages typically found in models of temporal processing.

Modelling within-channel temporal resolution

Models of temporal resolution assume that the internal representation of stimuli is 'smoothed' over time, so that rapid temporal changes are lost but slower ones are preserved. Several models of temporal resolution have the general form illustrated in Figure 4.1. There is an initial stage of bandpass filtering, reflecting the action of the auditory filters. For simplicity, only one filter is shown; in reality there is an array of parallel channels, each like that shown in the figure. Each filter is followed by a nonlinear device. This device may be thought of as crudely representing some aspects of the process of transduction from excitation at a particular point on the BM to activity in the auditory nerve. However, in most models, there has been little attempt to model accurately these peripheral pocesses. The output of the nonlinear device is fed through a 'smoothing' device, which can be implemented either as a lowpass filter (Viemeister 1979) or a sliding temporal integrator (Moore *et al.* 1988). Usually, this smoothing device is thought of as occurring after the auditory nerve; it is assumed to reflect a relatively central process. The output of the smoothing device is fed to a decision device.

The effect of auditory filtering

When a signal is passed through a bandpass filter, the time pattern of the signal is smeared or smoothed somewhat by the filter. Generally, the narrower the filter, the more is the smoothing. This is illustrated in Figure 4.2, which shows the response of a simulated auditory filter to a brief impulse. The filter was assumed to have either a normal bandwidth, or bandwidths two, four and eight times greater

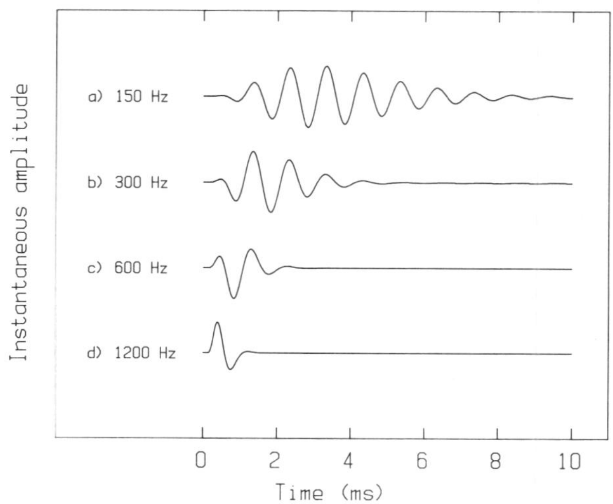

Fig. 4.2. The response to a brief impulse of a simulated auditory filter, and an auditory filter with a bandwidth two times, four times or eight times greater than normal, simulating moderate, severe and profound cochlear damage, respectively. All filters are centred at 1 kHz. The responses are not drawn to scale. The peak amplitude of the response actually increases as the filter bandwidth increases.

than normal, corresponding to increasing degrees of cochlear damage. The response, called the impulse response, clearly shortens in time as the filter becomes broader. The auditory filters have bandwidths that decrease progressively with decreasing centre frequency (Glasberg and Moore 1990); see chapter 2. One might expect, therefore, that the auditory filters would play some role in limiting temporal resolution, this effect being greater at low centre frequencies.

Many studies have addressed the question of whether temporal resolution does vary with centre frequency. Green (1973) measured the ability to distinguish two stimuli where one was the mirror image in time of the other (this is equivalent to playing one stimulus backwards in time). Such stimuli have identical long-term power spectra. Each stimulus consisted of a brief pulse of a sinusoid in which the level of the first half of the pulse was 10 dB different from that of the second half. Subjects were required to distinguish two signals, differing in whether the half with the high level was first or second. Green measured performance as a function of the total duration of each signal. The threshold was similar for centre frequencies of 2 and 4 kHz, and was between 1 and 2 ms. However, the threshold was slightly higher for a centre frequency of 1 kHz, being between 2 and 4 ms.

Several researchers have measured thresholds for detecting a gap in narrowband noise (Fitzgibbons 1983; Shailer and Moore 1983; Buus and Florentine 1985). When a temporal gap is introduced into a narrowband sound, energy 'splatter' occurs outside the nominal frequency range of the sound. To prevent the splatter being detected, the sounds are presented in a background sound, usually a noise, designed to mask the splatter. Gap thresholds have often been found to decrease monotonically with increasing centre frequency. At first sight this might be interpreted as indicating that temporal resolution improves with increasing frequency, as would be expected from the increasing bandwidths of the auditory filters. However, in these experiments, the bandwidth of the stimuli increased with increasing centre frequency, so the effect of centre frequency was confounded with the effect of bandwidth.

Noise bands have inherent fluctuations in amplitude, and the rapidity of these fluctuations increases with increasing bandwidth. Gap thresholds for noise bands are probably partly limited by the inherent fluctuations in the noise (Shailer and Moore 1983, 1985; Green 1985). Randomly occurring dips in the noise are 'confused' with the gap to be detected. The confusion is maximal for dips comparable in duration to the gap. In practice, this means that noise with a narrow bandwidth, and hence slow fluctuations, creates the greatest confusion and gives the largest gap thresholds. The data are consistent with this view: gap thresholds increase with decreasing noise bandwidth keeping either the centre frequency or the upper cutoff frequency fixed (Shailer and Moore 1983, 1985; Eddins *et al.* 1992; Glasberg and Moore 1992; Snell *et al.* 1994). Gap thresholds measured using noise bands of fixed width have often shown little effect of centre frequency (Shailer and Moore 1985; de Filippo and Snell 1986; Eddins *et al.* 1992). However, Snell *et al.* (1994) found that gap thresholds measured using a 1000-Hz wide band of noise were smallest for mid-range centre frequencies, and increased when the noise was centred at a low (500 Hz) or high (12,000 Hz) frequency. In summary, gap thresholds measured using bands of noise do not provide clear evidence of an improvement in temporal resolution with centre frequency. However, the gap thresholds are influenced by the inherent fluctuations in the noise, and the representation of these fluctuations in the auditory system may be affected by filtering in the auditory periphery.

Shailer and Moore (1987) studied the ability of subjects to detect a temporal gap in a sinusoid, which has no inherent fluctuations. To mask 'splatter' associated with the introduction of the gap, the sinusoid was presented in a continuous noise with a spectral notch at the frequency of the sinusoid. The results were strongly affected by the phase at which the sinusoid was turned off and on to produce the gap. Initially, only the simplest case will be considered here, called 'preserved phase' by Shailer and Moore. In this case the sinusoid was turned off at a positive-going zero crossing (i.e., as the waveform was about to change from negative to positive values) and it started (at the end of the gap) at the phase it would have had if it had continued without interruption. Thus, for the preserved-phase condition it was as if the gap had been 'cut out' from a continuous sinusoid. For this condition, the detectability of the gap increased monotonically with increasing gap duration.

Shailer and Moore (1987) found that the gap threshold was roughly constant at about 5 ms for centre frequencies of 400, 1000 and 2000 Hz. Recently, Moore *et al.* (1993a) measured gap thresholds for centre frequencies of 100, 200, 400, 800, 1000 and 2000 Hz, using a condition similar to the preserved-phase condition of Shailer and Moore. The gap thresholds were almost constant, at 6–8 ms over the frequency range 400–2000 Hz, but increased somewhat at 200 Hz, and increased markedly, to about 18 ms, at 100 Hz. Individual variability also increased markedly at 100 Hz.

Overall, the results of experiments using narrowband stimuli indicate that temporal resolution does not vary markedly with frequency, except at very low frequencies (200 Hz and below). This suggests in turn that the smoothing produced by the auditory filters does not play a major role, except perhaps at very low frequencies.

Two of the conditions in the experiment of Shailer and Moore (1987) did, however, show effects that could be attributed to 'ringing' in the auditory filter. In the condition that they called 'standard phase' the signal was turned off (to start the gap) at a positive-going zero crossing, and turned on again (at the end of the gap) at a positive-going zero crossing. An example of a psychometric function for the standard-phase condition is shown in Figure 4.3. The frequency of the sinusoid was 400 Hz. A two-alternative forced-choice task was used, so chance performance corresponds to 50% correct. The psychometric function is distinctly nonmonotonic. The gap is difficult to detect when its value is an integer multiple of the period (P) of the signal, i.e., 2.5 ms and 5 ms. Conversely, the gap is easy to detect when its value is $(n+0.5)P$, where $n = 0$ or 1. Nonmonotonic psychometric functions were also found for a frequency of 1000 Hz but not for a frequency of 2000 Hz.

Shailer and Moore (1987) explained these results in terms of ringing in the auditory filter. Their argument is illustrated in Figure 4.4, which shows responses of a simulated auditory filter with a centre frequency of 400 Hz to a series of stimuli from the standard-phase condition, with gap durations ranging from 1.2 to 3.7 ms. When the sinusoid is turned off at the start of the gap, the filter continues to respond or ring for a certain time. If the gap duration is 2.5 ms, corresponding to one whole period of the sinusoid, the sinusoid following the gap is in phase with the ringing response. In this case the output of the filter shows only a small dip, and gap detection should be difficult. This is exactly what is observed. For a gap duration of 1.2 ms or 3.7 ms, the sinusoid following the gap is out of phase with the ringing response. Now the output of the filter passes through zero before returning to its steady-state value. The resulting dip in the filter output is larger, and is much easier to detect. This explains why the psychometric function is nonmonotonic for the standard-phase condition. For the preserved-phase condition, the sinusoid following the gap is always in phase with the ringing response of the auditory filter. Thus, the dip in the output of the auditory filter increases monotonically with increasing gap duration, and the psychometric function is monotonic. The psychometric function at high frequencies is always monotonic, even for the standard-phase condition, since the auditory filter is sufficiently broad that ringing lasts only for a very short time.

In summary, the auditory filter can have a strong influence on the pattern of results for deterministic stimuli, especially at low frequencies. However, it appears

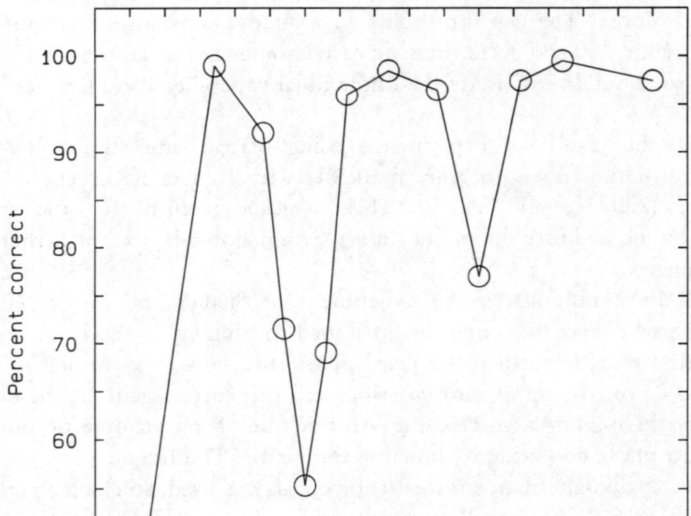

Fig. 4.3. The percentage correct detection of a gap in a 400-Hz sinusoid, plotted as a function of the gap duration. The gap started at a positive-going zero-crossing of the sinusoid and the sinusoid started after the gap at a positive-going zero-crossing, a condition referred to as standard phase.

to play only a minor role in limiting temporal resolution, except perhaps at very low frequencies.

The characteristics of the nonlinearity and the smoothing device

Although all the stages of the model can affect temporal resolution, it is often felt that the stage which is most directly related to temporal resolution is the lowpass filter or temporal integrator. Thus, it would be desirable to be able to determine the characteristics of this stage independently of the other stages. In practice, this is very difficult to do (Green and Forrest 1988).

Some recent experiments (Moore *et al.* 1988; Plack and Moore 1990) have attempted to determine the characteristics of the temporal integrator on the assumption that the nonlinearity has a square-law characteristic. In other words, the temporal integrator was assumed to act on a power-like quantity. The integrator itself was modelled as a weighting function, or 'window', which performs a running average of the power at the output of the auditory filter. The experimental data used to derive the window shape were thresholds for detection of a very brief tone pulse presented between two bursts of noise, measured as a function of the time interval from the end of the first burst to the centre of the tone pulse, and the

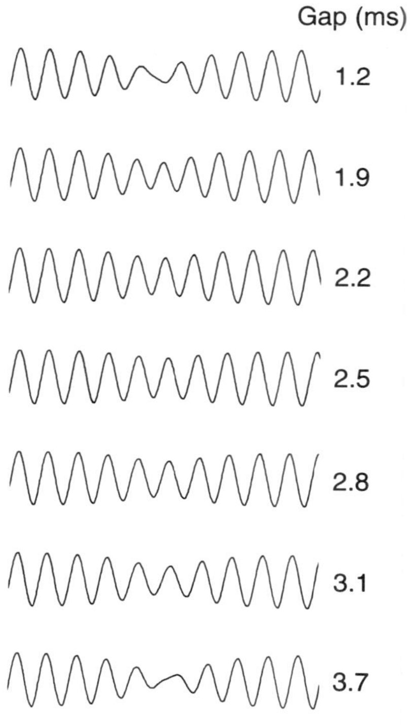

Fig. 4.4. Simulation of the output of an auditory filter centred at 400 Hz in response to stimuli in the standard-phase condition. The duration of the gap is indicated for each waveform.

centre of the tone pulse to the start of the second noise burst (combined forward and backward masking).

Some examples of temporal window shapes derived in this way are shown in Figure 4.5, taken from Plack and Moore (1990). In these examples, each side of the temporal window was modelled as the sum of two rounded-exponential functions. The shape of the temporal window is almost invariant with centre frequency, except for a slight broadening (associated with poorer temporal resolution) at low centre frequencies. The temporal window broadens somewhat as the sound level decreases. A simple summary measure of the temporal window is its equivalent rectangular duration (ERD). The ERDs found by Plack and Moore were typically about 8–9 ms.

One problem with this model is that it does not correctly account for the way that backward and forward masking combine. If a backward masker and a forward masker are equated for effectiveness when each is presented separately, and then the two maskers are combined, the resulting amount of masking is usually greater than would be predicted from a simple linear summation of the effects of the individual maskers (a 3 dB increase) (Cokely and Humes 1993; Oxenham and Moore 1994). To account for this effect, several workers have suggested models of temporal resolution in which there is a compressive nonlinearity prior to the temporal integrator (Penner 1980a; Penner and Shiffrin 1980; Moore *et al.* 1993b; Oxenham and Moore 1994). This is actually much more realistic than a square-law nonlinearity in modelling the transformation from the acoustic stimulus to neural activity; see chapters 1 and 3.

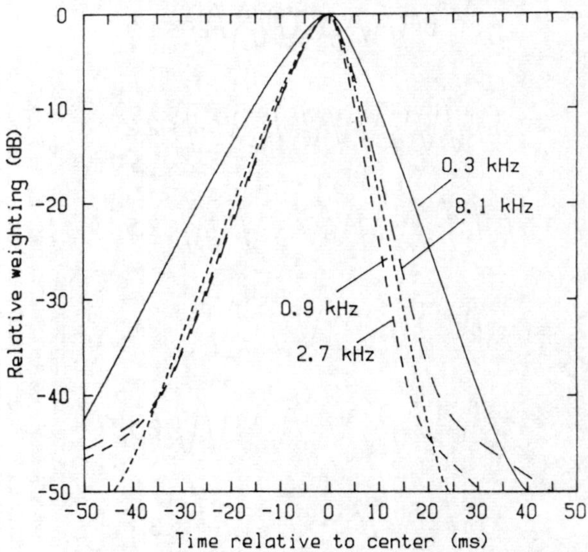

Fig. 4.5. Temporal window shapes derived by Plack and Moore (1990) for normally hearing subjects. Each curve represents a different centre frequency. Note that the shapes are plotted using a logarithmic (dB) ordinate.

Oxenham and Moore (1994) measured forward and backward masking separately and in combination for a very brief 6-kHz signal and a noise masker. They showed that the results could be used to separate the effects of the temporal integrator and the nonlinearity prior to the integrator. The results were fitted best by a nonlinearity where the rectified amplitude was raised to a power between 0.5 and 0.7. The inclusion of a compressive nonlinearity in the model has a marked effect on the derived temporal window. Specifically, the more compressive the nonlinearity, the broader the temporal window (Penner 1978, 1980a; Moore *et al.* 1993b). Oxenham and Moore, using rounded-exponentials to model the window shape, found ERDs of about 12–15 ms. When the window was modelled by exponential functions, the ERDs were smaller, typically about 8–10 ms. These values are broadly consistent with ERDs estimated in other ways (Moore *et al.* 1993b).

The physiological correlate of the compressive nonlinearity in the model described above is still somewhat uncertain. However, it can probably be partly related to the compressive nonlinearity that is observed in input–output functions of the BM in the normal cochlea; see chapter 1 and Oxenham and Moore (1995).

Temporal resolution in subjects with cochlear damage

Some measures of temporal resolution in subjects with cochlear damage appear to show reduced temporal resolution, while others do not. Several factors can affect the results, and not all of these are directly connected with temporal processing itself.

The influence of sound level

One important factor influencing measures of temporal resolution is the sound level used. Many measures of temporal resolution show that performance in normally hearing subjects worsens at low sensation levels (SLs) (Plomp 1964b; Shailer and Moore 1983; Buus and Florentine 1985; Fitzgibbons and Gordon-Salant 1987; Peters *et al.* 1995). This is not unique to temporal resolution; performance on many tasks worsens at low SLs, presumably because less neural information is available, or because of the greater effects of internal noise at low SLs. In the case of tasks measuring temporal resolution, the changes in performance with sound level may reflect mainly changes in the efficiency of central decision processes, rather than changes in the temporal integrator or temporal window (Peters *et al.* 1995). It is not generally possible to test hearing-impaired subjects at high SLs, because they have loudness recruitment; sounds with levels of 90–100 dB SPL appear as loud as they would to a normal listener, as described in chapter 3. On some measures of temporal resolution, such as the detection of gaps in bands of noise or the rate of recovery from forward masking, hearing-impaired subjects appear markedly worse than normal subjects when tested at the same SPLs, but only slightly worse at equal SLs (Fitzgibbons and Wightman 1982; Tyler *et al.* 1982a; Glasberg *et al.* 1987).

This is illustrated for the case of forward masking in Figure 4.6, adapted from Glasberg *et al.* (1987). They tested subjects with cochlear damage in one ear only.

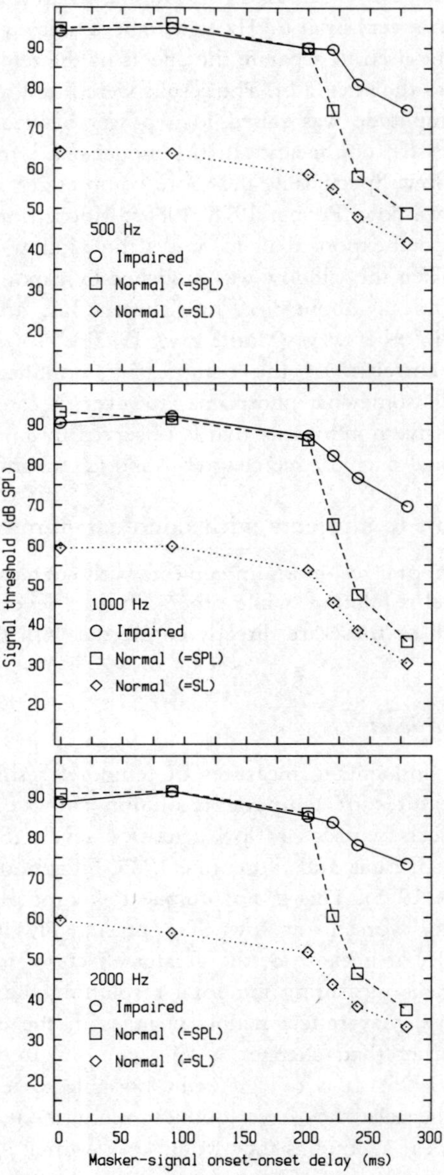

Fig. 4.6. The threshold for a brief sinusoidal signal presented at various times during and following a noise masker. The temporal position of the signal is plotted relative to the onset of the masker; times greater than 200 ms correspond to forward masking. Mean results are shown for the normal and impaired ears of five subjects with unilateral cochlear damage. Each panel shows results for a different signal frequency. The masker was presented at a single high level to the impaired ear (84 dB SPL). The masker was presented to the normal ear either at the same SPL or the same SL.

The brief sinusoidal signal was presented at various times during and following a noise masker. The masker was presented at a fixed high level to the impaired ear of each subject. In the normal ear it was presented both at the same SPL and at the same SL as for the impaired ear. The rate of recovery from forward masking can be considered as a measure of temporal resolution; the more rapidly the threshold drops as the time interval between the masker and signal increases, the better is temporal resolution.

It is clear from the figure that the rate of recovery from forward masking is much more rapid for the normal ear than for the impaired ear when the comparison is made at equal SPL. However, at equal SL, the difference is much reduced. This effect of level is not unexpected, since it is known that the rate of recovery from forward masking in normal ears depends strongly on sound level, as described in chapter 2. The slow rate of recovery from forward masking that is commonly found in people with cochlear damage probably depends on the low SL of the stimuli, rather than on an abnormality in temporal processing *per se.* Unfortunately, people with cochlear damage usually listen at low SLs, since loudness recruitment makes it impossible to present sounds at high SLs without discomfort occurring.

For deterministic stimuli that have no inherent random fluctuations, hearing-impaired subjects can actually perform a little better than normally hearing subjects when tested at equal SLs. This applies to the detection of gaps in sinusoids (Moore and Glasberg 1988c; Moore *et al.* 1989) and to the discrimination of Huffman sequences (Jesteadt *et al.* 1976); the latter are click-like sounds with identical power spectra but different phase spectra.

The influence of audible bandwidth

Another important consideration is the bandwidth available to the listeners. This can be clearly seen by consideration of studies measuring the temporal modulation transfer function (TMTF). The TMTF shows the amount of amplitude modulation required for detection of the modulation, plotted as a function of modulation rate (Viemeister 1979). It is generally assumed that the ability to detect modulation at high rates is limited by the temporal resolution of the ear. Several studies measuring TMTFs for broadband noise carriers showed that hearing-impaired listeners were generally less sensitive to high rates of modulation than normal listeners (Formby 1982; Lamore *et al.* 1984; Bacon and Viemeister 1985). However, this may have been largely a consequence of the fact that high frequencies were inaudible to the impaired listeners (Bacon and Viemeister 1985); most of the subjects used had greater hearing losses at high frequencies than at low, as is typical in cases of noise-induced hearing loss. When the broadband noise is lowpass filtered, as a crude simulation of the effects of threshold elevation at high frequencies, normally hearing subjects also show a reduced ability to detect modulation at high rates (Bacon and Viemeister 1985).

Bacon and Gleitman (1992) measured TMTFs for broadband noise using subjects with relatively flat hearing losses. They found that at equal (high) sound

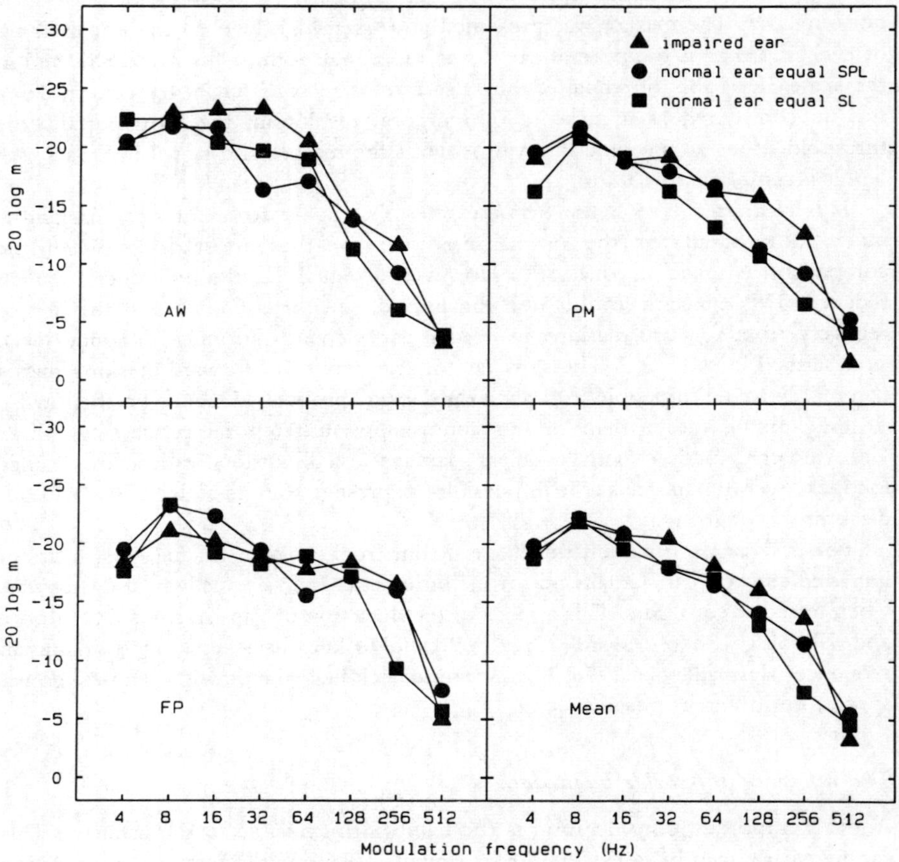

Fig. 4.7. Temporal modulation transfer functions (TMTFs) obtained using a bandpass noise carrier for the normal and impaired ears of three subjects with unilateral cochlear damage.

pressure levels (SPLs) performance was similar for hearing-impaired and normally hearing subjects. At equal (low) SLs, the hearing-impaired subjects tended to perform better than the normally hearing subjects. Moore *et al.* (1992d) controlled for the effects of listening bandwidth by measuring TMTFs for an octave-wide noise band centred at 2 kHz, using subjects with unilateral and bilateral cochlear hearing loss. Over the frequency range covered by the noise, the subjects had reasonably constant thresholds as a function of frequency, both in their normal and their impaired ears. This ensured that there were no differences between subjects or ears in terms of the range of audible frequencies in the noise. To ensure that subjects were not making use of information from frequencies outside the nominal passband of the noise, the modulated carrier was presented in an unmodulated broadband noise background. The results for the subjects with unilateral impairments are shown in Figure 4.7. It can be seen that performance is similar for the normal and impaired ears, both at equal SPL and equal SL, although there is a slight trend for the impaired ears to perform better at equal SL.

Studies of gap detection also show clear effects of the audible frequency range of the stimuli. For a broadband noise marker, gap thresholds become progressively larger as the audible frequency range of the stimuli is reduced by increasing high-frequency hearing loss (Florentine and Buus 1984; Buus and Florentine 1985; Salvi and Arehole 1985).

To summarise the results so far, subjects with cochlear damage often show reduced temporal resolution as a result of the low SL of the stimuli and/or the reduced audible bandwidth of the stimuli. When these factors are controlled for, hearing-impaired subjects often perform as well as, or even better than normal.

The influence of broadened auditory filters

Subjects with cochlear hearing loss usually have auditory filters that are broader than normal; see chapter 2. As mentioned earlier, one might expect that this would lead to improved temporal resolution. However, because the auditory filters in normal ears appear to play little role in limiting temporal resolution, except at very low frequencies, it has proved difficult to demonstrate improvements in temporal resolution resulting from broadened auditory filters.

One case where changes attributable to the auditory filters have been found is for the detection of temporal gaps in sinusoids. As described earlier, for the 'preserved phase' condition of Shailer and Moore (1987), psychometric functions for normal ears at low frequencies are nonmonotonic (see Figure 4.3). This was explained in terms of ringing in the auditory filters. For subjects with cochlear

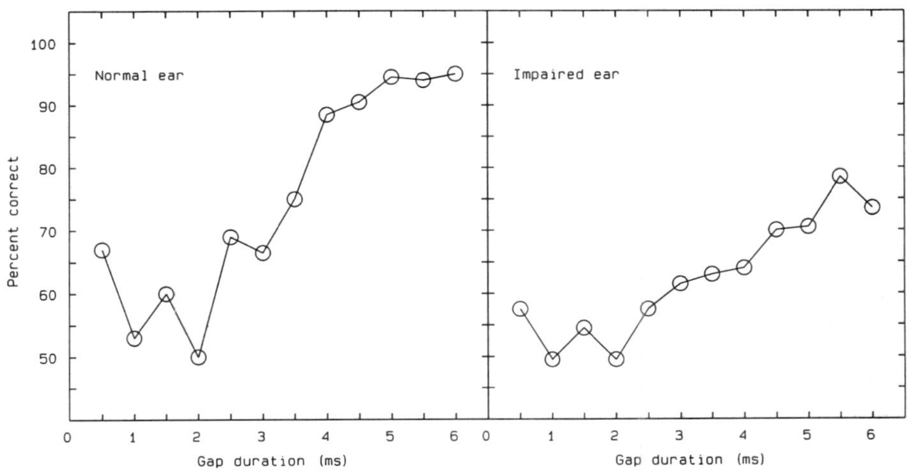

Fig. 4.8. Psychometric functions for gap detection in the standard-phase condition for the normal ear (left panel) and the impaired ear (right panel) of a subject with unilateral cochlear damage. Note that the function is non-monotonic for the normal ear but is almost monotonic for the impaired ear.

hearing loss, the psychometric functions are monotonic or nearly monotonic (Moore *et al.* 1989). An example is given in Figure 4.8. Moore *et al.* (1989) showed that this could be explained by the faster temporal response of the auditory filters, which resulted in a large dip in the filter output even when the gap corresponded to a small whole number of periods. Thus, the psychometric functions for impaired ears resemble those of normal ears at high frequencies (where the auditory filters are also broad); in both cases, performance appears to be limited by the more central temporal integration process.

The influence of changes in the compressive nonlinearity

For certain types of sounds, the temporal resolution of subjects with cochlear hearing loss seems to be worse than normal even when the stimuli are well above threshold and when all of the components of the stimuli fall within the audible range. This happens mainly for stimuli that contain slow random fluctuations in amplitude, such as narrow bands of noise. For such stimuli, subjects with cochlear damage often perform more poorly than normal in tasks such as gap detection (Fitzgibbons and Wightman 1982; Florentine and Buus 1984; Buus and Florentine 1985; Glasberg *et al.* 1987). However, gap detection is not usually worse than normal when the stimuli are sinusoids, which do not have inherent amplitude fluctuations (Moore and Glasberg 1988c; Moore *et al.* 1989). Glasberg *et al.* (1987) and Moore and Glasberg (1988c) suggested that the poor gap detection for narrowband noise stimuli might be a consequence of loudness recruitment, the abnormally rapid growth of loudness with increasing intensity that occurs commonly in cases of cochlear hearing loss; see chapter 3. For a person with recruitment, the inherent amplitude fluctuations in a narrowband noise would result in larger-than-normal loudness fluctuations from moment to moment, so that inherent dips in the noise might be more confusable with the gap to be detected.

This idea can also be expressed in terms of the model of temporal resolution described earlier. It seems likely that loudness recruitment is caused primarily by a reduction in or loss of the compressive nonlinearity found in the normal cochlea; see chapter 3. When cochlear damage occurs, the cochlea behaves in a more linear way, and the input–output function of the basilar membrane becomes less compressive, having a slope closer to unity (on log–log co-ordinates); see Figure 1.13.

To assess the idea that steeper input–output functions lead to impaired gap detection for stimuli with fluctuating envelopes, Glasberg and Moore (1992) processed the envelopes of narrow bands of noise so as to modify the envelope fluctuations. The envelope was processed by raising it to a power, N. For stimuli of constant amplitude, e.g. sinusoidal tones, the level (in dB) of stimuli processed in this way is a linear function of the level of the unprocessed stimuli, with slope N. This reproduces one of the features of loudness recruitment seen in subjects with unilateral hearing loss; for levels below about 90–100 dB SPL, the level of sound needed in the normal ear to match the loudness of a sound in the impaired ear is roughly a linear function of the level in the impaired ear; see Figure 3.2.

If N is greater than unity, this has the effect of magnifying fluctuations in the envelope, thus simulating the effects of recruitment; higher powers correspond to greater degrees of simulated recruitment. If N is less than unity, fluctuations in the envelope are reduced. This represents a type of signal processing that might be used to compensate for recruitment; it resembles the operation of a fast-acting compressor or automatic gain control (AGC) system; see chapter 8.

Values of N used were 0.5, 0.66, 1.0, 1.5 and 2. For N = 1, the stimuli were the same as unprocessed noise. A value of N of 2 simulates the type of recruitment typically found in cases of moderate to severe cochlear damage, where, for example, a 50-dB range of stimulus levels gives the same range of loudness as a 100-dB range of stimulus levels in a normal ear; see Figure 3.2.

Some examples of the envelopes of unprocessed and processed stimuli are shown in Figure 4.9. The envelopes are plotted on a logarithmic (dB) scale, as this seems more relevant to loudness perception than a linear amplitude scale. The bottom panel shows the envelope of a 'normal' noise band (N = 1) with a bandwidth of 10 Hz. The top panel shows the effect of squaring the envelope (N = 2), while the middle panel shows the result of raising the envelope to the power 0.5. The envelope fluctuations are obviously greatest in the top panel and smallest in the middle panel.

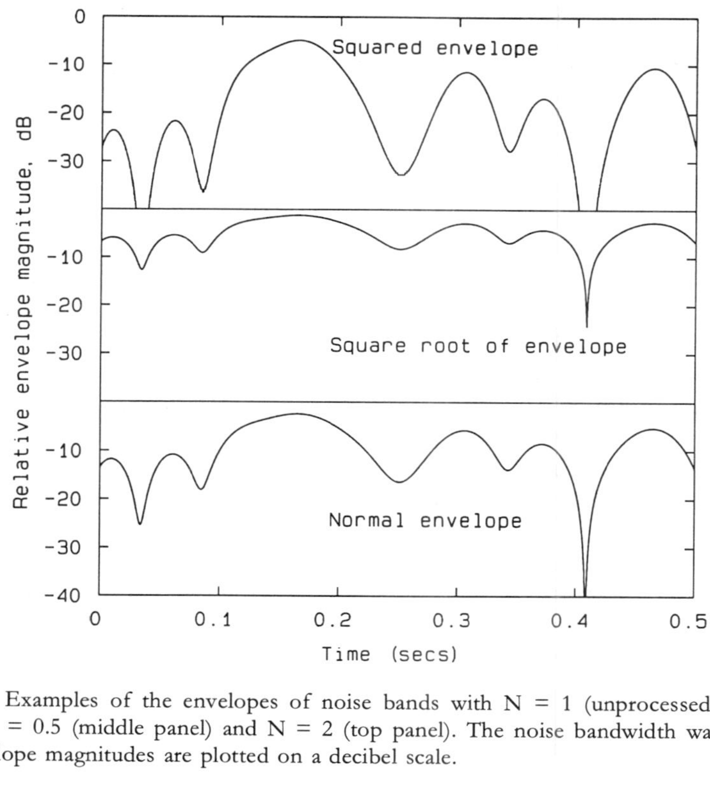

Fig. 4.9. Examples of the envelopes of noise bands with N = 1 (unprocessed, bottom panel), N = 0.5 (middle panel) and N = 2 (top panel). The noise bandwidth was 10 Hz. The envelope magnitudes are plotted on a decibel scale.

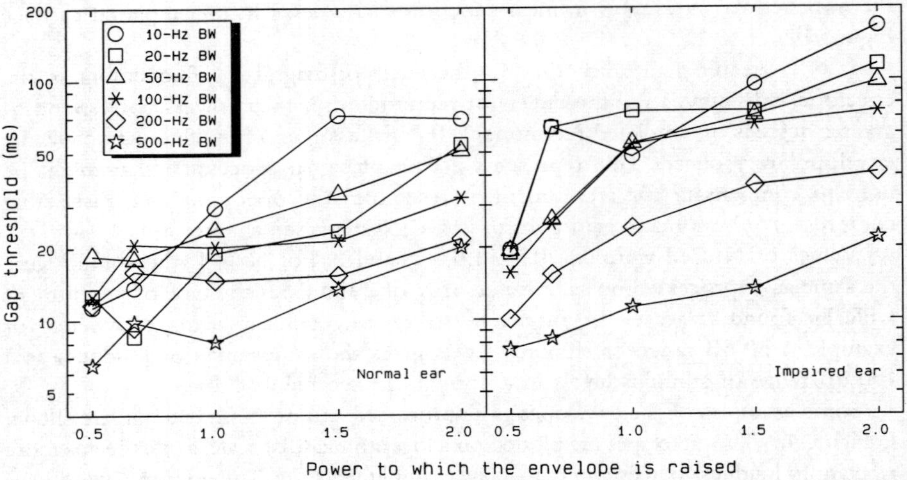

Fig. 4.10. Thresholds for detecting a gap in a noise band whose envelope had been processed to enhance or reduce fluctuations. Gap thresholds are plotted as a function of the power to which the envelope was raised, with noise bandwidth as parameter; the higher the power, the greater the fluctuations. Results are shown for each ear of a subject with unilateral cochlear hearing loss.

To prevent the detection of spectral splatter associated with the gap or with the envelope processing, the stimuli were presented in a continuous background noise. The spectrum of the noise was chosen so that it would be as effective as possible in masking the splatter while minimizing its overall loudness.

Figure 4.10 shows an example of results obtained using a subject with unilateral hearing loss of cochlear origin. The stimuli were presented at 85 dB SPL, a level which was well above the absolute threshold for both the normal and impaired ears (although the SL was lower in the impaired ear). The results for the normal ear were very similar to those of three normally hearing subjects who were also tested. Gap thresholds increased significantly with decreasing noise bandwidth. This is as expected, since the inherent fluctuations in the noise are slower, and more confusable with the gap to be detected, when the bandwidth is narrow (Shailer and Moore 1983; Moore 1989).

For all noise bandwidths, gap thresholds increased as N increased. This effect was particularly marked for the smaller noise bandwidths. There was a significant interaction between bandwidth and N, reflecting the fact that changes in gap threshold with N were greater for small bandwidths. This supports the idea that fluctuations in the noise adversely affect gap detection; greater fluctuations lead to worse performance, especially when the fluctuations are slow.

Gap thresholds were larger for the impaired than for the normal ear. The overall geometric mean gap threshold was 12.8 ms for the normal ear and 27.2 ms for the impaired ear. Performance for the normal ear with N = 2 was roughly similar to performance for the impaired ear with unprocessed noise bands (N = 1); geometric mean gap thresholds were 26.9 ms for the former and 26.5 ms for the latter. Thus, the simulation of recruitment in the normal ear was sufficient to produce impaired gap detection, comparable to that actually found in the impaired ear. This is consistent with the dynamic ranges inferred from audiometric data; the range from threshold to discomfort at 1 kHz was 90 dB in the normal ear and 45 dB in the impaired ear.

Reduction of fluctuations, by raising the envelope to a power less than one, produced a small improvement in performance for the normal ear. Values of N less than 1 gave a marked improvement for the impaired ear. Performance for the impaired ear with the envelope raised to the power 0.5 was comparable to, or even slightly better than, that for the normal ear with unprocessed stimuli; geometric mean thresholds were 11.6 ms for the former and 12.5 ms for the latter. This is again consistent with the fact that the dynamic range in the impaired ear was about half that in the normal ear. Thus, the impaired detection of gaps in noise bands occurring for an impaired ear can be restored to normal by appropriate compression of fluctuations in the envelopes of the stimuli.

For both normal-hearing and hearing-impaired subjects, the effects of changing N decreased with increasing noise bandwidth. One reason for this is that slow fluctuations can be followed by the auditory system, whereas rapid fluctuations are smoothed to some extent by the central temporal integration process described earlier. The rapid fluctuations of the wider noise bands are smoothed in this way, thus reducing their influence on gap detection.

The results suggest that, for most subjects with cochlear damage, recruitment, or equivalently, a reduction in the peripheral compressive nonlinearity, may provide a sufficient explanation for increased gap thresholds. Thus, it is not usually necessary to assume any abnormality in temporal processing occurring after the cochlea. However, one subject with a unilateral hearing loss tested by Glasberg and Moore showed higher gap thresholds in the impaired ear than would be expected just on the basis of loudness recruitment. This may have been due to the very low SL of the stimuli for that subject, or to some other factor affecting temporal resolution. Earlier reports have suggested that a few subjects show impairments in temporal resolution even using non-fluctuating stimuli (Jesteadt *et al.* 1976; Moore and Glasberg 1988c; Moore *et al.* 1989; Plack and Moore 1991). It is possible that the subjects showing this impaired resolution had damage to both outer hair cells (affecting the active process and the compressive nonlinearity) and inner hair cells (affecting the transduction process), or that they had a retrocochlear component to their hearing loss.

Temporal integration

Temporal integration in normally hearing people

It has been known for many years (Exner 1876) that the absolute threshold for detecting a sound depends upon the duration of the sound. For durations up to a few hundred milliseconds, the intensity required for threshold decreases as the duration increases. For durations exceeding about 500 ms, the sound intensity at threshold is roughly independent of duration. Many workers have investigated the relation between threshold and duration for tone pulses, over a wide range of frequencies and durations. The early work of Hughes (1946) and Garner and Miller (1947) indicated that, over a reasonable range of durations, the ear appears to integrate the intensity of the stimulus over time in the detection of short duration tone bursts. This is often called 'temporal integration'. In other words, the threshold corresponds to a constant energy rather than a constant intensity. If this were exactly true, the following formula would hold:

$$I \times t = \text{constant} \qquad \text{Eq. 4.1}$$

where I is the threshold intensity for a tone pulse of duration t. In practice the results are fitted better by the expression:

$$(I - I_L) \times t = I_L \times \tau = \text{constant} \qquad \text{Eq. 4.2}$$

where I_L is the threshold intensity for a long-duration tone pulse and τ is a constant representing the 'integration time' of the auditory system. Notice that in this formula it is not the product of time and intensity which is constant, but the product of time and the amount by which the intensity exceeds the value I_L. Garner and Miller (1947) interpreted I_L as the minimum intensity which is an effective stimulus for the ear. They assumed that only intensities above this minimum value are integrated linearly by the ear.

Thresholds as a function of duration are often plotted on dB versus log-duration coordinates. When plotted in this way, energy integration is indicated by the data falling on a straight line with a slope of −3 dB per doubling of duration. Although the average data for a group of subjects typically give a slope close to this value, the slopes for individual subjects can differ significantly from −3 dB per doubling. This suggests that it would be unwise to ascribe too much significance to the average slope. It seems very unlikely that the auditory system would actually integrate stimulus energy; it is almost certainly neural activity which is integrated (Zwislocki 1960; Penner 1972). It may also be the case that the auditory system does not actually perform an operation analogous to integration. Rather, it may be that the threshold intensity decreases with increasing duration partly because a longer stimulus provides more detection opportunities (more chances to detect the stimulus through repeated sampling). This idea is sometimes called 'multiple looks' (Viemeister and Wakefield 1991).

Temporal integration in people with cochlear damage

For people with cochlear damage, the change in threshold intensity with signal duration is often smaller than it is for normally hearing people. If the thresholds are plotted on dB versus log-duration coordinates, the slopes are usually much less in absolute value than the typical value of −3 dB/doubling found for normally hearing people. This is often described as reduced temporal integration (Gengel and Watson 1971; Pedersen and Elberling 1973; Elliott 1975; Chung 1981; Hall and Fernandes 1983; Carlyon *et al.* 1990). There is a trend for higher absolute thresholds to be associated with flatter slopes. In other words, the greater the hearing loss, the more reduced is the temporal integration.

Explanations for reduced temporal integration in people with cochlear damage

A number of explanations have been advanced to account for reduced temporal integration in people with cochlear damage. One explanation is that it is connected with the higher sound level at threshold. Perhaps temporal integration simply reduces as the sound level increases. This idea has been tested by measuring temporal integration in normally hearing subjects whose thresholds are elevated by a background of noise. In other words, temporal integration has been measured for masked threshold rather than for absolute threshold. In some experiments the noise has been spectrally shaped so that masked thresholds for the normal listeners matched those of specific hearing-impaired listeners (Florentine *et al.* 1988). The results show that temporal integration in normally hearing subjects is not markedly altered by the presence of broadband background noise (Garner and Miller 1947; Chung 1981; Hall and Fernandes 1983; Florentine *et al.* 1988). Hence, higher sound levels cannot account for reduced temporal integration in people with cochlear damage.

A second explanation has been in terms of the detection of spectral changes associated with the change in duration (Elliott 1975; Hall and Fernandes 1983). As the duration of a tone is decreased, its spectrum becomes broader, another example of 'spectral splatter'. The spectral energy becomes spread towards both lower and higher frequencies. Even for long-duration sounds, splatter occurs at the start and finish of the sound, especially when the sound is turned on and off abruptly. In people with normal hearing, it is very unlikely that the splatter would be detectable for tones close to absolute threshold, since the energy in the splatter is much less than the energy in the main on-frequency part of the spectrum. However, in a person with cochlear damage it is common for the absolute threshold to be more elevated at high frequencies than at low frequencies. If the person is trying to detect a high-frequency tone, the splatter may fall in a frequency region where their threshold is lower than at the test-tone's nominal frequency. Hence, the absolute threshold may be determined by detection of the splatter rather than by detection of the energy around the nominal test frequency. For fixed rise and fall times, the energy in the splatter is hardly affected by the steady state duration. Hence, splatter detection could lead to reduced temporal integration.

Although this explanation seems plausible, the experimental evidence suggest that it is not, in fact, correct. Even in people with relatively 'flat' losses, for whom the absolute threshold does not vary much with frequency, reduced temporal integration is observed. Also, when normally hearing subjects are tested in the presence of noise that has been spectrally shaped so that masked thresholds for the normal subjects match those of specific hearing-impaired subjects, temporal

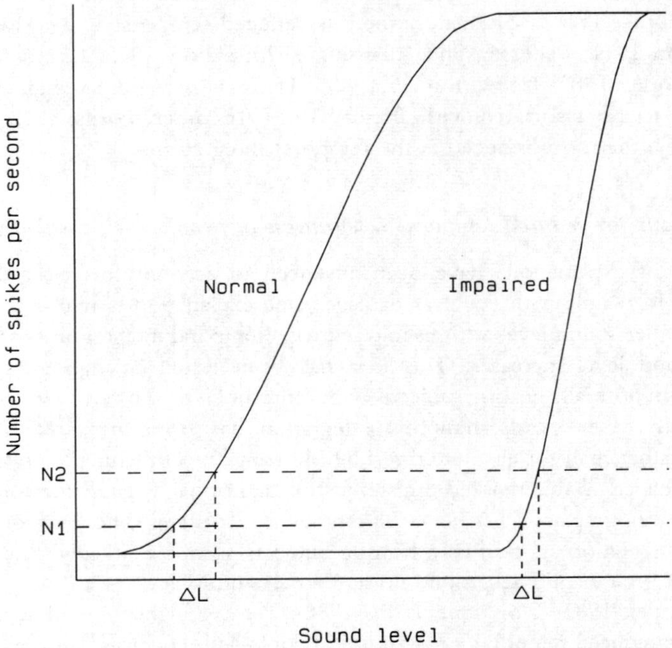

Fig. 4.11. Schematic illustration of rate-versus-level functions in single neurones of the auditory nerve for a normal ear (left curve) and an impaired ear (right curve). The horizontal dashed lines indicate the mean firing rate needed for threshold for a long-duration sound (lower line, rate N1) and a short-duration sound (upper line, rate N2) on the assumption that threshold corresponds to a fixed total number of spikes.

integration remains greater than observed for the hearing-impaired subjects (Florentine *et al.* 1988). This is true even in cases where the loss occurs mainly at high frequencies. Finally, Carlyon *et al.* (1990) measured temporal integration for a single brief tone pulse and for ten successive such pulses. The spectral splatter associated with the train of pulses is very similar to that for a single pulse. The normal subjects showed a difference in threshold between one and ten pulses of about 8 dB when the inter-pulse interval was less than 20 ms. In contrast, subjects with cochlear damage showed a threshold difference of only 2–3 dB, indicating reduced temporal integration. Taken together, these results make it very unlikely that detection of spectral splatter plays a significant role in reduced temporal integration.

It seems likely that the main cause of reduced temporal integration in people with cochlear damage is a reduction or complete loss of the compressive nonlinearity on the BM. This leads to steeper input–output functions on the BM (see Figure 1.13) and to steeper rate-versus-level functions in the auditory nerve. According to the models of temporal integration proposed by Zwislocki (1960) and by Penner (1972) this will automatically lead to reduced temporal integration. Figure 4.11, adapted from Moore (1991), illustrates schematically two rate-versus-level functions: the left-hand curve shows a typical function for a low-threshold neurone in a normal auditory system; the right-hand curve shows a typical function for a neurone in an auditory system with cochlear damage. The curve is shifted to the right, reflecting a loss of sensitivity, and is steeper, reflecting loss of the compressive nonlinearity on the BM.

Consider now how steeper rate-versus-level functions can lead to reduced temporal integration. Assume that, to a first approximation, the threshold for detecting a sound requires a fixed number of neural spikes to be evoked by that sound. Assume also, for the sake of simplicity, that the neurones involved in detection at absolute threshold are relatively homogeneous in terms of their input–output functions. The lower dashed horizontal line in Figure 4.11 indicates the number of neural spikes per second, N1, needed to achieve absolute threshold for a long-duration sound; in practice of course, the absolute threshold depends upon the activity of many neurones, but if they are all similar, then the argument can be illustrated by considering just one. If the duration of the sound is decreased by a factor R, then the level has to be increased to restore the total number of spikes evoked by the sound. Assume that the higher spike rate needed for the shorter-duration sound is N2, where N2 = R × N1. For example, if the duration is halved, the spike rate has to be increased by a factor of two to achieve the same total spike count. The increase in level, L, needed to achieve this increased rate is greater for the normal than for the impaired ear, because the rate-versus-level function is steeper for the impaired ear, and this explains the reduced temporal integration.

The argument given above is somewhat over-simplified because the firing rate in response to a tone burst is not uniform over time, but shows adaptation; the firing rate is highest at the onset of the sound and decreases over time. Hence, rate-versus-level functions depend somewhat on the duration of the stimuli used to determine them. However, adaptation is small for stimuli that are close to the detection threshold.

One problem with the argument given above is that, in normal ears, the input–output functions on the BM become steeper, and almost linear, at very low sound levels; see Figure 1.13. Hence, the input–output functions should be similar in steepness for a normal ear tested at a low (near-threshold) level and an impaired ear tested at a higher (but still near-threshold) level. However, the exact level at which the input–output function becomes linear in normal ears varies across studies. In some studies significant nonlinearity can still be observed at levels as low as 20 dB SPL. Furthermore, it is not known whether a low-level linear part of the input–output function occurs in humans, or, if it does, over what range of levels it occurs. For the moment, the reduced temporal integration observed for people with cochlear damage seems to be best explained in terms of a steeper growth of response on the BM.

Perceptual consequences of abnormal temporal processing in people with cochlear damage

Consequences of abnormal temporal resolution

It has been argued above that the central temporal integration mechanism (lowpass filter or sliding temporal window) is probably normal in people with cochlear damage. However, the nonlinearity preceding the integrator is less compressive in ears with cochlear damage than in normal ears. For stimuli with inherent slow amplitude fluctuations (such as narrow bands of noise) this can lead to poorer temporal resolution, since the inherent fluctuations become more confusable with the temporal feature to be detected. However, for deterministic stimuli (such as sinusoids) or for broadband noise stimuli, the reduced compression can actually lead to better performance in impaired than in normal ears, when the comparison is made at equal SLs. Unfortunately, most sounds in everyday life are characterised by unpredictable fluctuations in amplitude from moment to moment. For such sounds, people with cochlear damage will have more difficulty than normal in following the temporal structure of the sounds. In addition, temporal resolution may be poor because the sounds are at low SLs and/or because the audible bandwidth of the stimuli is restricted. All of these factors can lead to problems in understanding speech and in discriminating and identifying music and environmental sounds.

Consequences of reduced temporal integration

One consequence of reduced temporal integration is that the loss of sensitivity to weak sounds experienced by people with cochlear damage is less severe for short sounds than for long sounds. Consider, as an example, two sounds with durations 400 ms and 10 ms. For a normally hearing person the level required for detection of these two sounds might be, for example, 4 dB SPL and 20 dB SPL, respectively; the shorter sound has to be about 16 dB higher in level to reach the absolute threshold. For a person with moderate cochlear damage, the threshold for detecting the longer sound, might be 54 dB SPL, i.e. 50 dB higher than normal. However, the threshold for detecting the shorter sound might be 60 dB SPL, which is only 40 dB higher than normal. Thus the 'loss' relative to normal hearing is 10 dB less for the shorter sound than for the longer sound.

5. Pitch perception and frequency discrimination in normally hearing and hearing-impaired people

Introduction to the perception of pitch

Pitch may be defined as 'that attribute of auditory sensation in terms of which sounds may be ordered on a musical scale' (American Standards Association 1960). In other words, variations in pitch give rise to a sense of melody. Pitch is related to the repetition rate of the waveform of a sound; for a pure tone this corresponds to the frequency, and for a periodic complex tone to the fundamental frequency. There are, however, exceptions to this simple rule. Since pitch is a subjective attribute, it cannot be measured directly. Assigning a pitch value to a sound is generally understood to mean specifying the frequency of a sinusoid having the same subjective pitch as the sound. Sometimes a periodic complex sound, such as a pulse train, is used as a matching stimulus.

Traditional theories of pitch perception

For many years there have been two competing theories of pitch perception. One, the 'place' theory of hearing, is based on the fact that sound undergoes a limited-resolution spectral analysis in the cochlea, so that different frequencies (or frequency components in a complex sound) excite different places along the BM, and hence neurones with different CFs. The place theory assumes that the pitch of a sound is related to the excitation pattern produced by that sound; for a pure tone the pitch is generally assumed to correspond to the position of maximum excitation.

An alternative to the place theory, called the 'temporal' theory, suggests that the pitch of a sound is related to the time pattern of the neural impulses evoked by that sound. Nerve impulses tend to occur at a particular phase of the cochlear-filtered waveform, and thus the intervals between successive neural impulses approximate integer multiples of the period of the waveform, as described in chapter 1. The temporal theory cannot work at very high frequencies, since phase locking does not occur for frequencies above about 5 kHz. However, the tones produced by musical instruments, the human voice, and most everyday sound sources have fundamental frequencies below this range.

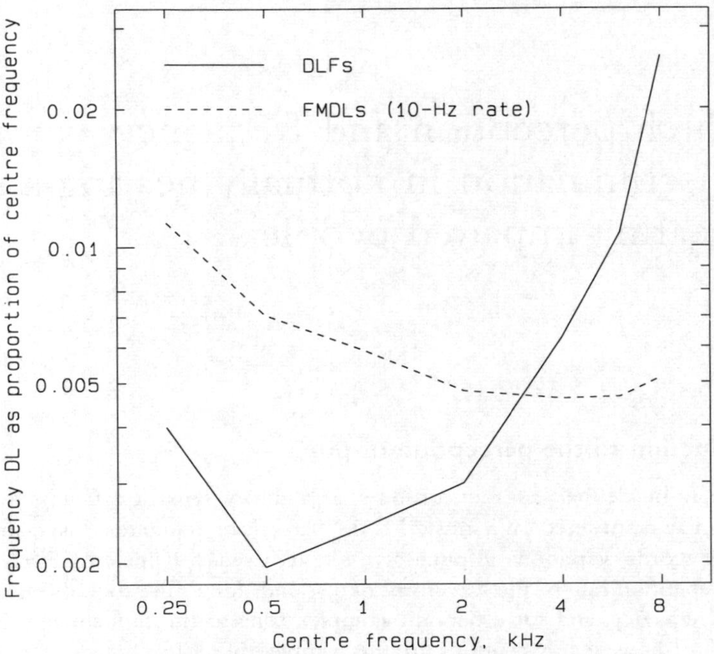

Fig. 5.1. Thresholds for detecting differences in frequency between steady pulsed tones (DLFs) and for detecting frequency modulation (FMDLs), plotted as a percentage of the centre frequency and plotted against centre frequency. The modulation rate for the FMDLs was 10 Hz.

The perception of the pitch of pure tones by normally hearing subjects

The frequency discrimination of pure tones

It is important to distinguish between frequency selectivity and frequency discrimination. The former refers to the ability to resolve the frequency components of a complex sound, as described in chapter 2. The latter refers to the ability to detect changes in frequency over time; these changes are usually heard as changes in pitch. The smallest detectable change is called the difference limen (DL). There have been two common ways of measuring frequency discrimination. One measure involves the discrimination of two successive steady tones with slightly different frequencies. The subject is required to indicate whether the first or second tone is higher in frequency. This measure will be called the DLF (difference limen for frequency). A second measure uses tones which are frequency modulated at a low rate. The amount of modulation required for detection of the modulation is determined. This measure will be called the FMDL (frequency modulation difference limen).

Early studies of frequency discrimination mainly measured FMDLs (Shower and Biddulph 1931; Zwicker 1952). Recent studies have concentrated more on the

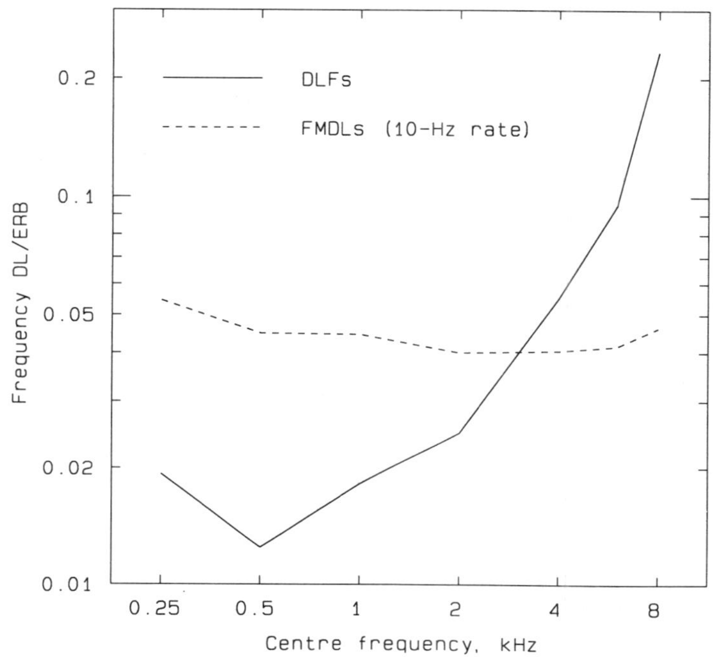

Fig. 5.2. DLFs and FMDLs plotted relative to the ERB of the auditory filter at each centre frequency, and plotted as a function of centre frequency. The modulation rate for the FMDLs was 10 Hz.

measurement of DLFs. An example of results obtained with both types of experiments is given in Figure 5.1 (data from Sek and Moore, 1995). Expressed in Hz, both DLFs and FMDLs are smallest at low frequencies, and increase monotonically with increasing frequency. Expressed as a proportion of centre frequency, as in Figure 5.1, DLFs are smallest for middle frequencies, and are larger for very high and very low frequencies. FMDLs vary less with frequency than DLFs. Both DLFs and FMDLs tend to get somewhat smaller as the sound level increases.

Place models of frequency discrimination (Henning 1967; Siebert 1970; Zwicker 1970) predict that frequency discrimination should be related to frequency selectivity; the sharper the tuning of peripheral filtering mechanisms, the smaller should be the frequency DL. It follows from this that the frequency DL should vary with frequency in roughly the same way as the ERB of the auditory filter (see chapter 2). In fact, this prediction fails for DLFs (Moore 1974; Moore and Glasberg 1986d; Sek and Moore 1995), but works reasonably well for FMDLs (Zwicker 1970; Moore and Glasberg 1989), especially if the modulation rate is reasonably high. This is illustrated in Figure 5.2, which shows the ratio DLF/ERB and FMDL/ERB for centre frequencies from 250 to 8000 Hz (Sek and Moore 1995); the modulation rate for the FMDLs was 10 Hz. For the FMDLs, the ratio is almost independent of frequency. For the DLFs, the ratio varies markedly with frequency.

At low frequencies, DLFs are usually smaller than predicted by place models, but at high frequencies, above 4–5 kHz, they are not. This is consistent with the idea that DLFs are determined by temporal information for frequencies up to about 4–5 kHz, and by place information above that. Moore and Sek (1995; Sek and Moore 1995) suggested that FMDLs for modulation rates of 10 Hz and above were determined by place mechanisms. For rates below 10 Hz, they suggested that both place and temporal mechanisms played a role.

The perception of musical intervals

Two tones which are separated in frequency by an interval of one octave (i.e. one has twice the frequency of the other) sound similar. They are judged to have the same name on the musical scale (for example, C or D). This has led several theorists to suggest that there are at least two dimensions to musical pitch. One aspect is related monotonically to frequency (for a pure tone) and is known as 'tone height'. The other is related to pitch class (i.e. name note) and is called 'tone chroma' (Bachem 1950).

If subjects are presented with a pure tone of a given frequency, f_1, and are asked to adjust the frequency, f_2, of a second tone so that it appears to be an octave higher in pitch, they will generally adjust f_2 to be roughly twice f_1. However, when f_1 lies above 2.5 kHz, so that f_2 would lie above 5 kHz, octave matches become very erratic (Ward 1954). It appears that the musical interval of an octave is only clearly perceived when both tones are below 5 kHz.

Other aspects of the perception of pitch also change above 5 kHz. A sequence of pure tones above 5 kHz does not produce a clear sense of melody (Attneave and Olson 1971). Also, subjects with absolute pitch (the ability to assign name notes without reference to other notes) are very poor at naming notes above 4–5 kHz (Ohgushi and Hatoh 1991).

These results are consistent with the idea that the pitch of pure tones is determined by different mechanisms above and below 5 kHz, specifically, by temporal mechanisms at low frequencies and place mechanisms at high frequencies. It appears that the perceptual dimension of tone height persists over the whole audible frequency range, but tone chroma only occurs in the frequency range below 5 kHz.

The pitch perception of complex tones

The phenomenon of the missing fundamental

For complex tones the pitch does not, in general, correspond to the position of maximum excitation on the BM. A striking illustration of this is provided by the 'phenomenon of the missing fundamental' (Ohm 1843; Schouten 1940). Consider, as an example, a sound consisting of short impulses (clicks) occurring 200 times per second. This sound has a low pitch, which is very close to the pitch of a

200-Hz pure tone, and a sharp timbre. It contains harmonics with frequencies at integer multiples of 200 Hz (200, 400, 600, 800 . . . Hz). However, if the sound is filtered so as to remove the 200-Hz component, the pitch does not alter; the only result is a slight change in timbre. Indeed, all except a small group of mid-frequency harmonics can be eliminated, and the low pitch is still heard, although the timbre becomes markedly different.

Schouten (1940, 1970) called this low pitch associated with a group of high harmonics the 'residue'. Several other names have been used to describe residue pitch, including 'periodicity pitch', 'virtual pitch', and 'low pitch'. This book will use the term residue pitch. Schouten pointed out that the residue is distinguishable, subjectively, from a fundamental component which is physically presented or from a fundamental which may be generated (at high sound levels) by nonlinear distortion in the ear. Thus it seems that the perception of a residue pitch does not require activity at the point on the BM which would respond maximally to a pure tone of similar pitch. This is confirmed by a demonstration of Licklider (1956) that the low pitch of the residue persists when low-frequency noise is present that would mask any component at the fundamental frequency. Even when the fundamental component of a complex tone is present, the pitch of the tone is usually determined by harmonics other than the fundamental. Thus the perception of residue pitch should not be regarded as unusual. Rather, residue pitches are normally heard when listening to complex tones.

Discrimination of the pitch of complex tones

When the repetition rate of a complex tone changes, all of the components change in frequency by the same ratio, and a change in residue pitch is heard. The ability to detect such changes in pitch is better than the ability to detect changes in a sinusoid at the fundamental frequency (Flanagan and Saslow 1958) and it can be better than the ability to detect changes in the frequency of any of the sinusoidal components in the complex tone (Moore *et al.* 1984b). This indicates that information from the different harmonics is combined or integrated in the determination of residue pitch. This can lead to very fine discrimination; changes in repetition rate of about 0.2% can be detected for fundamental frequencies in the range 100–400 Hz.

Analysis of a complex tone in the peripheral auditory system

A simulation of the analysis of a complex tone in the peripheral auditory system is illustrated in Figure 5.3. In this example, the complex tone is a periodic pulse train, containing many equal-amplitude harmonics. The lower harmonics are partly resolved on the BM, and give rise to distinct peaks in the pattern of activity along the BM. At a place tuned to the frequency of a low harmonic, the waveform on the BM is approximately a sinewave at the harmonic frequency. In contrast, the higher harmonics are not resolved, and do not give rise to distinct peaks on the BM. The waveform at places on the BM responding to higher harmonics is complex, and has a repetition rate equal to the fundamental frequency of the sound.

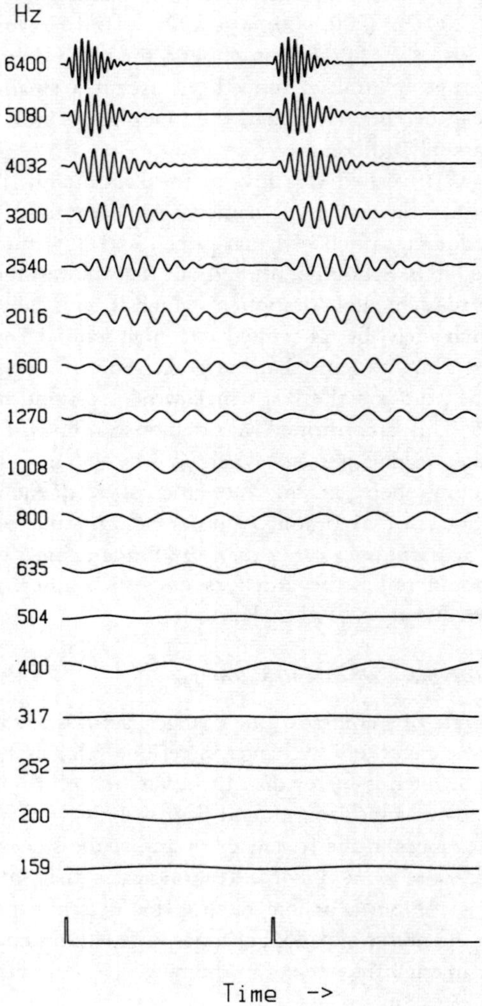

Fig. 5.3. Simulation of responses at different places on the BM to a periodic impulse with rate 200 periods per second. The numbers on the left-hand side indicate the CF of the place whose response is shown to the right.

Theories of pitch perception for complex tones

Several theories have been proposed to account for residue pitch. Theories prior to 1980 may be divided into two broad classes. The first, spectral theories, propose that the perception of the pitch of a complex tone involves two stages. The first stage is a frequency analysis which determines the frequencies of some of the individual sinusoidal components of the complex tone. These frequencies can only be determined accurately for the lower harmonics (about the first five to eight) that are resolved in the peripheral auditory system (Plomp 1964a; Moore *et al.* 1984b). The second stage is a pattern recognizer which determines the pitch of the complex from the frequencies of the resolved components (Goldstein 1973; Terhardt 1974). In essence the pattern recognizer tries to find the harmonic series giving the best match to the resolved frequency components; the fundamental frequency of this harmonic series determines the perceived pitch. For these theories, the lower resolvable harmonics are essential for pitch determination.

The alternative, temporal, theories assume that pitch is based on the time pattern of the waveform at a point on the BM responding to the higher harmonics. Pitch is assumed to be related to the time interval between corresponding points in the fine structure of the waveform close to adjacent envelope maxima (Schouten *et al.* 1962). Nerve firings tend to occur at these points (i.e. phase locking occurs), so this time interval will be present in the time pattern of neural impulses. For these theories, the upper unresolved harmonics should determine the pitch.

Spectral theories are supported by the finding that the lower, resolved harmonics give a clearer residue pitch, and are more important in determining residue pitch, than the upper unresolved harmonics (Plomp 1967; Ritsma 1967). This is described by the concept of dominance: 'if pitch information is available along a large part of the basilar membrane the ear uses only the information from a narrow band. This band is positioned at 3–5 times the pitch value. Its precise position depends somewhat on the subject.' (Ritsma 1970). The data of Moore *et al.* (1984b, 1985b) show that there are large individual differences in which harmonics are dominant, and for some subjects the first two harmonics play an important role. Other data show that the dominant region is not fixed in terms of harmonic number, but depends somewhat on absolute frequency (Plomp 1967; Patterson and Wightman 1976). For high fundamental frequencies (above about 1000 Hz), the fundamental is usually the dominant component, while for very low fundamental frequencies, around 50 Hz, harmonics above the fifth may be dominant (Moore and Glasberg 1988b; Moore and Peters 1992).

Temporal theories are supported by the finding that a residue pitch can be heard when only high unresolvable harmonics are present (Ritsma 1962, 1963; Moore 1973b; Moore and Rosen 1979; Houtsma and Smurzynski 1990). However, this pitch is often rather weak. Temporal theories are also supported by the finding that the relative phase of the components in a complex tone can affect pitch perception. Changes in phase can change the temporal structure of the tone, but have little effect on the auditory representation of the lower, resolved harmonics. Thus, spectral theories predict that relative phase should not influence pitch, while temporal theories predict that relative phase should affect pitch, pitch being more distinct for phase relations producing 'peaky' waveforms after auditory filtering (waveforms with high crest factors).

For tones containing many harmonics, phase has only small effects on the value of the pitch heard (Patterson 1973), but it does affect the clarity of pitch (Lundeen and Small 1984). For tones containing only a few high harmonics, phase can affect both the pitch value and the clarity of pitch (Moore 1977; Shackleton and Carlyon

1994). These results suggest that the temporal structure of complex sounds does influence pitch perception.

The evidence reviewed above indicates that neither spectral nor temporal theories can account for all aspects of the pitch perception of complex tones. This has led several workers to propose theories in which both spectral and temporal mechanisms play a role; these are referred to as spectro-temporal theories. The initial place/spectral analysis in the cochlea is followed by an analysis of the time pattern of the waveform at each place or of the neural spikes evoked at each place (Moore 1982, 1989; Srulovicz and Goldstein 1983; Patterson 1987; Meddis and Hewitt 1991). The model proposed by Moore is illustrated in Figure 5.4. The sound is passed through an array of bandpass filters, each corresponding to a specific place on the BM. The time pattern of the neural impulses at each CF is determined by the cochlear-filtered waveform. The inter-spike intervals at each CF are determined. Then, a device compares the time intervals present at different CFs, and searches for common time intervals. The device may also integrate information over time. In general the time interval which is found most often corresponds to the period of the fundamental component and the perceived pitch corresponds to the reciprocal of this interval. Spectro-temporal theories can account for most existing data on the pitch perception of complex tones, and so are more satisfactory than either spectral or temporal theories.

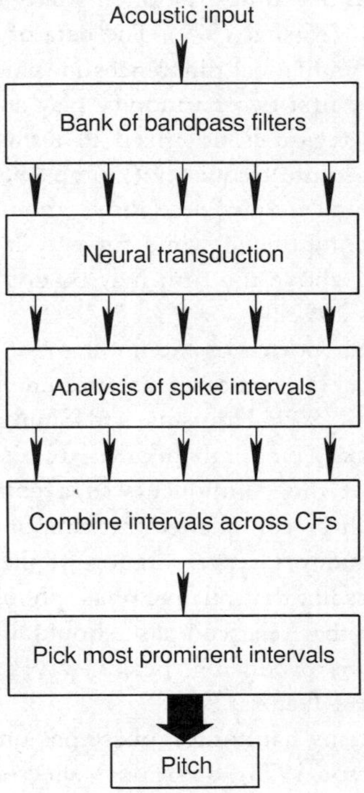

Fig. 5.4. A schematic diagram of the spectro-temporal model of pitch perception for complex tones described in Moore (1989).

Frequency discrimination of pure tones by people with cochlear damage

People with cochlear damage usually have auditory filters that are broader than normal; see chapter 2. According to the place theory, this should lead to poorer frequency discrimination than normal. According to the temporal theory, there should not necessarily be a relationship between frequency selectivity and frequency discrimination. However, frequency discrimination could be adversely affected by the reduced precision of phase locking that can occur in cases of cochlear damage; see chapter 1.

Several studies have measured DLFs in subjects with cochlear damage (Gengel 1973; Tyler *et al.* 1983; Hall and Wood 1984; Freyman and Nelson 1986, 1987, 1991; Moore and Glasberg 1986c; Moore and Peters 1992; Simon and Yund 1993). The results have generally shown that frequency discrimination is adversely affected by cochlear damage. However, there is considerable variability across subjects and the size of the DLF has not been found to be strongly correlated with the absolute threshold at the test frequency. Simon and Yund (1993) measured DLFs separately for each ear of subjects with bilateral cochlear damage and found that DLFs could be markedly different for the two ears at frequencies where absolute thresholds were the same. They also found that DLFs could be the same for the two ears when absolute thresholds were different.

Tyler *et al.* (1983) compared DLFs and frequency selectivity measured using psychophysical tuning curves (see chapter 2). They found a low correlation between the two. They concluded that frequency discrimination was not closely related to frequency selectivity, suggesting that place models were not adequate to explain the data. Moore and Peters (1992) measured DLFs for four groups of subjects: young normally hearing, young hearing impaired, elderly with near-normal hearing, and elderly hearing impaired. The auditory filters of the subjects had been measured in earlier experiments using the notched-noise method (see chapter 2), for centre frequencies (f_c) of 100, 200, 400 and 800 Hz. The DLFs for both impaired groups were higher than for the young normal group at all f_cs (50–4000 Hz). The DLFs at a given f_c were generally only weakly correlated with the sharpness of the auditory filter at that f_c, and some subjects with broad filters at low frequencies had near-normal DLFs at low frequencies. These results suggest a partial dissociation of frequency selectivity and frequency discrimination of pure tones.

Freyman and Nelson (1986, 1987) attempted to evaluate a specific place model proposed by Zwicker (1956, 1970). This model is based on the concept of the excitation pattern, as described in chapter 2. A change in frequency results in a shift of the whole excitation pattern along the tonotopic axis, as illustrated in Figure 5.5. The model assumes that the change in frequency can be detected if the change in excitation level at any point on the pattern exceeds a criterion amount, ΔL, assumed by Zwicker to be about 1 dB. Since excitation patterns at moderate to high sound levels are asymmetric, with a steeper low-frequency skirt, the biggest change in excitation level occurs on the low-frequency side of the pattern. Zwicker

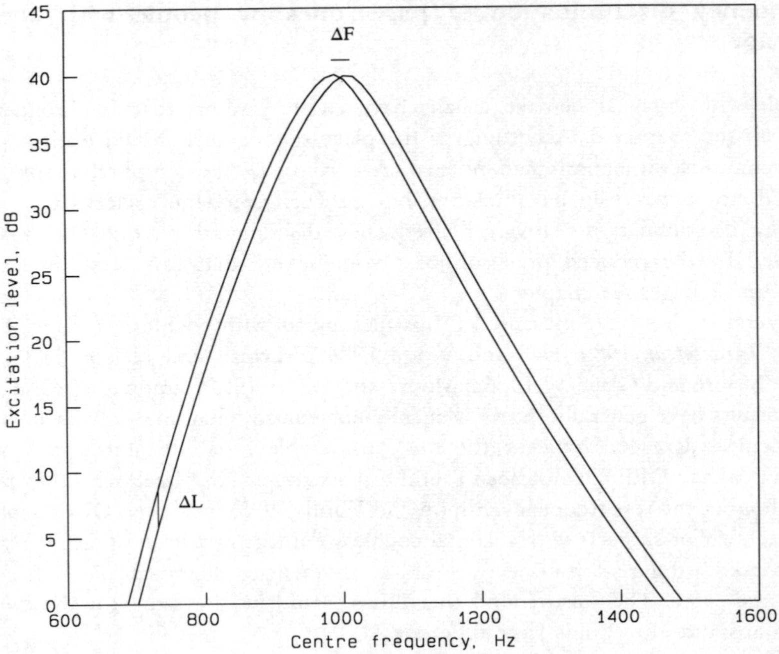

Fig. 5.5. Schematic illustration of an excitation-pattern model for frequency discrimination. Excitation patterns are shown for two sinusoidal tones differing slightly in frequency. It is assumed that the difference in frequency, Δf, can be detected if the excitation level changes anywhere by more than a criterion amount (ΔL).

originally proposed the model to account for FMDLs, but other researchers, including Nelson and Freyman, have attempted to apply it to DLFs.

Following Moore (1973a), Freyman and Nelson (1986) argued that for a tone with a very short duration, the physical broadening of the spectrum of the sound (spectral splatter) should limit the slope of the excitation pattern. Hence, for durations below a critical duration, frequency discrimination should be independent of the frequency selectivity of the subject. However, for longer durations, where the physical spectrum is narrower, the frequency selectivity of the subject should play a stronger role, and frequency discrimination should be poorer in subjects with reduced frequency selectivity.

The results obtained by Freyman and Nelson were generally in agreement with these predictions. Subjects with cochlear damage had larger DLFs than normally hearing subjects for long and medium durations, but the DLFs for normal and hearing-impaired subjects did not differ significantly for very short durations. Similar results were obtained by Hall and Wood (1984).

Freyman and Nelson (1986) estimated the slopes of the low-frequency sides of the excitation patterns of their subjects by measuring masking patterns and psychophysical tuning curves in forward masking; the high-frequency slopes of the PTCs were used to estimate the low-frequency slopes of the excitation patterns.

From these slopes they were able to estimate the 'critical duration' for each subject and signal frequency at which the physical slope of the spectrum for a short-duration tone equals the slope of the excitation pattern for a long-duration tone. For the hearing-impaired subjects, the critical durations were often less than 5 ms; for a centre frequency of 2000 Hz they were always less than 5 ms. According to the excitation-pattern model, this means that performance should be limited by the frequency selectivity of the subject rather than by the physical slope of the spectrum for all durations down to 5 ms. However, at 2000 Hz, the DLFs of the hearing-impaired subjects were similar to those of the normally hearing subjects for a duration of 11 ms, which is not entirely consistent with the excitation-pattern model.

Another aspect of the results is hard to account for in terms of the excitation-pattern model. Freyman and Nelson calculated the value of the change in excitation level required for threshold at long durations, ΔL, by multiplying the estimated excitation-pattern slope by the DLF at long durations. For stimuli at high SPLs, the value of ΔL would not be expected to be greatly different for normal and hearing-impaired subjects, since intensity discrimination thresholds, DLIs, are similar for the two groups (see chapter 3). However, the mean values of ΔL calculated by Freyman and Nelson were markedly smaller for the hearing-impaired subjects (0.62 dB) than for the normally hearing subjects (1.32 dB). Also, the data showed a clear increase in ΔL with increasing centre frequency, which would not be expected on the basis of intensity discrimination data. Given these difficulties, these data cannot be taken as strong support for the excitation-pattern model, although the effects of duration are broadly consistent with the model.

Moore and Glasberg (1986c) attempted to evaluate the excitation-pattern model in a different way. They measured DLFs in subjects with moderate unilateral and bilateral cochlear losses. They also estimated auditory filter shapes in the same subjects using the notched-noise method described in chapter 2. This allowed them to estimate the slope of the low-frequency side of the excitation pattern. Finally, they estimated the criterion change in excitation level, ΔL, by measuring the intensity discrimination of pulsed tones (the DLI); see chapter 3 for details of this measure. The DLIs were measured in the presence of a high-pass noise intended to mask the upper side of the excitation pattern. This was done to ensure that the same side of the excitation pattern was involved as for the frequency discrimination measures. The stimuli were centred at three frequencies, 0.5, 1.0 and 2.0 kHz, and had a level of 80 dB SPL. The absolute thresholds of the subjects were relatively uniform over this frequency range.

The DLIs were similar for the normal and impaired ears. However, the slopes of the auditory filters were less for the impaired than for the normal ears, and the DLFs were larger for the impaired than for the normal ears. For both the normal and impaired ears, the DLFs were generally smaller than predicted by the excitation-pattern model.

Overall, the results of the experiments reviewed above do not provide strong support for the excitation-pattern model. An alternative way of accounting for the fact that cochlear damage results in larger-than-normal DLFs is in terms of loss of neural synchrony (phase locking) in the auditory nerve; see chapter 1. Goldstein and Srulovicz (1977) described a model for frequency discrimination based on an optimal processor that used information from the inter-spike intervals in the auditory nerve. This model was able to account for the way that DLFs depend on frequency and duration for normally hearing subjects. Wakefield and Nelson (1985) showed that a simple extension to this model, taking into account the dependence of phase locking on sound level, allowed the model to predict the effects of level on DLFs. They also applied the model to DLFs measured as a function of level in subjects with high-frequency hearing loss, presumably resulting from cochlear damage. They were able to predict the results of the hearing-impaired subjects by assuming that neural synchrony was reduced in neurones with CFs corresponding to the region of hearing loss. Of course, this does not prove that loss of synchrony is the cause of the larger DLFs, but it does demonstrate that loss of synchrony is a plausible candidate.

Yet another possibility is that the central mechanisms involved in the analysis of phase-locking information make use of differences in the preferred time of firing of neurones with different CFs; these time differences arise from the propagation time of the travelling wave on the BM (Loeb *et al.* 1983; Shamma 1985). The propagation time along the BM can be affected by cochlear damage, and this could disrupt the processing of the temporal information by central mechanisms.

Detection of frequency modulation by people with cochlear damage

There have been relatively few studies measuring FMDLs in hearing-impaired people. This is a pity, since practice effects are generally much smaller for FMDLs than for DLFs (Moore 1976). The values of FMDLs for untrained subjects are not much larger than those of highly trained subjects, whereas DLFs can change markedly with training.

Zurek and Formby (1981) measured FMDLs in ten subjects with sensorineural hearing loss (assumed to be mainly of cochlear origin) using a 3-Hz modulation rate and frequencies between 125 and 4000 Hz. Subjects were tested at an SL of 25 dB, a level above which performance was found (in pilot studies) to be roughly independent of level. The FMDLs tended to increase with increasing hearing loss at a given frequency. For a given degree of hearing loss, the worsening of performance with increasing hearing loss was greater at low frequencies than at high frequencies.

Zurek and Formby suggested two possible explanations for the greater effect at low frequencies. The first is that that two mechanisms are involved in coding frequency, a temporal mechanism at low frequencies and a place mechanism at high frequencies. The temporal mechanism may be more disrupted by hearing loss than the place mechanism. An alternative possibility is that absolute thresholds at low frequencies do not provide an accurate indicator of the extent of cochlear damage, since these thresholds may be mediated by neurones with CFs above the test frequency; this point is discussed in more detail in the following section.

As part of the experiment of Moore and Glasberg (1986c) described in the previous section, FMDLs and AMDLs (see chapter 3) were also measured, using a 4-Hz modulation rate. The AMDLs, together with the estimated slopes of the auditory filters, were used to predict the FMDLs on the basis of Zwicker's excitation-pattern model. In contrast to the DLFs, which were generally smaller than predicted by the model, the obtained FMDLs were reasonably close to the predicted values.

The fact that the obtained DLFs were smaller than predicted by the excitation-pattern model could be explained by a systematic error in estimating the auditory-filter slopes. However, Moore and Glasberg pointed out that it was possible to test whether the model could explain both DLFs and FMDLs without using the estimated slope values. For a given ear at a given test frequency, the value of the slope should be the same regardless of whether a DLF or an FMDL is being measured. Thus, if the excitation-pattern model applies to both types of discrimination, the ratio FMDL/DLF should equal the ratio AMDL/DLI. In fact, these two ratios were essentially uncorrelated ($r = -0.06$). Moore and Glasberg concluded that the excitation-pattern model cannot account for both DLFs and FMDLs. It seems likely that FMDLs can be explained by some form of excitation-pattern model (Moore and Sek 1994; Sek and Moore 1995). However, DLFs appear to depend on some other mechanism.

Grant (1987) studied FM detection in three normally hearing subjects and three subjects with profound hearing losses. The sinusoidal carrier was modulated in frequency by a triangle function 3 times per second. Stimuli were presented at 30 dB SL for the normal subjects and at a 'comfortable listening level' (110–135 dB SPL) for the impaired subjects. For all carrier frequencies (100 to 1000 Hz), FMDLs were larger for the hearing–impaired than for the normally hearing subjects. Grant also measured FMDLs when the stimuli were simultaneously amplitude modulated by a lowpass noise (cutoff frequency 3 Hz). The random amplitude fluctuations produced by this modulation would be expected to impair the use of cues for FM detection based on changes in excitation level. Consistent with the predictions of the excitation-pattern model, the random amplitude modulation led to increased FMDLs. However, the increase was much greater for the impaired than for the normally hearing subjects.

It is possible that, at low modulation rates, normally hearing subjects can extract information about frequency modulation both from changes in excitation level and from phase locking (Moore and Sek 1995; Sek and Moore 1995). The random amplitude modulation disrupts the use of changes in excitation level, but does not markedly affect the use of phase locking cues. The profoundly hearing-impaired subjects of Grant appear to have been relying mainly or exclusively on changes in excitation level. Hence, the random amplitude modulation had severe adverse effects on the FMDLs.

In conclusion, FMDLs for hearing-impaired people can be accounted for reasonably well in terms of excitation-pattern models. The reduced frequency selectivity typically associated with cochlear loss leads to larger-than-normal FMDLs.

The perception of pure-tone pitch in the absence of functioning hair cells with CFs at the test frequency

In some people with cochlear damage restricted to low-frequency regions of the cochlea, it appears that there are no functioning IHCs with CFs corresponding to the frequency region of the loss. The detection of low-frequency tones is mediated by neurones with high CFs. One way of demonstrating this is by the measurement of psychophysical tuning curves (PTCs); see chapter 2. If the signal to be detected has a frequency corresponding to the region of the hearing loss, and if there are no functioning hair cells in this region, the tip of the tuning curve lies well above the signal frequency. In other words, a masker centred well above the signal in frequency is more effective than a masker centred close to the signal frequency (Thornton and Abbas 1980; Florentine and Houtsma 1983; Turner *et al.* 1983). For example, Florentine and Houtsma (1983) studied a subject with a moderate to severe unilateral low-frequency loss of cochlear origin. For a 1-kHz signal, the tip of the PTC fell between 2.2 and 2.85 kHz, depending on the exact level of the signal.

The perception of pitch in such subjects is of considerable theoretical interest. A low-frequency pure tone cannot produce maximum neural excitation at the CF corresponding to its frequency, since there are no neural responses at that CF. The peak in the neural activity pattern must occur at CFs higher than the frequency of the signal. If the place theory is correct, this would be expected to lead to marked upward shifts in the pitch of the tone. In fact, this does not happen.

Florentine and Houtsma (1983) obtained pitch matches between the two ears of their unilaterally impaired subject. They presented the stimuli at very low SLs, to minimise the spread of excitation along the BM. Pitch shifts between the two ears were small. Turner *et al.* (1983) studied six subjects with low-frequency cochlear losses, three of whom showed PTCs with tips close to the signal frequency (presumably having functioning IHCs with CFs close to the signal frequency) and three of whom showed PTCs with tips well above the signal frequency. Pitch perception was studied either by pitch matching between the two ears (for subjects with unilateral losses) or by octave matching (for subjects with bilateral losses, but with some musical ability). The subjects whose PTCs had tips above the signal frequency gave results similar to those of the subjects whose PTCs had tips close to the signal frequency; no distinct pitch anomalies were observed.

These results are hard to explain in terms of the traditional place theory. They show that a pure tone can evoke a low pitch even when there are no functioning hair cells or neurones with CFs corresponding to that pitch. The results are more readily explained in terms of the temporal theory; the pitch of the low-frequency tone may be coded in the temporal pattern of neural responses in neurones with CFs above the signal frequency.

There have been a few reports of people with hearing losses that increase abruptly at high frequencies who appear to have no functioning IHCs tuned to high frequencies. These subjects report that high-frequency sinusoids do not have a distinct pitch, but sound like noises (Moore *et al.* 1985c; Murray and Byrne 1986).

Presumably, in these cases, neither place coding nor temporal coding mechanisms for pitch can operate effectively. Interestingly, subjects with this type of loss are helped only to a limited extent by hearing aids which attempt to restore audibility of high frequencies; they are helped more by aids which low-pass filter the signal to remove components in the frequency region of high-frequency loss (Moore *et al.* 1985c; Murray and Byrne 1986).

Pitch anomalies in the perception of pure tones

Although people with low-frequency hearing loss often perceive the pitch of low-frequency tones in a more or less 'normal' way, cochlear damage does sometimes lead to changes in perceived pitch. For people with unilateral cochlear damage, or asymmetrical hearing losses, the same tone presented alternately to the two ears may be perceived as having different pitches in the two ears. This effect is given the name diplacusis. Sometimes different pitches are perceived even when the hearing loss is the same in the two ears. The magnitude of the shift can be measured by getting the subject to adjust the frequency of the tone in one ear until its pitch matches that of the tone in the other ear.

According to the place theory, cochlear damage might result in pitch shifts for two reasons. The peak in the neural excitation pattern evoked by a tone may be shifted away from a region of hearing loss, because of a reduction of effective excitation level in that frequency region. Hence the perceived pitch should shift away from the frequency region of hearing loss. Early studies of diplacusis (de Mare 1948; Webster and Schubert 1954) were generally consistent with this prediction, showing that when a sinusoidal tone is presented in a frequency region of hearing loss, the pitch shifts towards a frequency region where there is less hearing loss. For example, in a person with a high-frequency hearing loss, the pitch was reported to be shifted downwards. However, there are clearly cases where the pitch does not shift as predicted, as described in the previous section.

An alternative way in which pitch shifts might occur is by shifts in the position of the peak excitation on the BM; such shifts can occur even for a 'flat' hearing loss. Chapter 1 described work showing that the tips of neural tuning curves were often shifted downwards in cases of moderate to severe cochlear damage.

This means that the maximum excitation at a given place is produced by a lower frequency than normal. Hence, for a given frequency, the peak of the BM response in an impaired cochlea would be shifted towards the base, i.e. towards places normally responding to higher frequencies. This leads to the prediction that the perceived pitch should be shifted upwards. Several studies have found that this is usually the case. For example, Gaeth and Norris (1965) and Schoeny and Carhart (1971) reported that pitch shifts were generally upwards regardless of the configuration of loss. However, it is also clear that individual differences can be substantial, and subjects with similar patterns of hearing loss (absolute thresholds as a function of frequency) can show quite different pitch shifts.

Burns and Turner (1986) measured changes in pitch as a function of intensity, by obtaining pitch matches between a tone presented at a fixed level (midway, in dB, between the absolute threshold and 100 dB SPL) and a tone of variable level. The tones were presented alternately to the same ear. Normally hearing subjects usually show small shifts in pitch with intensity in this type of task; the pitch of low-frequency tones shifts downwards with increasing intensity, while the pitch of high-frequency tones shifts upwards (Verschuure and van Meeteren 1975). The shifts are rarely greater than about 3%. The hearing-impaired subjects of Burns and Turner often showed abnormally large pitch-intensity effects, with shifts up to 10%. A common pattern was an abnormally large negative pitch shift with increasing level for low-frequency tones.

Burns and Turner (1986) obtained several other measures from their subjects, including psychophysical tuning curves (PTCs) in forward masking, DLFs, diplacusis, and octave judgements. There was a tendency for increased DLFs and increased pitch-matching variability in frequency regions where the PTCs were broader than normal. The exaggerated pitch-level effects occurred both in frequency regions where PTCs were broader than normal, and (sometimes) in regions where both absolute thresholds and PTCs were normal. The results of the diplacusis measurements and octave matches indicated that the large pitch-intensity effects were mainly a consequence of large increases in pitch at low levels; the pitch returned to more 'normal' values at higher levels.

As pointed out by Burns and Turner, these results are difficult to explain by the place theory. There is no evidence to suggest that peaks in BM responses or in neural excitation patterns are shifted at low levels but return to 'normal' positions at high levels. Also, even in subjects with similar configurations of hearing loss, the pitch shifts and changes in pitch with level can vary markedly. Furthermore, as pointed out earlier, low-frequency pure tones can evoke low pitches even in people who appear to have no IHCs or neurones tuned to low frequencies.

The results are also problematic for the temporal theory. There is no obvious reason why systematic shifts in pitch should occur as a result of cochlear damage or of changes in level. Unfortunately, there seem to be no physiological data concerning the effects of level on phase locking in ears with cochlear damage. As pointed out earlier, it is possible that the central mechanisms involved in the analysis of phase-locking information make use of the propagation time of the travelling wave on the BM (Loeb *et al.* 1983; Shamma 1985). This time can be affected by cochlear damage, and this could disrupt the processing of the temporal information by central mechanisms.

Frequency discrimination of complex tones by people with cochlear damage

Studies of the pitch discrimination of complex tones in people with cochlear damage have implications for pitch theories. According to spectral theories, the pitch of a complex tone is determined primarily by resolved harmonics. If the auditory filters are broader than normal, as is usually the case in people with cochlear damage, then this will make it more difficult to resolve harmonics, especially when the harmonics are of moderate harmonic number. For example,

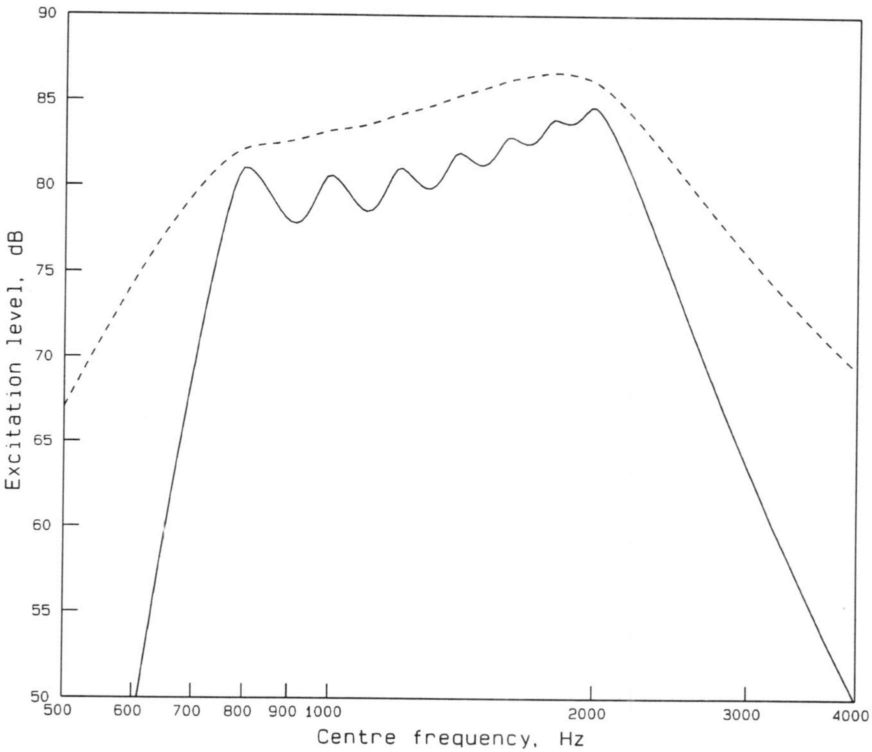

Fig. 5.6. Excitation patterns for a harmonic complex tone containing harmonics 4–10 of a 200-Hz fundamental. Each harmonic has a level of 80 dB SPL. Excitation patterns are shown for a normal ear (solid curve), and for an impaired ear (dashed curve) in which the auditory filters are three times as broad as normal.

for a fundamental frequency (F0) of 200 Hz, the fourth and fifth harmonics would be quite well resolved in a normal auditory system, but would be poorly resolved in an ear where the auditory filters were, say, three times broader than normal. This is illustrated in Figure 5.6, which shows excitation patterns for a complex tone composed of the fourth to tenth harmonics of a 200-Hz fundamental, for a normal auditory system (solid curve), and for an impaired auditory system (dashed curve) in which the auditory filters are three times broader than normal. The former shows distinct ripples corresponding to the lower harmonics, whereas the latter does not. The spectral theories predict that discrimination of changes in F0 of such a tone should be much poorer for the impaired than for the normal auditory system.

According to spectro-temporal theories, the pitches of complex tones can be extracted from higher unresolved harmonics as well as from lower resolved harmonics. Pitch discrimination might be somewhat impaired by broadened filters in an ear with cochlear damage, because the temporal information conveying pitch is more ambiguous (Rosen and Fourcin 1986); in response to a complex tone, the temporal waveform at the output of a broadened filter is generally more complex than that at the output of a normal filter. However, for complex tones with many harmonics, this effect should be small; spectro-temporal theories assume that information can be combined across different frequency regions to resolve ambiguities. On the other hand, it is also possible that phase locking (neural synchrony) is abnormal in people with cochlear damage, in which case pitch discrimination could be markedly impaired.

Hypothetically, then, of subjects with broad auditory filters, some might show reasonably good pitch discrimination, while others (those with abnormal phase locking) might show marked impairments. The spectro-temporal theories also predict that pitch discrimination by subjects with broader-than-normal auditory filters might be more affected by the relative phases of the components, since even the lower harmonics would interact at the outputs of the auditory filters.

The pitch discrimination of complex tones by hearing-impaired people has been the subject of several studies (Hoekstra and Ritsma 1977; Rosen 1987; Moore and Glasberg 1988d; 1990; Moore and Peters 1992; Arehart 1994). Most studies have required subjects to identify which of two successive harmonic complex tones had the higher F0. The threshold determined in such a task will be described as a DLC. These studies have revealed the following:

(1) There was considerable individual variability, both in overall performance and in the effects of harmonic content.
(2) For some subjects, when F0 was low, DLCs for complex tones containing only low harmonics (1–5) were markedly higher than for complex tones containing higher harmonics, suggesting that pitch was conveyed largely by the higher, unresolved harmonics.
(3) For some subjects, DLCs were larger for complex tones with lower harmonics (1–12) than for tones without lower harmonics (4–12 and 6–12) for F0s up to 200 Hz. In other words, adding lower harmonics made performance worse. This may happen because, when auditory filters are broader than normal, adding lower harmonics can create more complex waveforms at the outputs of the auditory filters, making temporal analysis more difficult.
(4) The DLCs were mostly only weakly correlated with measures of frequency selectivity. There was a slight trend for large DLCs to be associated with poor frequency selectivity, but the relationship was not a close one. Some subjects with very poor frequency selectivity had reasonably small DLCs.
(5) There can be significant effects of component phase. In several studies, DLCs have been measured with the components of the harmonic complexes added in one of two phase relationships, all cosine phase or alternating cosine and sine phase. The former results in a waveform with prominent peaks and low amplitudes between the peaks. The latter results in a waveform with a much flatter envelope. The DLCs tended to be larger for complexes with components added in alternating sine/cosine phase than for complexes with components added in cosine phase. However, the opposite effect was sometimes found. The direction of the phase

effect varied in an unpredictable way across subjects and across type of harmonic complex.

The variability in the phase effect may arise from variability in the properties of the auditory filters across subjects and across centre frequencies. According to spectro-temporal theories, the time patterns of the waveforms at the outputs of the auditory filters are important for determining pitch. These waveforms are determined by the magnitude and phase response of the auditory filters, and these may vary markedly across subjects and centre frequencies depending on the specific pattern of cochlear damage.

Some workers (Buunen *et al.* 1974) have suggested that the effects of component phase on pitch can be explained in terms of combination tones, particularly the tone, $2f_1$-f_2; see chapter 1. Changing the phases of the components in a complex tone may affect the relative levels of the combination tones, which in turn might affect pitch. However, this explanation seems unlikely to apply to results from subjects with cochlear damage, since the levels of combination tones are lower in these subjects than in normal subjects (Leshowitz and Lindstrom 1977). Furthermore the phase effects are generally larger for impaired than for normal subjects. The effects of phase on the DLCs most likely reflect a sensitivity to the time structure of the waveforms at the outputs of the auditory filters, as proposed by spectro-temporal theories of pitch.

Overall, these results suggest that people with cochlear damage depend relatively more on temporal information and less on spectral information than normally hearing people. The results lend support to spectro-temporal theories of pitch perception. The variability in the results across subjects, even in cases where the audiometric thresholds are similar, may occur partly because of individual differences in the auditory filters and partly because loss of neural synchrony is greater in some subjects than others. Subjects in whom neural synchrony is well preserved may have good pitch discrimination despite having broader-than-normal auditory filters. Subjects in whom neural synchrony is adversely affected may have poor pitch discrimination regardless of the degree of broadening of their auditory filters.

Perceptual consequences of altered frequency discrimination and pitch perception

The perception of pitch plays an important role in the ability to understand speech. In all languages, the pitch patterns of speech indicate which are the most important words in an utterance, they distinguish a question from a statement and they indicate the structure of sentences in terms of phrases. In tone languages, such as Mandarin Chinese, Zulu and Thai, pitch can affect word meanings. Pitch also conveys non-linguistic information about the gender, age and emotional state of the speaker. Supplementing lip reading (speechreading) with an auditory signal containing information only about voice pitch can result in a substantial improvement in the ability to understand speech (Risberg 1974; Rosen *et al.* 1981; Grant *et al.* 1985). The use of a signal that conveys information about the presence or absence of voicing (i.e. about whether a periodic complex sound is present or not) gives less improvement than when pitch is signalled in addition. It seems likely that reduced ability to discriminate pitch changes, as occurs in people with cochlear hearing loss would reduce the ability to use pitch information in this way.

For complex tones, people with cochlear damage are often more affected by the relative phases of the components than are normally hearing people. When a hearing-impaired person is reasonably close to a person speaking, and when the room is reasonably 'dead', the waveforms reaching the listener's ears when a voiced sound is produced will typically have one major peak per period. These peaky waveforms may evoke a distinct pitch sensation. On the other hand, when the listener is some distance from the speaker, and when the room is reverberant, the phases of the components become essentially random (Plomp and Steeneken 1973) with the result that the waveforms are less peaky. In this case, the evoked pitch may be less clear. The ability of hearing-impaired listeners to extract pitch information in everyday situations may be over-estimated by studies using headphones or conducted in rooms with sound-absorbing walls.

The existence of pitch anomalies (diplacusis and exaggerated pitch-intensity effects) may affect the enjoyment of music. There have been few, if any, studies on diplacusis for complex sounds, but it is likely to occur to some extent. One person studied in our laboratory was a Professor of music who had a unilateral cochlear loss. He reported that he typically heard different pitches in his normal and impaired ear, and that musical intervals in his impaired ear sounded distorted. Other subjects have reported that some musical notes do not produce a distinct pitch, and that they get no pleasure from listening to music.

6. Sound localization and binaural hearing in normal and hearing-impaired people

There are several advantages associated with having two ears. Firstly, differences in the amplitude or time of arrival of sounds at the two ears provide cues that contribute greatly to the ability to localize sound sources. Secondly, the ability to detect signals in noise can be improved by comparison of the stimuli reaching the two ears. Thirdly, when listening to a target sound such as speech in the presence of background noise, the target-to-noise ratio may be much higher at one ear than at the other ear (for example, if the speech comes from the left and the noise from the right, the speech-to-noise ratio will be higher at the left ear than at the right). Under these circumstances, people are able to make use of the ear receiving the higher target-to-noise ratio. Finally, even when the signals reaching the two ears are identical (diotic stimuli), the ability to discriminate or identify the signals is often slightly better than when the signals are delivered to one ear only (monaural stimuli). These advantages can be reduced by cochlear damage, but this does not always happen. This chapter reviews these various aspects of binaural and spatial hearing, comparing results for normally hearing and hearing-impaired people.

The localization of sinusoids

Cues for localization

Consider a sinusoidal sound source located to one side of the head. The sound reaching the farther ear is delayed in time and is less intense relative to that reaching the nearer ear. There are thus two possible cues as to the location of the sound source. However, these cues are not equally effective at all frequencies. Low-frequency sounds have a wavelength which is long compared with the size of the head, and thus the sound diffracts very well around the head. The result is that little or no 'shadow' is cast by the head. On the other hand, at high frequencies, where the wavelength is short compared with the dimensions of the head, little diffraction occurs. A 'shadow', almost like that produced by a beam of light, occurs. Interaural differences in intensity are negligible at low frequencies, but may be 20 dB or more at high frequencies. This is illustrated in Figure 6.1, adapted from Feddersen *et al.* (1957).

Interaural differences in time range from 0 (for a sound straight ahead) to about 690 μs for a sound at 90° azimuth (directly opposite one ear). This is illustrated in

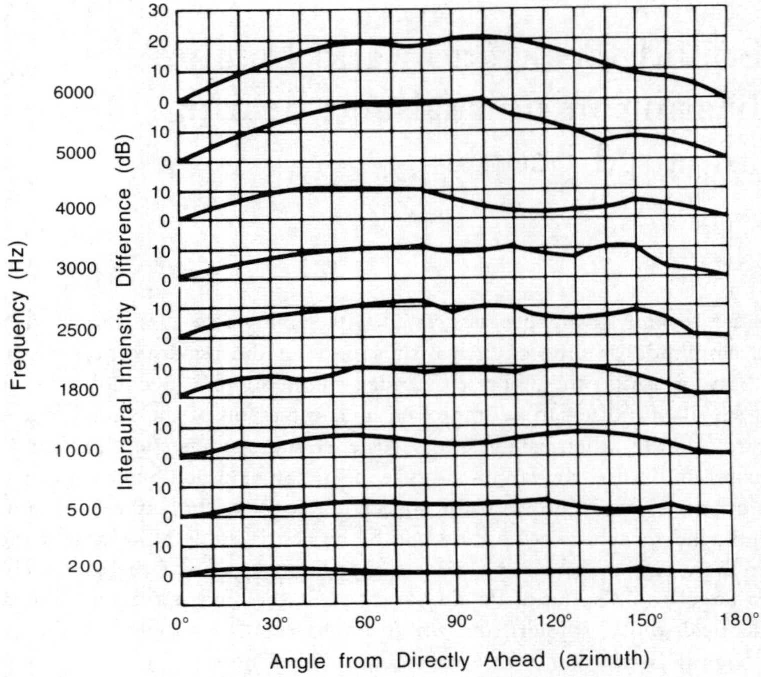

Fig. 6.1. Interaural intensity differences (IIDs) for sinusoidal stimuli plotted as a function of azimuth; each curve is for a different frequency. Adapted from Feddersen *et al.* (1957).

Figure 6.2, adapted from Feddersen *et al.* (1957). For a sinusoidal tone, a time difference is equivalent to a phase difference between the two ears. For low-frequency tones, this cue provides effective information about the location of the sound. However, for higher-frequency sounds, whose wavelength is comparable with or less than the path distance between the two ears (about 23 cm), the phase difference provides an ambiguous cue. For example, for a high-frequency sinusoid, say around 10 kHz, there may be many cycles of phase difference between the two ears. The auditory system has no way of determining which cycle in the left ear corresponds to a given cycle in the right ear. Ambiguities start to occur when the half-wavelength of the sound is about 23 cm, i.e. when the frequency of the sound is about 750 Hz. A sinusoid of this frequency lying to one side of the head (90° azimuth) produces waveforms at the two ears which are in opposite phase (phase difference between the two ears of 180°). The location of the sound source is now ambiguous, since the waveform at the right ear might be either a half-cycle behind that at the left ear or a half-cycle ahead. Head movements, or movements of the sound source, may resolve this ambiguity, so that there is no abrupt upper limit in the ability to use phase differences between the two ears. However, phase differences become highly ambiguous for frequencies above about 1500 Hz.

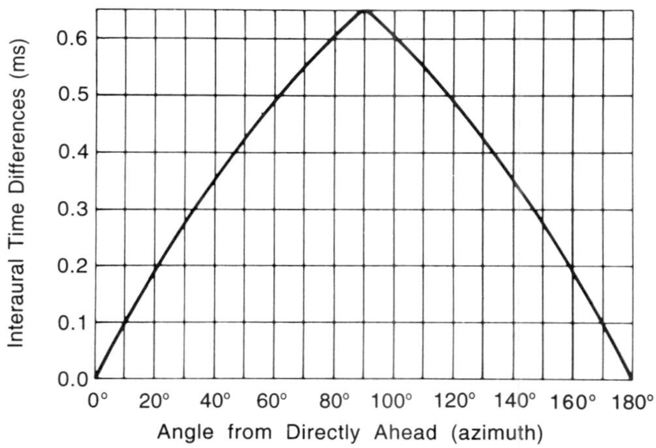

Fig. 6.2. Interaural time differences (IIDs) plotted as a function of azimuth. Adapted from Feddersen *et al.* (1957).

The idea that sound localization is based on interaural time differences at low frequencies and interaural intensity differences at high frequencies has been called the 'duplex theory' and it dates back to Lord Rayleigh (1907). While it appears to hold for pure tones, it is not strictly accurate for complex sounds.

Performance of normally hearing people in localization and lateralization

The term 'localization' refers to judgements of the direction and distance of a sound source. Sometimes, when headphones are worn, the sound image is located inside the head. The term 'lateralization' is used to describe the apparent location of a sound source within the head. Headphones allow precise control of interaural differences and eliminate effects related to room echoes. Thus lateralization may be regarded as a laboratory version of localization which provides an efficient means of studying direction perception.

There are two aspects to performance in localization of sounds. The first aspect is concerned with how well the perceived direction of a sound source corresponds to its actual direction. For normally hearing people, the perceived direction generally corresponds reasonably well with the actual direction, although for sinusoidal stimuli errors sometimes occur in judging whether a sound is coming from in front or behind, or from above or below the horizontal (Stevens and Newman 1936); this point is discussed in more detail later on. The second aspect of localization is concerned with how well subjects can detect a small shift in position of a sound source. This aspect measures the resolution of the auditory system. When resolution is studied using stimuli presented via loudspeakers, the smallest detectable change in angular position, relative to the subject, is referred to as the minimum audible angle (MAA). Studies of localization using sinusoids have usually used tone bursts with gradual onsets and offsets, to minimize cues related to the interaural timing of the envelope; envelope cues are discussed in more detail later in this chapter.

Figure 6.3 shows the MAA for sinusoidal signals, plotted as a function of frequency (Mills 1958, 1972). Each curve shows results for a different reference direction; the task was to detect a shift in position around that direction. The MAA is smallest for a reference direction of 0, i.e. for sounds coming from directly in front of the subject. A shift of only about 1° can be detected for frequencies below 1000 Hz. Performance worsens around 1500 Hz. This is consistent with the duplex theory; at 1500 Hz phase differences between the two ears are ambiguous cues for localization, and interaural intensity differences are small. Performance worsens markedly when the reference direction is moved away from 0 azimuth. Indeed, for reference directions of 60° and 75°, the MAA was so large that it could not be determined when the frequency was around 1500 Hz.

When resolution is studied using earphones, it is possible to study the effectiveness of interaural intensity differences (IIDs) alone or interaural time differences (ITDs) alone. The discriminability of interaural differences is usually measured in a two-alternative forced-choice task. The stimuli delivered in the two observation intervals differ in interaural amplitude or time. For example, one stimulus might be identical at the two ears, while the other stimulus might have an ITD ΔT. The task of the subject is to say whether the first stimulus was to the left or the right of the second stimulus. In other words, the task is to identify a shift in location associated with a change in interaural amplitude or timing.

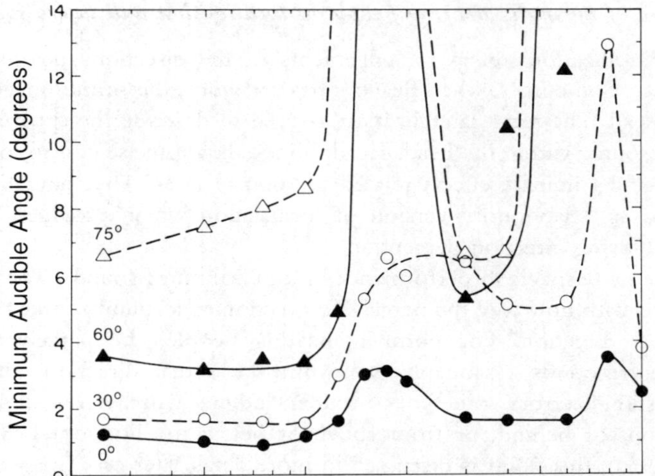

Fig. 6.3. The minimum audible angle (MAA) for sinusoidal signals, plotted as a function of frequency; each curve shows results for a different reference direction. Data from Mills (1958, 1972).

Thresholds for detecting changes in ITD are smallest when the reference ITD is zero, corresponding to a sound heard in the centre of the head (Yost 1974). In this case, a change in ITD of about 10μs can be detected for a frequency of 900 Hz. Such a change would be produced by moving a sound source through an angle of about 1° relative to the subject; this corresponds well with the MAA value described above. The smallest detectable ITD increases somewhat at lower frequencies, although the threshold is roughly constant at about 3° when it is expressed as the smallest detectable change in relative phase at the two ears. Above 900 Hz, the threshold ITD increases markedly, and above 1500 Hz changes in ITD are essentially undetectable. The threshold ITD increases for all frequencies when the reference ITD is greater than zero.

Thresholds for detecting changes in IID are also smallest when the reference IID is zero. In this case, changes in IID of about 1 dB can be detected across a wide range of frequencies, although performance worsens slightly for frequencies around 1000 Hz (Mills 1960; Yost and Dye 1988). When the reference IID is 15 dB, as would occur for a sound well to one side of the head, the threshold change in IID varies between 1.3 dB (at low and high frequencies) and 2.5 dB (around 1000 Hz).

In summary, the resolution of the binaural system, which determines the ability to detect changes in the position of a sound source, is best for sounds that come from directly ahead (0 azimuth). Resolution at low frequencies is based on the use of ITDs. Changes in ITD cannot be detected for frequencies above 1500 Hz. Changes in IID can be detected over the whole audible frequency range, but, in practice, IIDs sufficiently large to provide useful cues to sound location occur only at high frequencies.

Performance of hearing-impaired people in localization and lateralization

There have been few studies of localization and lateralization of sinusoids by hearing-impaired subjects; most studies have used complex stimuli (see below). Nordlund (1964) measured free-field localization of sinusoids with frequencies 500, 2000 and 4000 Hz. He reported both the mean error (a measure of systematic errors or biases), and the standard deviation (a measure of resolution). For subjects with cochlear losses in both ears, only one out of thirteen showed any abnormal results (based on a 99.9% confidence interval). For subjects with unilateral or highly asymmetric cochlear losses, seven out of nine showed at least one abnormal result. However, even for these subjects, the majority of results were within the normal range.

Häusler *et al.* (1983) reported limited measurements on subjects with unilateral cochlear losses (mainly Ménière's syndrome). Stimuli were presented via earphones. Thresholds for detecting changes in ITD were sometimes very large, but few specific details were given.

Hall *et al.* (1984b) measured ITD thresholds for a 500-Hz sinusoid at a level of 70 dB SPL. They tested six normally hearing subjects and ten subjects with mild-to-moderate symmetrical cochlear hearing losses. The ITD thresholds were markedly larger for the impaired subjects (mean 176 μs) than for the normally hearing subjects (mean 65 μs). The ITD thresholds tended to increase with increasing absolute threshold at 500 Hz, and three subjects with absolute thresholds less than 40 dB SPL had near-normal ITD thresholds. The poor performance of the subjects with higher absolute thresholds could have been partly due to the low sensation level (SL) of the stimuli.

Smoski and Trahiotis (1986) measured thresholds for detecting changes in ITD using 500-Hz sinusoids delivered by earphones. They used four subjects with mainly high-frequency cochlear losses caused by noise exposure or viral infections. At equal sound pressure level (80 dB SPL), the hearing-impaired subjects had higher ITD thresholds than the two normally hearing subjects tested. However, at an equal SL of 25 dB, ITD thresholds did not differ greatly for the normal and hearing-impaired subjects.

In summary, the limited data available on the localization and lateralization of sinusoids suggest that bilateral symmetric cochlear damage does not lead to marked abnormalities, except when the stimuli are at low SLs. Asymmetrical or unilateral damage more often leads to abnormalities. In most studies, abnormalities in localization were not closely related to audiometric thresholds, although sometimes absolute thresholds and ITD thresholds have been found to be correlated. Sometimes abnormal localization is found in frequency regions where absolute thresholds are normal.

The localization of complex sounds

The role of transients and across-frequency comparisons

All sounds which occur in nature have onsets and offsets, and many also change their intensity or their spectral structure as a function of time. Interaural differences in the time of arrival of these transients provide cues for localization which are not subject to the phase ambiguities which occur for steady sinusoidal tones. Also, for sounds that cover a reasonable frequency range, phase ambiguities can be resolved by comparisons across frequency; the ITD that is common across all frequency channels must be the 'true' ITD (Grantham 1995; Stern and Trahiotis 1995).

Performance of normally hearing subjects

Klump and Eady (1956) measured thresholds for discriminating ITDs using stimuli delivered via headphones. They compared three types of stimuli: band-limited noise (containing frequencies in the range 150–1700 Hz); 1000-Hz pure tones with gradual rise and fall times; and clicks of duration 1 ms. For a reference ITD of 0, the threshold ITDs were 9 μs, 11 μs and 28 μs, respectively. Thus the greatest acuity occurred for the noise stimulus. The single click gave rise to the poorest performance. However, threshold ITDs for click trains can be as small as 10 μs (Dye and Hafter 1984) when the click rate is reasonably low (200 clicks per second or less). For bursts of noise (lowpass filtered at 5000 Hz), the ability to detect changes in ITD improves with duration of the bursts for durations up to about 700 ms, when the threshold change in ITD reaches an asymptotic value of about 6 μs (Tobias and Zerlin 1959).

Yost *et al.* (1971) investigated what frequencies were most important for the discrimination of ITDs in click trains. They did this by filtering the click trains, and by adding filtered noise to mask the energy in certain frequency regions. They found that discrimination deteriorated for clicks which were highpass filtered, so that only energy above 1500 Hz was present, but was largely unaffected by lowpass filtering. Masking with a lowpass noise produced a marked disruption, while a highpass noise had little effect. Thus discrimination of lateral position on the basis of time delays between the two ears depends largely on the low-frequency content of the clicks, although somewhat poorer discrimination is possible with only high-frequency components.

Henning (1974) investigated the lateralization of high-frequency sinusoids which were amplitude modulated. He found that the detectability of changes in ITD in the envelope of a 3900-Hz carrier modulated at a frequency of 300 Hz was about as good as the detectability of changes in ITD of a 300-Hz sinusoid. However, there were considerable differences among subjects; the threshold ITDs had values of 20, 50 and 65 μs for three different subjects (all stimuli had 250-ms durations and 50-ms rise-fall times). Henning found that time delay of the envelope rather than time delay of the 'fine structure' within the envelope determines the lateralization. The signals could be lateralized on the basis of time delays in the envelope even when the carrier frequencies were different in the two ears. Thus it seems that for complex signals containing only high-frequency components, listeners extract the envelopes of the signals and compare the relative timing of the envelopes at the two ears. However, lateralization performance is best when the carrier frequencies are identical, and poor lateralization results when the complex waveforms at each ear have no frequency component in common.

Performance of people with cochlear damage

A survey of studies of localization and lateralization in hearing-impaired people, for studies up to 1981, has been given by Durlach *et al.* (1981). A wide variety of stimuli were used in the studies, but the majority used either wideband noise or filtered noise. Durlach *et al.* concluded that many of the studies were hard to interpret because they did not distinguish between systematic errors in localization and poor resolution. Nevertheless, there was a clear trend for poor localization and lateralization to occur in people with unilateral or asymmetrical cochlear damage. Subjects with symmetrical cochlear losses often showed near-normal performance, especially when tested at reasonably high sound levels.

Häusler *et al.* (1983) studied sound localization and lateralization in hearing-impaired subjects using broadband noise as a stimulus. They measured MAAs for stimuli presented in free-field at various azimuths, and ITDs and IIDs for stimuli presented via earphones. Stimuli were presented at levels ranging from 85 to 100 dB SPL. Some subjects with bilateral sensorineural losses (presumably cochlear in origin) showed MAAs within the normal range, both for stimuli at 0 azimuth, and for stimuli to one side. These subjects nearly always had good speech discrimination scores. Other subjects with bilateral losses showed somewhat larger MAAs than normal, especially for stimuli located to the side. These subjects usually had poor speech discrimination scores. Subjects with unilateral or asymmetric losses (mainly Ménière's syndrome) tended to have larger MAAs than normal, especially for sounds towards the side of the impaired ear, but a few subjects showed performance within the normal range.

Subjects with bilateral sensorineural losses usually showed thresholds for the detection of changes in ITD and IID that were within the normal range, although a few showed larger ITDs than normal. Subjects with unilateral or asymmetric sensorineural losses (Ménière's) showed threshold ITDs that were normal or slightly larger than normal. However, threshold IIDs were mostly larger than normal.

Hawkins and Wightman (1980) measured thresholds for detecting changes in ITD and IID for narrow bands of noise centred at 500 and 4000 Hz, using eight subjects with moderate cochlear losses, six of whom had symmetrical losses. The remaining two had unilateral losses caused by Ménière's syndrome. The stimuli were presented at 85 dB SPL. For most subjects, ITD thresholds were much higher than normal at 4000 Hz (greater than 250 μs as compared to 40–80 μs for normally hearing subjects). At 500 Hz, ITD thresholds were more variable, with two subjects showing performance within the normal range (12–29 μs) and the remainder showing thresholds in the range 33 μs to unmeasurable. The IID thresholds were often close to normal, except for the subjects with unilateral losses. Abnormally large ITDs were sometimes found when both IIDs and absolute thresholds were normal.

Smoski and Trahiotis (1986) measured thresholds for detecting a change in ITD using narrowband noises centred at 500 and 4000 Hz and an amplitude modulated (AM) 4000-Hz sinusoidal carrier. Stimuli were delivered by earphones. They used four subjects with mainly high-frequency cochlear losses caused by noise exposure or viral infections. At equal sound pressure level (80 dB SPL), the hearing-impaired subjects had higher ITD thresholds than the two normally hearing subjects tested. The difference was small for the 500-Hz stimulus, but was large for the 4000-Hz stimuli. For example, for the 4000-Hz AM stimulus, the threshold ITD averaged 25 μs for the normally hearing subjects, and about 250 μs for the hearing-impaired subjects. However, at an equal SL of 25 dB, ITD thresholds were much larger (200–600 μs), but did not differ greatly for the normal and hearing-impaired subjects.

Kinkel *et al.* (1991) measured thresholds for detecting changes in ITD and IID of narrow bands of noise presented via earphones at centre frequencies of 500 Hz and 4000 Hz. They used 15 normally hearing subjects and 49 subjects with hearing loss, presumed to be mainly of cochlear origin. Stimuli were presented at 75 dB SPL or at the 'most comfortable level', whichever was the higher. The ITD thresholds were, on average, much larger for the hearing-impaired than for the normally hearing subjects, both at 500 Hz (210 μs versus 38 μs) and at 4000 Hz (530 μs versus 81 μs), although some hearing-impaired subjects had ITDs within the normal range. The average IID thresholds were also larger for the hearing-impaired than for the normally hearing subjects, both at 500 Hz (4.7 dB versus 2.6 dB) and at 4000 Hz (5.1 dB versus 2.2 dB). However, many hearing-impaired subjects had IID thresholds within the normal range.

Gabriel *et al.* (1992) measured thresholds for detecting changes in ITD and IID for narrowbands of noise presented via earphones at about 30 dB SL. The centre frequency of the noise was varied from 250 to 4000 Hz in one-octave steps. They used three subjects with symmetrical cochlear losses. Both ITDs and IIDs were generally larger than normal, although results varied markedly across subjects. One subject with a flat loss showed essentially no sensitivity to changes in ITD, except at 500 Hz, where the threshold was 100 μs. That subject also had unusually large IID thresholds (3–8 dB as compared to about 1 dB for normally hearing subjects). Even for two subjects with similar audiograms and similar causes of hearing loss (noise induced), performance differed markedly both in the values of the thresholds and in their pattern across frequency.

It is clear from these studies that binaural performance can vary markedly across subjects. Subjects with unilateral or asymmetric losses tend to show larger than normal thresholds for detecting changes in ITD and IID. Subjects with symmetrical losses sometimes show normal or near-normal performance for broadband noise stimuli. However, they often show impaired performance for narrowband stimuli. It is possible, as pointed out by Colburn and Trahiotis (1992), that good performance for a restricted frequency range may be enough to ensure good performance for broadband stimuli.

Reasons for large ITD and IID thresholds in people with cochlear damage

The poor discrimination of ITDs, when it occurs, may be the result of several factors. Firstly, it may be partly related to the relatively low SL of the stimuli; ITD discrimination in normally hearing subjects worsens markedly below about 20 dB SL (Häusler *et al.* 1983). Secondly, it may result from abnormalities in the travel time of the travelling wave along the BM or in the phase of spike initiation, and from differences in travel time or phase of spike initiation between the two ears (Ruggero and Rich 1987; Ruggero *et al.* 1993). Thirdly, it may be the result of abnormalities in phase locking (see chapter 1).

Abnormalities in IID discrimination may also have multiple causes. As for ITD discrimination, they may result from the relatively low SL of the stimuli. Secondly, they may result from abnormal intensity coding, and from differences in intensity coding in the two ears; see chapter 3. In this context it is noteworthy that IID discrimination in normally hearing subjects can be markedly impaired by putting an earplug in one ear (Häusler *et al.* 1983).

The cone of confusion, head movements, and pinna cues

If the influence of the pinnae is ignored, then the head may be regarded as a pair of holes separated by a spherical obstacle. If the head is kept stationary, then a given ITD will not be sufficient to define uniquely the position of the sound source in space; there is a cone of confusion such that any sound source on the surface

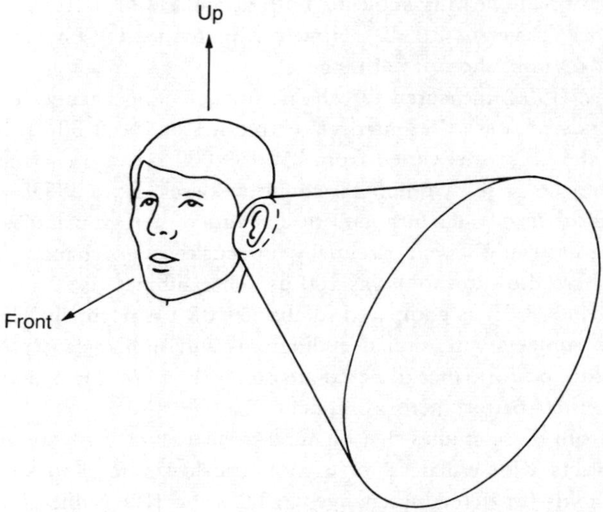

Fig. 6.4. Illustration of the cone of confusion for a specific ITD. All points on the surface of the cone give rise to that same ITD.

of this cone would give rise to the same interaural time difference (see Mills, 1972, and Figure 6.4). A similar ambiguity arises for IIDs.

Ambiguities related to the cone of confusion, or to the location of a sound source in the vertical direction, may be resolved by head movements. If the head is rotated about a vertical axis by, say, 20°, and this results in a 20° shift in the apparent lateral position of the auditory image in relation to the head, then the sound source is located in the horizontal plane. If the rotation of the head is accompanied by no change in the auditory image, then the sound is located either directly above or directly below the head. Intermediate shifts in the location of the auditory image lead to intermediate vertical height judgements (Wallach 1940).

Even when the head is fixed, or when the duration of a sound is too short to allow useful information to be gained from head movements, ambiguities associated with the cone of confusion do not seem to pose a problem in everyday situations. The ambiguities are resolved by information provided by the pinnae. The pinnae affect the spectra of sounds reaching the eardrum, introducing a complex pattern of peaks and dips. The spectral pattern varies systematically with the direction of the sound source (Blauert 1983; Wightman and Kistler 1989). The spectral changes produced by the head and pinna can be used to judge the location of a sound source. Since it is the spectral patterning of the sound which is important, the information provided by the pinnae is most effective when the sound has spectral energy over a wide frequency range. High frequencies, above 6 kHz, are especially important, since it is only at high frequencies that the wavelength of sound is sufficiently short for it to interact strongly with the pinna.

Resolution using pinna cues by normal and hearing-impaired subjects

Häusler *et al.* (1983) measured MAAs in the vertical direction for sounds coming from straight ahead, using broadband noise as a stimulus. Stimuli were presented at levels ranging from 85 to 100 dB SPL. One ear was plugged, so presumably the only cue available was the spectral patterning provided by the pinna and head. Subjects with normal hearing had MAAs in the range 1–10°. Subjects with bilateral cochlear hearing loss fell into two groups. One group had MAAs within the normal range and also had good speech discrimination. The other group had MAAs that were so large that they could not be measured, and had poor speech discrimination. It is not clear whether this poor performance was due to low audibility of the high frequencies that carry pinna cues, or poor resolution of the spectral features introduced by the pinnae. For subjects with unilateral losses due to Ménière's syndrome, MAAs were within the normal range for the normally hearing ear. Some of the impaired ears also showed MAAs within the normal range, while others showed slightly larger than normal MAAs.

In summary, hearing-impaired subjects can differ markedly in their ability to make use of the high-frequency spectral cues provided by the pinna. Some subjects appear to be completely unable to use these cues, while others use them almost normally.

General conclusions on sound localization

The auditory system is capable of using a great variety of physical cues to determine the location of a sound source. Time and intensity differences at the two ears, changes in the spectral composition of sounds due to head shadow and pinna effects, and changes in all of these cues produced by head or sound source movements, can all influence the perceived direction of a sound source. In laboratory studies usually just one or two of these cues are isolated. In this way it has been shown that sometimes a single cue may be sufficient for accurate localization of a sound source. For real sound sources, such as speech or music, all of the cues described above may be available simultaneously. In this situation, the multiplicity of cues makes the location of the sound sources more definite and more accurate.

Hearing-impaired people show considerable individual differences in their ability to localize sounds. Often, in studies measuring the horizontal MAA for broadband sounds at high levels, performance is nearly normal, especially in cases of symmetrical losses. In this situation several cues are available—ITDs, IIDs and pinna cues—and an ability to use any one of these, or any combination, is sufficient to give good performance. In studies using earphones, where usually only one cue is present at a time, the performance of hearing-impaired subjects is often poorer than normal, especially when narrowband stimuli are used.

Binaural masking level differences (MLDs)

MLDs for normally hearing subjects

The masked threshold of a signal can sometimes be markedly lower when listening with two ears than when listening with one (Hirsh 1948). Consider the situation

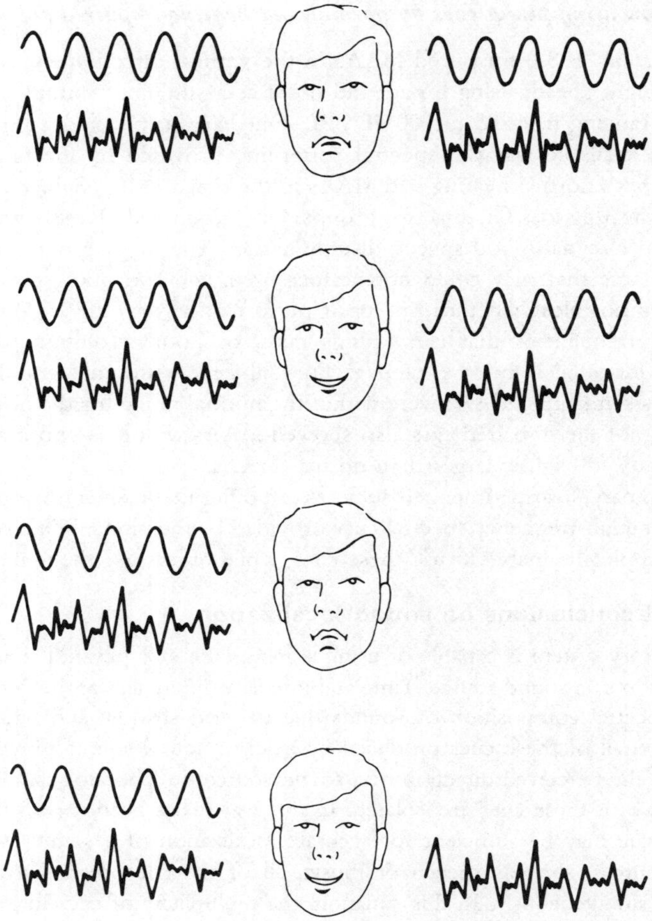

Fig. 6.5. Illustration of two situations in which binaural masking level differences (MLDs) occur. In conditions (a) and (c) detectability is poor, while in conditions (b) and (d), where the interaural relations of the signal and masker are different, detectability is good (hence the smiling faces).

shown in Figure 6.5a. White noise from the same noise generator is fed to both ears via stereo headphones. Pure tones signals, also from the same signal generator, are fed separately to each ear and mixed with the noise. Thus the stimuli at the two ears are identical. Assume that the level of the tone is adjusted until it is just masked by the noise, i.e. it is at its masked threshold, and let its level at this point be L_0 dB. Assume now that the signal is inverted in phase (equivalent to a phase shift of 180° or π radians) in one ear only (see Figure 6.5b). The result is that the tone becomes audible again. The tone can be adjusted to a new level, L_π, so that it is once again at its masked threshold. The difference between the two levels, $L_0 - L_\pi$ (dB) is known as a masking level difference (MLD), and its value may be as large as 15 dB at low frequencies (around 500 Hz), decreasing to 2–3 dB for frequencies above 1500 Hz. Thus, simply by inverting the signal waveform at one ear the signal becomes considerably more detectable.

An example which is perhaps even more startling is given in Figure 6.5c. The noise and signal are fed to one ear only, and the signal is adjusted to be at its masked threshold. Now the noise alone is added at the other ear; the tone becomes audible once again (Figure 6.5d). Further, the tone disappears when it, too, is added to the second ear, making the sounds at the two ears the same. Notice that it is important that the same noise is added to the non-signal ear; the noises at the two ears must be correlated or derived from the same noise generator. Release from masking is not obtained when an independent noise (derived from a second noise generator) is added to the non-signal ear.

The phenomenon of the MLD is not limited to pure tones. Similar effects have been observed for complex tones, clicks and speech sounds. Whenever the phase or level differences of the signal at the two ears are not the same of those of the masker, the ability to detect and identify the signal is improved relative to the case where the signal and masker have the same phase and level relationships at the two ears. Such differences only occur in real situations when the signal and masker are located in different positions in space. Thus, the detection and discrimination of signals, including speech, is better when the signal and masker are not coincident in space than when they are coincident (for example when they come from the same loudspeaker).

To describe the conditions in experiments measuring MLDs, it is customary to use the symbols N (for noise) and S (for signal), each being followed by a suffix denoting relative phase at the two ears. A phase inversion is equivalent to a phase shift of 180° or π radians. Thus N_0S_π refers to the condition where the noise is in phase at the two ears and the signal is inverted in phase. N_u means that the noise is uncorrelated at the two ears. The suffix m indicates monaural presentation, i.e. presentation to one ear only. Table 6.1 gives the magnitude of the MLD for a variety of combinations of signal and noise. Four conditions for which there is no binaural advantage, N_0S_0, N_mS_m, N_uS_m and $N_\pi S_\pi$, all give about the same 'reference' threshold. The MLDs for the conditions shown in the table are obtained by expressing thresholds relative to this reference threshold.

In addition to improving the detectability of tones, conditions which produce MLDs also favour other aspects of the ability to discriminate signals. For example, when speech signals are presented against noisy backgrounds, speech intelligibility is better under conditions when the speech and noise do not have the same interaural phase (Licklider 1948). However, the advantage for intelligibility is not as large as the advantage for detection. For single words in broadband white noise, the speech-to-noise ratio required for 50% intelligibility is typically about 6 dB lower for N_0S_π than for N_0S_0, whereas the threshold for detecting the words is about 13 dB lower (Levitt and Rabiner 1967).

MLDs for people with cochlear damage

A survey of studies of the MLD using hearing-impaired subjects was presented by Durlach *et al.* (1981). While there was considerable variability in the results across

Table 6.1 Values of the MLD for various interaural phase relationships of the signal and masker. These results are typical for broadband maskers and low-frequency signals.

Interaural condition	MLD in dB
N_uS_π	3
N_uS_0	4
$N_\pi S_m$	6
N_0S_m	9
$N_\pi S_0$	13
N_0S_π	15

studies, generally it was found that cochlear hearing loss leads to reduced MLDs, even when the hearing loss is reasonably symmetrical. For example, Quaranta and Cervellera (1974) reported abnormally small MLDs in 86% of cases. However, the relative sizes of the MLDs in different conditions (see Table 6.1) were often similar to normal. In some cases with asymmetric hearing losses, the pattern of results can be very different from normal. For example, in the study of Schoeny and Carhart (1971), thresholds for the condition N_0S_m were lower (better) when the signal was delivered to the better-hearing ear than when it was delivered to the ear with poorer hearing, even though the N_mS_m thresholds were similar for the two ears.

Several more recent studies have confirmed that MLDs are typically smaller than normal in subjects with cochlear hearing loss (Hallet al.1984b; Jerger *et al.* 1984; Staffel *et al.* 1990; Kinkel *et al.* 1991). These studies have shown a trend for smaller MLDs in subjects with higher absolute thresholds, although the association is not generally strong, and subjects with similar absolute thresholds can have very different MLDs. MLDs also tend to be smaller the more asymmetrical is the loss (Jerger *et al.* 1984).

Possible reasons for smaller MLDs in people with cochlear damage

In normally hearing subjects, MLDs increase with increasing sound level, so the reduced MLDs in hearing-impaired subjects could be partly a consequence of the low SL of the stimuli; the loudness recruitment associated with cochlear damage prevents the use of high SLs. However, this cannot be a complete explanation, since reduced MLDs for subjects with cochlear hearing loss occur when the stimuli are at SLs where normally hearing subjects show large MLDs (Quaranta and Cervellera 1974). Also reduced MLDs occur when the relative levels of the stimuli at the two ears are adjusted so that an in-phase stimulus produces an image centred in the head (Quaranta and Cervellera 1974).

Hall *et al.* (1984b) suggested that the small MLDs found for hearing-impaired subjects might be partly a consequence of poor coding of temporal fine structure. They tested six normally hearing subjects and ten subjects with mild-to-moderate cochlear hearing losses. They found a significant correlation between the MLD at

500 Hz and ITD thresholds for 500-Hz sinusoids, supporting their suggestion. Kinkel *et al.* (1991) also found a correlation between the MDL at 500 Hz and the ITD threshold at 500 Hz, but this correlation was not statistically significant after the effects of age and absolute threshold were partialled out (Kinkel and Kollmeier 1992).

Staffel *et al.* (1990) suggested that the small MLDs found for hearing-impaired subjects might be partly a consequence of asymmetry of the auditory filters at the two ears at a given centre frequency. This asymmetry would effectively reduce the correlation of the noise at the outputs of corresponding auditory filters in the two ears; recall that MLDs do not occur when the noise is uncorrelated at the two ears. To test this hypothesis, they measured N_0S_0 and N_0S_π thresholds as a function of masker bandwidth, using a 500-Hz signal and noise centred at 500 Hz. Six normally hearing subjects and 18 subjects with cochlear hearing loss were tested; ten of the latter had distinctly asymmetric hearing losses. Staffel *et al.* reasoned that interaural asymmetry of the auditory filters would have little effect for very small masker bandwidths, but would have an increasing effect as bandwidth increased. However, the results did not support this hypothesis. The MLDs of the hearing-impaired subjects were smaller than normal both for a masker with a very small bandwidth (25 Hz) and for maskers with much wider bandwidths (400 and 800 Hz). Thus, while auditory-filter asymmetry may play a small role in reducing MLDs in hearing-impaired subjects, it does not seem to be a major factor.

In summary, the causes of the reduced MLDs found for people with cochlear damage are not fully understood. The reduced SL of the stimuli, and reduced abilities to discriminate changes in interaural time and intensity may all play a role.

Head shadow effects

Results for normally hearing subjects

Most studies of the MLD have used conditions where performance cannot be improved simply by attending to one ear only. Hence, these studies have been specifically concerned with the benefit of binaural processing, where information from the two ears is combined and compared. However, when listening for a signal in background noise in everyday listening situations, it is often the case that the signal-to-noise ratio is much better at one ear than at the other. The differences in signal-to-noise ratio occur as a result of the head-shadow effects illustrated in Figure 6.1, and as a result of filtering by the pinnae. An advantage of having two ears is that the listener can effectively 'select' the ear giving the higher signal-to-masker ratio.

Bronkhorst and Plomp (1988) studied the effects of ITDs and head shadow on the intelligibility of speech in noise, under binaural listening conditions. The sounds were recorded using a realistic model of a human head and torso (KEMAR; see Burkhard and Sachs 1975). The speech was presented from directly in front of KEMAR, while the noise was presented at seven azimuths ranging from 0 (frontal) to 180°. The noise had the same long-term average spectrum as the speech. The recorded sounds were digitally processed to derive two signals, one containing only ITDs (identical intensity at the two ears at all frequencies) and the other containing only IIDs due to head shadow and these stimuli were presented via earphones. The speech-to-noise ratio required for 50% of sentences to be understood (the speech reception threshold, SRT) was determined for each noise azimuth. The decrease in SRT, relative to the case where both speech and noise came from 0 azimuth, is called the Binaural Intelligibility Level Difference (BILD). The BILD due to ITDs was between 3.9 and 5.1 dB (for noise azimuths between 30 and 150°), while the BILD due to IIDs was 3.5 to 7.8 dB. When both ITDs and IIDs were present (i.e. when the unprocessed stimuli were used), the improvements were larger still, ranging from 5.8 to 10.1 dB. However, the overall effect was not as great as would be obtained if the BILDs gained from ITDs and IIDs simply added. The presence of IIDs decreased the effectiveness of the masking release due to ITDs. In additional experiments where the stimulus to one ear was turned off, they showed that the advantage gained from IIDs mainly depends on the ear receiving the highest speech-to-noise ratio. However, this advantage decreases when the noise in the other ear is fairly loud.

In summary, spatial separation of speech and background noise can lead to a BILD of up to 10 dB. Most of this effect (7–8 dB) is due to the fact that the speech-to-noise ratio is improved at one ear by head shadow effects. A small part (2–3 dB) is due to binaural processing of ITDs.

Results for hearing-impaired subjects

Bronkhorst and Plomp (1989) carried out similar experiments to those described above using seventeen subjects with symmetrical hearing loses and seventeen subjects with asymmetrical losses (differences in threshold between the two ears, averaged over 500, 1000 and 2000 Hz, ranging from 5 to 31 dB). Most subjects were diagnosed as having mild to moderate cochlear hearing losses. The noise level was adjusted for each subject so as to be as far as possible above absolute threshold without being uncomfortably loud. When the speech and noise both came from 0 azimuth, the SRTs were, on average, 2.5 dB higher than found for normally hearing subjects. The hearing-impaired subjects showed 2.6–5.1 dB less binaural gain than normal when the noise azimuth was changed to 90°. In other words, in this condition SRTs were 5.1–7.6 dB higher than normal, a considerable difference.

The BILDs due to IIDs alone ranged from 0 dB to normal values of 7 dB or more. The size of the BILD depended on the high-frequency loss in the ear receiving the higher speech-to-noise ratio; greater high-frequency losses were associated with a reduced advantage. This makes sense, since head-shadow effects are greatest at high frequencies, and if those high frequencies are inaudible, little advantage can be gained. The average BILD due to ITDs alone was nearly normal (4.2 dB as compared to 4.7 dB for normally hearing subjects) for subjects with symmetrical hearing losses. However, subjects with asymmetrical losses showed smaller BILDs, averaging 2.5 dB. When ITDs were introduced in stimuli already containing IIDs, the gain was 2–2.5 dB for both groups, comparable to what was obtained for normally hearing subjects.

In summary, subjects with cochlear hearing loss are generally less able than normal to take advantage of spatial separation of speech and interfering noise. When tested under conditions where speech and noise are spatially separated, they perform more poorly, relative to normal, than when the speech and noise come from the same position in space. The disadvantage appears to arise mainly from the inaudiblity of high frequencies in the ear at which the speech-to-noise ratio is highest.

Diotic summation

In many tasks, detection and discrimination performance is better when listening with two ears than with one, even when the same stimulus is delivered to the two ears. This is given the general name diotic summation. For example, the absolute threshold is slightly lower for diotic than for monaural stimulation (Shaw *et al.* 1947), and thresholds for the detection of changes in frequency or intensity are also lower for diotic stimulation (Jesteadt *et al.* 1977a).

Of perhaps more interest is the fact that the intelligibility of speech in noise is usually greater for diotic stimulation than for monaural stimulation. Davis *et al.* (1990) estimated that, for normally hearing subjects, the diotic advantage in intelligibility for key words in simple sentences was about 9% when the baseline performance in the monaural condition was about 70%, although an earlier study had suggested that the advantage was larger at around 20% when monaural performance was around 50% (Davis and Haggard 1982). Plomp and Mimpen (1979) reported that the SRT for sentences presented in noise with the same long-term average spectrum as the speech was 1.4 dB lower for diotic presentation than for monaural presentation. This corresponds to an improvement in intelligibility in difficult listening situations of about 20%.

People with cochlear hearing impairment also show better speech intelligibility for diotic stimulation than for monaural stimulation. Laurence *et al.* (1983) measured SRTs in noise of eight subjects with moderate to severe cochlear losses under three conditions: unaided, with linear hearing aids, and with two-channel compression hearing aids (see chapter 8 for more details). For each condition they compared three cases: listening with both ears (either unaided or binaurally aided), listening with the left ear only, and listening with the right ear only. In the latter two cases, the unused ear was either plugged and muffed or fitted with a hearing aid that was turned off. For all three conditions, there was a significant advantage of binaural versus monaural listening, even when the speech and noise came from the same loudspeaker directly in front of the subject (this gives essentially diotic stimulation, at least for unaided listening). There was no significant interaction between condition (unaided versus linear aiding versus compression aiding) and case (monaural versus binaural listening). Thus the advantage of using two ears was similar for unaided and aided conditions. On average, for the case where the speech and noise came from directly in front, the SRT was about 2 dB lower when listening binaurally than when listening with the better ear. For the speech material they used, this is equivalent to an improvement in intelligibility of about 22%. A similar average diotic advantage for subjects with cochlear damage was reported by Moore *et al.* (1992b).

In summary, performance on many tasks, including the understanding of speech in noise, is better using two ears than using one, even when the stimuli at the two ears are essentially the same. This diotic advantage occurs for both normally hearing people and people with cochlear damage. If anything, it may be larger for hearing-impaired people.

Perceptual consequences of abnormal binaural and spatial hearing in people with cochlear damage

The most obvious consequence of abnormal binaural and spatial hearing is difficulty in localizing sound sources. Some people with cochlear damage have essentially no ability to use spectral cues provided by pinna transformations. This may happen either because the cues are inaudible, or because the patterns of spectral peaks and dips cannot be resolved. When pinna cues are lacking, this creates difficulty in deciding whether a sound comes from in front or behind, and from above or below. It should be noted that pinna cues are drastically altered or removed altogether by hearing aids; hearing aids alter the spectral patterns at the eardrum and usually do not amplify sounds in the frequency range above 6 kHz where pinna cues are most effective. Hence, hearing aid users are likely to suffer from difficulty in resolving the cone of confusion.

Some people with cochlear damage have higher than normal thresholds for detecting changes in ITD and IID. This applies especially to people with asymmetrical losses, and to sounds with narrow bandwidths. This means that the precision with which the azimuth of a sound source can be located is reduced, making it more difficult to orient to a sound and to decide what physical object gave rise to that sound.

Many studies comparing the intelligibility of speech in noise for normally hearing and hearing-impaired subjects have used speech and noise coming from the same loudspeaker. Such studies underestimate the difficulty experienced by hearing-impaired people in everyday life, as they fail to take into account the reduced ability of people with cochlear damage to take advantage of spatial separation of a desired sound and one or more interfering sounds. This reduced ability shows up both in studies of the MLD using earphones and in studies using stimuli presented in a free field. The disadvantage in free field depends partly on reduced binaural processing abilities, and partly on reduced audibility of high-frequency sounds at the ear receiving the higher signal-to-background ratio. For normally hearing subjects, spatial separation of speech and background noise can reduce the SRT by up to 10 dB. For people with moderate cochlear damage the advantage is 3–5 dB less. This is equivalent to a substantial loss in intelligibility.

7. Speech perception by people with cochlear damage

Introduction

One of the commonest complaints of people with cochlear hearing loss is difficulty with speech communication. The extent and nature of the difficulty depends partly on the severity of the hearing loss. People with mild or moderate losses can usually understand speech reasonably well when they are in a quiet room with only one person talking. However, they have difficulty when more than one person is talking at once, or when background noise or reverberation are present. People with severe or profound losses usually have difficulty even when listening to a single talker in a quiet room, and they generally have severe problems when background noise is present. Hence their ability to understand speech relies heavily on lip reading and on the use of context.

There has been considerable controversy in the literature about the reasons for these difficulties in understanding speech. Some researchers have suggested that the difficulties arise primarily from reduced audibility; absolute thresholds are higher than normal, so the amount by which speech is above threshold, and the proportion of the speech spectrum which is above threshold, are both less than for normal listeners (Humes *et al.* 1987; Zurek and Delhorne 1987; Lee and Humes 1993). Other researchers (Plomp 1978; Dreschler and Plomp 1980, 1985; Glasberg and Moore 1989) have argued that the difficulty in understanding speech arises at least partly from deficits in the ability to discriminate sounds which are well above the absolute threshold. Many of these deficits have been reviewed in earlier chapters. The evidence reviewed below indicates that, for mild losses, audibility is the single most important factor. However, for severe to profound losses, poor discrimination of suprathreshold (audible) stimuli is also of major importance.

The magnitude of the noise problem

Plomp (1994) reviewed several studies which measured the Speech Reception Threshold (SRT) for sentences presented in a continuous background noise. The SRT was defined as the speech-to-noise ratio in dB required for 50% of sentences to be identified completely correctly. The noise had the same long-term average spectrum as the speech; such noise is referred to as speech-shaped noise. For high noise levels, people with cochlear damage had higher SRTs than normally hearing people. The increase in SRT varied from about 2.5 dB for people with mild hearing losses caused by noise exposure or associated with aging, to about 7 dB for people with moderate to severe losses caused by Ménière's syndome or by unknown pathologies. At first sight, these numbers do not appear very large. However, for these speech materials, each 1-dB change in speech-to-noise ratio corresponds to a 14–19% change in intelligibility around the 50% point. Thus, even an elevation in SRT of 2.5 dB is sufficient to create a substantial loss of intelligibility in difficult listening situations.

The elevation in SRT can be much greater when a fluctuating background noise or a single competing talker is used instead of a steady noise. Normally hearing subjects are able to take advantage of temporal and spectral 'dips' in the interfering sound to achieve a much lower SRT than when steady background noise is used (Duquesnoy 1983; Festen and Plomp 1990; Hygge *et al.* 1992; Baer and Moore 1994; Moore *et al.* 1995). For normally hearing people, the SRT when the background is a single talker is 7 to 18 dB lower than when the background is speech-shaped noise. People with cochlear damage appear to be less able than normally hearing people to take advantage of the temporal and spectral dips. For the hearing impaired, SRTs are not greatly different for a steady noise background and a single talker background (Duquesnoy 1983; Festen and Plomp 1990; Hygge *et al.* 1992). Hence, when the background is a single talker, the SRT is 12 dB or more higher for people with cochlear damage than for normally hearing people. This represents a very large deficit.

Finally, as described in chapter 6, people with cochlear damage are less able than normally hearing people to take advantage of spatial separation of the target speech and the interfering sound(s). This can lead to a further elevation in SRT, relative to that found for normally hearing subjects, of about 7 dB.

In summary, in some listening situations common in everyday life, such as trying to listen to one person when another person is talking, people with cochlear damage may require speech-to-background ratios 16 dB or more higher than normal (Duquesnoy 1983). This represents a very substantial problem. However, the majority of laboratory experiments show a less severe problem, as they have used a background sound consisting of steady speech-shaped noise coming from the same direction as the target speech.

The role of audibility

The Articulation Index

There is no doubt that audibility is crucial for speech intelligibility; if part of the speech spectrum is below the absolute threshold or is masked by background sound, then information is lost, and intelligibility will suffer to some extent. The Articulation Index (AI) provides a way of quantifying the role of audibility (French and Steinberg 1947; Fletcher 1952; Kryter, 1962; Pavlovic 1984). The AI is based on the assumption that speech intelligibility is uniquely related to a quantity that, for a normally hearing person, can be calculated from the long-term average spectra of the speech and background sound reaching the ear of the listener. The AI is defined by the equation:

$$AI = P\int_0^{\infty} I(f)W(f)df, \qquad \text{Eq. 7.1}$$

where I(f) is a function, called the 'importance function', which characterises the relative importance of different frequencies to speech intelligibility, W(f) is a weighting function (with a value between zero and unity) which expresses the proportion of the information given by I(f) that is actually delivered under the conditions of testing, and P is a 'proficiency factor' related to the precision of the talker's enunciation and the experience of the listener with that talker. I(f) varies depending on the nature of the speech material used, for example whether it is composed of single words or sentences (Pavlovic 1987). W(f) depends on the spectra of the speech and the background, and on the spectral levels relative to the absolute threshold.

In practice, the expression in Eq. 7.1 is often approximated by dividing the frequency region from about 200 to 7000 Hz into a number of discrete bands. In the original approach of French and Steinberg (1947) 20 bands were used and their widths were adjusted so that each was of equal importance. Hence, each band had an equal weighting, W, of 0.05. However, more recent approaches have used 1/3-octave or one-octave wide bands, each of which is assigned a different weighting. For example, Kryter (1962) divided the range 180 to 5600 Hz into 15 1/3-octave wide bands. Equation 7.1 then becomes:

$$AI = P\sum_{i=1}^{15} I_i W_i \qquad \text{Eq. 7.2}$$

It is usually assumed that the speech in each band covers a 30-dB range of levels when measured using 125-ms samples. The speech peaks, specified as the level exceeded 1% of the time, have levels 12 dB above the level corresponding to the root-mean-square power of the speech. The valleys have levels 18 dB below this mean level. Basically, W_i is the proportion of the 30-dB dynamic range in the ith band that is above both the absolute threshold and the masked threshold imposed by the background sound.

To predict intelligibility, the empirical relationship between the value of the AI and intelligibility must first be determined for the specific speech material used and with a representative group of normally hearing subjects. The resulting 'intelligibility-articulation transfer function' (Fletcher 1952) then includes the effects of the proficiency factor P. Provided the subjects in a given experiment have a similar amount of training to the subjects used to determine the transfer function, the transfer function can then be used to predict intelligibility from the AI.

Several researchers have examined the question of whether the AI can be used to predict speech intelligibility for hearing-impaired listeners. Obviously, in this case, the absolute thresholds of the individual listeners must be used in calculating the weighting factors W_i. If the AI is successful in this respect, without any modification, this would imply that audibility is the main factor limiting intelligibility. While a few researchers have reported accurate predictions using the unmodified AI (Aniansson 1974; Lee and Humes 1993), most studies have shown that speech intelligibility is worse than would be predicted by the AI (Fletcher 1952; Dugal *et al.* 1978; Pavlovic 1984; Pavlovic *et al.* 1986; Smoorenburg 1992), especially for listeners with moderate or severe losses. The predictions are often quite accurate for those with mild losses.

An example of the results of this type of experiment is given in Figure 7.1; the data are from Pavlovic (1984). The speech materials were word lists presented under various conditions of filtering (broadband, lowpass and highpass) either with or without background white noise at a speech-to-noise ratio of 10 dB. Sixteen subjects with noise-induced hearing loss were used. For the eight subjects with the mildest losses (thresholds better than 50 dB HL at 4000 Hz), the mean scores across subjects for the eight different conditions, indicated by the numbers in the left panel of the figure, are close to the predictions based on the AI (solid curve). For the eight subjects with more severe losses (thresholds 55 dB HL or worse at 4000 Hz), the mean scores, shown in the right panel, fall consistently below the predicted values.

Overall, the results from studies using the AI suggest that, while audibility is of major importance, it is not the only factor involved, at least for people with moderate to severe cochlear losses. Suprathreshold discrimination abilities also need to be taken into account. Additionally, it should be noted that the AI does not give accurate predictions of speech intelligibility under conditions where the background noise is fluctuating (e.g. when there is a single background talker) or when reverberation is present.

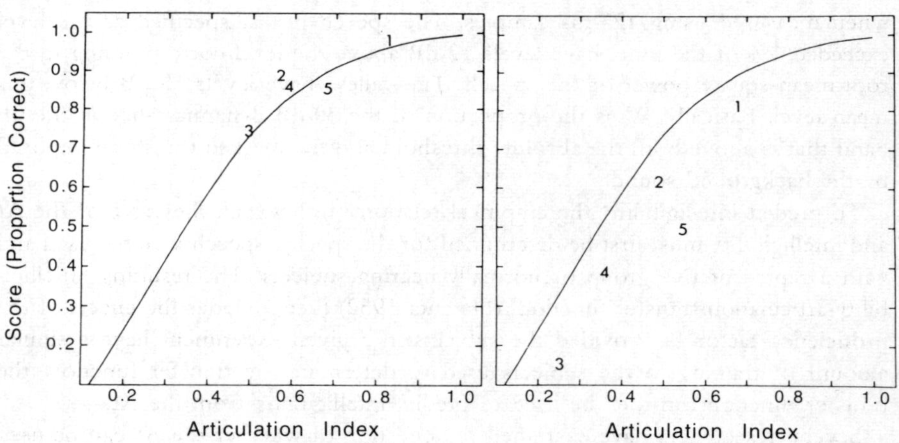

Fig. 7.1. Results of Pavlovic (1984) comparing speech recognition scores of hearing-impaired subjects with predictions based on the AI. Each number represents the mean score across subjects for a specific condition of filtering/background noise. For subjects with mild losses, the predictions are accurate (left panel); for subjects with more severe losses, the obtained scores fall below the predicted values (right panel).

The intelligibility of speech in noise at high overall levels

Another way of evaluating the importance of audibility is to measure the SRT in noise as a function of overall noise level. If the performance of hearing-impaired subjects is limited by part of the speech spectrum being below absolute threshold, then the SRT, expressed as a speech-to-noise ratio, should decrease progressively with increasing noise level; as the noise level is increased, the speech level has to be increased also, and so more and more of the speech spectrum should lie above absolute threshold. Furthermore, the SRT for hearing-impaired subjects should approach that for normally hearing subjects at sufficiently high noise levels.

One study, using 20 elderly subjects with mild hearing losses (mean threshold about 20 dB HL at medium frequencies, increasing to 40 dB HL at 4000 Hz), reported results consistent with these predictions (Lee and Humes 1993). However, the results of most other studies have not shown the predicted pattern: the SRT for hearing-impaired subjects remains approximately constant for noise levels above a certain value, and the SRT at high noise levels remains greater for hearing-impaired than for normally hearing subjects (Plomp 1978, 1986; Smoorenburg 1992).

Overall, these results lead to the same conclusions as those derived from studies using the AI. For subjects with moderate to severe losses, factors other than audibility contribute to the limited ability of hearing-impaired subjects to understand speech in noise.

Comparison of detection and recognition for speech in noise

Turner *et al.* (1992) measured psychometric functions (percent correct as a function of signal level) for the detection and recognition of stop consonants presented in white noise. They used two normally hearing subjects and three subjects with 'flat' moderate cochlear loss. They found that *detection* of the consonants occurred at the same speech-to-noise ratio for the normal and hearing-impaired subjects. However, for a given level of recognition, the hearing-impaired subjects required higher speech-to-noise ratios. They concluded that '. . . the poorer-than-normal speech recognition in noise exhibited by some hearing-impaired listeners is not due to a deficit in detecting the speech signal in noise. Instead, their poorer speech recognition performance in noise is due to their inability to efficiently utilize audible speech cues'. Some caution is needed, however, in drawing strong conclusions from these results. Detection can be based on audibility of a very limited part of the spectrum of the speech, but recognition of speech requires information to be audible over a wider frequency range.

The intelligibility of speech in quiet at high overall levels

As described earlier, hearing-impaired people with mild-to-moderate cochlear hearing losses do not generally have difficulty in understanding connected discourse in a quiet non-reverberant room. However, they may have some difficulty for isolated nonsense syllables. Subjects with severe losses can have considerable difficulty with speech in quiet. Turner and Robb (1987) tried to determine whether this difficulty could be explained in terms of audibility. They studied the identification of synthetic consonant–vowel syllables, composed of one of the six stop consonants /b, d, g, p, t, k/ followed by the vowel /a/. A model of filtering in the peripheral auditory system was used to estimate the portion of the speech spectrum that was above the threshold of audibility for a given presentation level. Several presentation levels were used for each subject. They tested four normally hearing subjects and five subjects with moderate-to-severe hearing losses.

For the normally hearing subjects, recognition improved monotonically as the audible portion of the stimulus increased, and performance was perfect when most of the spectrum was above threshold. For four out of the five hearing-impaired subjects, recognition scores were consistently lower than for the normally hearing subjects at a given level of audibility. For these subjects, scores remained below 100%, even in cases where audibility was close to 100%. For the remaining subject, the hearing loss at low frequencies was too severe for even 50% audibility to be achieved. Overall, these results strongly suggest that reduced audibility is not sufficient to explain the relatively poor consonant recognition of the hearing-impaired subjects. It is noteworthy, however, that even presentation levels of 100 dB SPL were not sufficient to provide 100% audibility for subjects with severe losses (although appropriate frequency-dependent amplification could ensure 100% audibility at overall levels below 100 dB SPL).

Simulation of hearing loss by selective filtering or masking

Yet another approach for studying the effects of audibility is to subject the stimuli to frequency-selective attenuation (filtering) so as to imitate the effect of a hearing loss on audibility. Say, for example, that a hearing-impaired subject has absolute thresholds of 30, 40, 45, 50, 70 and 70 dB HL at 250, 500, 1000, 2000, 4000 and 6000 Hz, respectively. The filter would be designed to attenuate by 30 dB at 250 Hz, 40 dB at 500 Hz, 45 dB at 1000 Hz, etc. The filtered stimuli are presented to normally hearing subjects. The filtering has the effect of matching the audiogram for the impaired ear (listening to unfiltered stimuli) and for the normal ears (listening to filtered stimuli). If audibility is the main cause of difficulty in speech understanding experienced by the hearing-impaired subject, then performance should be similar for the hearing-impaired subject listening to unfiltered speech and normally hearing subjects listening to filtered speech.

Only a few studies have used this approach. Sher and Owens (1974) compared consonant recognition in quiet for subjects with hearing loss above 2000 Hz and for normally hearing subjects listening to stimuli that were low-pass filtered at 2040 Hz. The filtering did not exactly simulate the reduced audibility for the hearing-impaired subjects. There were no significant differences between the two groups either in overall scores or in the patterns of consonant confusion.

Walden *et al.* (1981) used eight subjects with unilateral hearing losses. Consonant recognition in quiet was compared between the two ears. However, rather than using filtering to match audiograms in the two ears, they matched loudness in the two ears using tones at a suprathreshold level (60 dB HL in the normal ear). This meant that the filtering/attenuation of the stimuli presented to the normal ear was less than would be required to match the audiograms in the two ears. Large individual differences were observed, but, on average, consonant recognition scores were 21% lower for the impaired than for the normal ears. This happened despite the fact that the proportion of the speech that was above threshold was greater for the impaired than for the normal ears (because the filtering/attenuation for the normal ears was less than would be required to match audibility). This strongly suggests that some factor other than audibility contributed to the relatively poor performance for the impaired ears.

Fabry and van Tasell (1986) used six subjects with unilateral cochlear loss, filtering the stimuli to match the audiograms of the normal and impaired ears. Several of the subjects had absolute thresholds that were normal or near-normal at low frequencies, but increased markedly at high frequencies. They measured the identification of consonant–vowel nonsense syllables in quiet. For two subjects, scores were similar for unprocessed stimuli presented to the impaired ear and filtered stimuli presented to the normal ear. Patterns of errors were also similar for the two ears. For three subjects, performance was better for the *impaired* than for the normal ears, by an average of about 8%. This may have happened because of the unfamiliarity of the filtered stimuli presented to the normal ears. Another possibility is that, for speech in quiet, loudness recruitment can actually have a small beneficial effect by increasing the loudness of sounds presented at low sensation levels (Gatehouse and Haggard 1987); see the next section for further discussion of this point. For the remaining subject, the score was 11% worse for the impaired than for the normal ear.

Unfortunately, there do not seem to have been any studies of this type examining the intelligibility of speech in noise. Thus, it is not known whether selective filtering to match the attenuative component of a hearing loss would produce equivalent performance to that found in hearing-impaired subjects.

Another approach to this problem uses masking noise with normal listeners to simulate the effects of the elevated thresholds associated with hearing impairment. The noise is spectrally shaped so that the masked audiograms of the normal listeners match the unmasked audiograms of the hearing-impaired listeners. This technique has been used by a number of different investigators (Fabry and Van Tasell 1986; Humes *et al.* 1987; Zurek and Delhorne 1987; Humes and Roberts 1990; Dubno and Schaefer 1992). Generally, speech intelligibility performance for the noise-masked normal ears has been reasonably close to that of the hearing-impaired subjects whose absolute thresholds were simulated. However, this technique is limited to the simulation of mild-to-moderate hearing losses; the simulation of severe losses would require unacceptably intense noise.

A problem with this technique is that it does not simulate the loss of audibility alone. The noise also produces an effect resembling loudness recruitment (see chapter 3). Indeed, some researchers have suggested that noise may be regarded as simulating the combined effects of threshold elevation and loudness recruitment (Humes and Roberts 1990). However, the nature of the recruitment may be different from that produced by cochlear hearing loss (Phillips 1987). More generally, the background noise may affect not only the detection thresholds, but also the perception of suprathreshold sounds. This idea is supported by the observation that using masking noise to match the audiograms of normal and impaired listeners has greater effects on speech intelligibility than using selective filtering, as described earlier (Fabry and Van Tasell 1986).

Comparison of speech intelligibility for conductive and cochlear losses

Conductive hearing loss has the effect of attenuating sounds, but it does not produce any substantial changes in the perception or discrimination of sounds that are presented at suprathreshold levels. Therefore, comparisons of performance between people with conductive and cochlear losses of similar magnitude can provide some insight into the role of supra-threshold factors in cochlear hearing loss. Gatehouse and Haggard (1987) measured the intelligibility of isolated words in quiet as a function of presentation level, using subjects either with 'pure' sensorineural losses of varying severity (presumably mainly cochlear losses) and subjects with varying degrees of conductive loss (sometimes in combination with sensorineural loss). They showed that, for a given degree of hearing loss, subjects with conductive loss showed poorer performance than subjects with cochlear loss at low stimulus levels; at high levels the reverse occurred.

They interpreted their results as indicating a beneficial effect of loudness recruitment (in subjects with cochlear losses) for stimuli that are at low sensation levels; the recruitment has the effect of increasing the loudness of the speech, making the speech information more usable. However, at high levels, the benefit of recruitment is offset by the poor suprathreshold discrimination abilities of those with cochlear loss, so they perform more poorly than those with conductive loss. Gatehouse and Haggard emphasized that the beneficial effect of recruitment at low levels is only observed for speech in quiet. For speech in noise, people with cochlear loss perform more poorly than people with conductive loss, even at low presentation levels.

Conclusions on the role of audibility

Taken together, the results reviewed above strongly suggest that one or more factors other than audibility contribute to the difficulties of speech perception experienced by those with moderate or greater cochlear losses. This is especially true in situations where the stimuli are presented at high levels and/or in background noise. In other words, the difficulties arise partly from abnormalities in perception of sounds that are above the threshold of audibility. For those with mild losses, audibility may be the dominant factor.

Correlational studies of psychoacoustic abilities and speech perception

If it is accepted that the speech perception difficulties of people with moderate or greater cochlear losses are partly caused by abnormalities in the perception of sounds that are above the threshold for detection, the question naturally follows: what psychoacoustical factors have the most influence on speech intelligibility. One method for studying this problem is to examine statistical relationships between measures of these abilities in hearing-impaired subjects. Typically, subjects have been given a battery of psychoacoustical and speech perceptual tests. Ideally, a large number of subjects should be tested (for statistical validity), the subjects should be given practice on each test until their performance is stable, and sufficient data should be gathered to give a reliable and accurate score on each test. Unfortunately, this would take an enormous amount of time and, in practice, compromises are inevitable. Either a large number of subjects can be tested, but with little time for practice on each test or for the execution of each test; or fewer subjects can be tested, with each given more training and more time per test.

Several researchers have conducted correlational studies (Dreschler and Plomp 1980, 1985; Patterson *et al.* 1982; Tyler *et al.* 1982a; Festen and Plomp 1983; Horst 1987; Glasberg and Moore 1989; van Rooij and Plomp 1990; Lutman 1991). Most studies have measured SRTs in noise and have assessed whether the SRTs can be 'accounted for' (in a statistical sense) by performance on various psychoacoustic tests. The studies agree that a substantial part of the variability in SRTs is not explained by absolute thresholds. Most studies also agree that suprathreshold abilities such as frequency selectivity (Horst 1987) or temporal resolution (Tyler *et al.* 1982a) can account for a significant proportion of the variance in the SRTs. However, the effects of these variables are difficult to separate from the effects of absolute threshold, and their correlation with SRTs in noise has sometimes been found to be non-significant after the effect of absolute threshold has been partialled out (Kendall and Stuart 1967). This does not necessarily mean that these psychoacoustic variables are unimportant for speech intelligibility. It simply means that the variables are closely coupled to the absolute threshold.

I will consider in more detail a study by Glasberg and Moore (1989) which used a relatively small number of highly practiced subjects. Most previous studies used subjects with a wide range of audiometric configurations; both the average degree of hearing loss and the slope of the audiogram varied considerably across subjects. This causes a number of problems: (1) When testing with speech stimuli, the proportion of the speech energy which is above absolute threshold varies considerably from one subject to another, except at very high sound levels. These variations in the audibility of speech can obscure the effects of other psychoacoustic factors; (2) Steeply sloping audiograms can make it difficult to obtain and interpret psychoacoustical measures of frequency selectivity. Glasberg and Moore used subjects with a relatively narrow range of absolute thresholds (30–65 dB HL), at least over the frequency range 500–2000 Hz. In addition, most subjects had relatively uniform losses as a function of frequency. All the impaired ears were tested at relatively high sound levels, chosen so that the stimuli were generally 20 dB or more above absolute threshold.

Glasberg and Moore used nine subjects with unilateral cochlear impairments; performance using the normal ear acted as a control for performance in the impaired ear, and the normal ear was compared with the impaired ear both at equal

SL and at equal SPL. One possible drawback of using such subjects is that the impaired ear may become 'lazy' or 'neglected' in some sense, giving poorer discrimination abilities than might be expected from the pure-tone audiogram (Hood 1984). In addition, the pathologies producing unilateral loss may not be typical of hearing losses in general. Hence, Glasberg and Moore also tested six subjects with bilateral losses of cochlear origin.

Psychoacoustic tests were generally conducted at three centre frequencies, 0.5, 1.0 and 2.0 kHz. Most subjects had absolute thresholds for their impaired ears in the range 40 to 60 dB HL at these frequencies, but a few had thresholds as low as 30 dB HL or as high as 80 dB HL at one of the test frequencies. The measures used included the following:

(1) SRTs in quiet (abbreviated SQ), and in speech-shaped noise with a level of 60 dB SPL (S60) and 75 dB SPL (S75).
(2) The mean absolute threshold at 0.5, 1 and 2 kHz (ABS), and the dynamic range (DR) measured as the difference between the highest comfortable level and the absolute threshold, averaged over the same three frequencies.
(3) The shape of the auditory filter, estimated using the notched-noise method (see chapter 2). Two summary measures were used: the bandwidth (ERB) and the mean attenuation of the auditory filter at frequencies 40% below and above the centre frequency (ATT4).
(4) The frequency difference limen for pulsed sinusoids (DLF) and for pulsed complex tones (CPX).
(5) The threshold for detecting a temporal gap in a band of noise (NG).

The SRTs were higher for the impaired than for the normal ears, both in quiet and in noise. The elevation in quiet could be largely accounted for by the higher absolute thresholds for the impaired ears. Taking the results for all ears together, the SQ was highly correlated with the ABS ($r = 0.96$, $p < 0.001$). For the impaired ears only, the corresponding correlation was $r = 0.82$ ($p < 0.001$).

The level of the 75-dB noise was sufficient to raise the SRTs well above those measured in quiet, and, at this noise level, the SRTs were higher for the impaired ears. The mean S75 for the normal ears (standard deviations in brackets) was −0.9 dB (2.0). For the impaired ears of the subjects with unilateral impairments the mean S75 was 7.1 dB (2.5). Thus the impaired ears required, on average, an 8 dB higher speech-to-noise ratio to achieve 50% intelligibility. For the subjects with bilateral impairments the mean S75 was 1.3 dB (4.3). Taking the results for all ears together, the S60 was highly correlated with ABS ($r = 0.89$, $p < 0.001$), but the correlation was lower, although still highly significant, for the S75 ($r = 0.62$ $p < 0.001$,). For the impaired ears only these correlations reduced to $r = 0.74$ ($p < 0.001$) and $r = 0.56$ ($p < 0.01$), respectively. This indicates that, for noise levels sufficient to raise the SRT well above that measured in quiet, a significant proportion of the variance in the SRTs was not accounted for by variations in absolute threshold.

The better performance for the bilaterally impaired subjects might have been a consequence of the fact that their hearing losses were, on average, less than those for the impaired ears of the unilaterally impaired subjects. The bilaterally impaired subjects also tended to perform better on the psychoacoustic tasks described below, which may indicate that the effects of the pathology were more severe for those with unilateral impairments. Five of the subjects with unilateral losses had Ménière's disease, which may have particularly severe effects on the ability to understand speech.

While the S75 was correlated with ABS, it was more highly correlated with three measures of suprathreshold discrimination, namely DLF, CPX and NG. This was true both for the results of all ears and for the impaired ears only. This is consistent with the hypothesis that, in high levels of background noise, the ability to understand speech is determined more by suprathreshold discrimination abilities than by absolute sensitivity.

Principal components analysis (PCA) was used to analyse the inter-relationships among scores for the different tests. This method represents the scores for the different tests by points in a geometrical space, with one dimension for each test. The first principal component is determined by finding the direction in the space which explains as much as possible of the variation between subjects, i.e. the direction in which the scores are most widely separated. Stated differently, the first principal component is the linear combination of observed variables (scores on the different tests) that maximally separates subjects by maximizing the variance of their component scores (Tabachnick and Fidell 1983). The second principal component is orthogonal to the first, and is chosen to account for as much as possible of the remaining variance in the data. Subsequent components are derived in a similar way.

The results are presented by plotting the correlation between the original test scores and the principal components. Tests which are closely related appear as clusters in such a plot. Figure 7.2 shows the results of a PCA based only on the S75 and on the psychoacoustic measures whose scores showed a correlation greater than 0.45 with the S75. Most of the points lie very close to the circle indicating that the first two components explain most of the variance in the data for these tests. The SQ and ABS form a cluster which is somewhat separated from the points for the other tests, including the S75. This suggests that absolute threshold is the primary determinant of the SQ, but not the S75. The point for the S75 lies quite close to those for three of the tests: NG, DLF and CPX. The measures of sharpness of the auditory filter also lie reasonably close (ATT4 is at the opposite side of the circle since a large SRT is associated with a small value of ATT4). This suggests that the S75 is primarily determined by suprathreshold discrimination abilities rather than by absolute sensitivity.

However, caution is needed in interpreting the results. PCA analysis is based on the assumption that the relative importance of different psychoacoustical abilities is the same for all subjects. This may well not be the case. For example, a subject with particularly poor frequency selectivity but good temporal resolution may come to rely very heavily on temporal cues rather than spectral cues in speech. Thus the relative importance of different cues will vary across subjects.

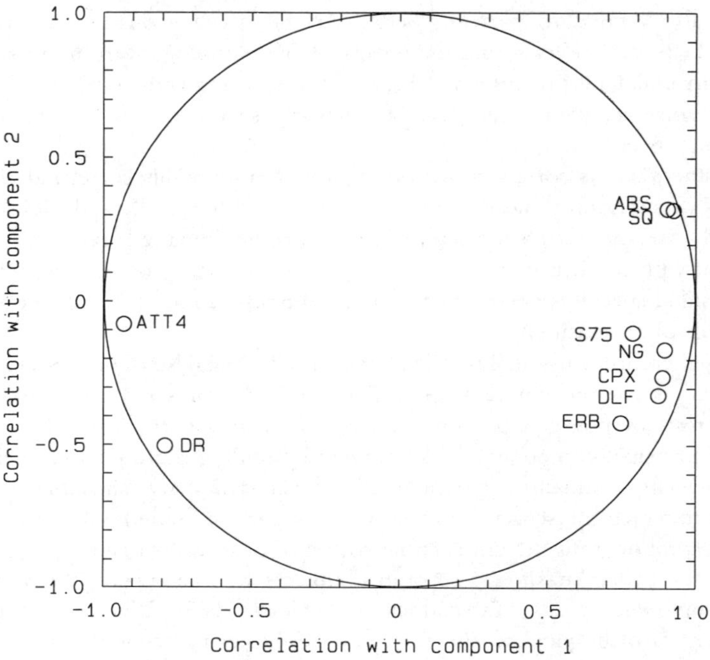

Fig. 7.2. Results of a Principal Components Analysis (PCA) conducted by Glasberg and Moore (1989). The correlation of each of the tests with the first two principal components is plotted.

Overall, the results of studies using the correlational approach have been somewhat inconclusive. They have provided evidence that the intelligibility of speech in noise for subjects with moderate or greater cochlear losses is influenced by suprathreshold discrimination abilities, but they have not provided a clear indication of the relative importance of the various psychoacoustic factors that might be involved.

Assessing the effects of frequency selectivity on vowel and consonant perception

Some studies have attempted to relate measures of frequency selectivity in specific frequency regions to the intelligibility of speech sounds for which important information is carried in those frequency regions. This more focussed approach can yield useful insights into the importance of frequency selectivity.

Consonant perception

Preminger and Wiley (1985) measured psychophysical tuning curves (see chapter 2) for a 500-Hz signal and a 4000-Hz signal in subjects with cochlear hearing loss of various configurations. Losses were classified as high frequency, flat, or low frequency; there were two subjects in each group. The test stimuli were consonant–vowel syllables which were categorized into three groups on the basis of the predominant spectral energy in the consonant parts of the sounds; the three groups were low frequency (e.g. w, b, m, l), high frequency (e.g. t, d, k, z, s), and diffuse (e.g. v, f). The subjects with high-frequency loss had broadened PTCs at 4000 Hz, but normal PTCs at 500 Hz. These subjects achieved higher performance for low-frequency consonants than for high-frequency consonants. The subjects with flat hearing losses showed almost no frequency selectivity at 4000 Hz (the PTCs were 'flat') and they both performed poorly at identifying high-frequency consonants. One subject also had a very broad PTC at 500 Hz, and that subject performed poorly at identifying low-frequency consonants. The other subject showed some tuning at 500 Hz and achieved better identification of low-frequency consonants. For the subjects with low-frequency loss, the relation between PTC tuning and consonant identification was not so clear.

Thibodeau and van Tasell (1987) measured frequency selectivity at 2000 Hz by measuring the percent correct detection of a 2000-Hz sinusoid as a function of the width of a spectral notch in a noise, the notch being centred at 2000 Hz. Two normally hearing subjects and seven subjects with moderate flat sensorineural (probably cochlear) losses were used. They also measured the ability to discriminate two synthetic stop-vowel syllables, /di/ and /gi/, which were identical except for spectral transitions in the range 1800–2500 Hz. Discrimination was measured both in broadband noise and in noise with a spectral notch around 2000 Hz. There was a significant correlation between scores on the two tasks; subjects with poorer frequency selectivity were also poorer at discriminating the syllables.

These results indicate that effects of reduced frequency selectivity on consonant discrimination can be observed when the information in the speech is suitably restricted. However, natural speech contains information over a wide frequency range, making it much harder to show specific effects of reduced frequency selectivity.

Vowel perception

Vowel sounds are characterized by spectral prominences (corresponding to vocal tract resonances) at certain frequencies. These are called formants, and the pattern of frequencies at which the formants occur is thought to play an important role in determining the perceived vowel quality or identity. The excitation pattern evoked by a vowel can be regarded as an internal representation of the spectral shape of the vowel. This is illustrated in Figure 7.3. The top panel shows the spectrum of a synthetic vowel /I/ on a linear frequency scale while the middle panel shows the same spectrum on an ERB scale (see chapter 2). The bottom panel shows the excitation pattern for the vowel plotted on an ERB scale. This pattern was calculated as described in chapter 2 for a normal auditory system. Note that the calculation did not take into account the effects of suppression, which would be expected to enhance the contrast between peaks and valleys in the excitation pattern (Houtgast 1974; Moore and Glasberg 1983b).

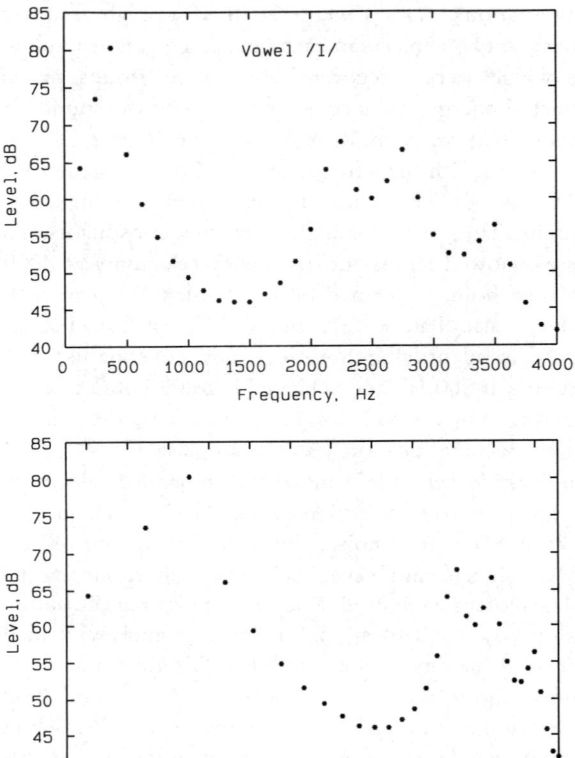

Fig. 7.3. The top panel shows the spectrum of the synthetic vowel /I/, plotted on a linear frequency scale. The middle panel shows the spectrum plotted on an ERB scale. The bottom panel shows the excitation pattern for that vowel, calculated for a normal ear, and plotted on an ERB scale.

Several aspects of the excitation pattern are noteworthy. Firstly, the lowest three peaks in the excitation pattern do not correspond to formant frequencies, but rather to individual lower harmonics; these harmonics are resolved in the normal peripheral auditory system, and can be heard out as separate tones under certain conditions (Plomp 1964a; Moore and Ohgushi 1993). Hence the centre frequency of the first formant is not directly represented in the excitation pattern; it must be inferred from the relative levels of the peaks corresponding to the individual lower harmonics.

A second noteworthy aspect of the excitation pattern is that the second, third and fourth formants, which are clearly separately visible in the original spectrum, are not well resolved. Rather, the second and third formants form a single prominence in the excitation pattern, with only a small dip to indicate that two formants are present. The fourth formant appears as a small 'shoulder' on the upper side of this prominence.

Figure 7.4 shows excitation patterns for the same vowel, but calculated for impaired auditory systems in which the auditory filters were assumed to have ERBs twice as great as normal (top panel) or four times as great as normal (bottom panel); these degrees of broadening are typical of moderate and severe cochlear hearing losses, respectively. It is obvious that spectral details are less well represented in these excitation patterns; the peaks and dips corresponding to the lower harmonics are less clear, and the second, third and fourth formants are represented by only a single broad prominence. Indeed, in the lower panel, there is only a small, 2–3 dB, peak to indicate the presence of the second, third and fourth formants.

Given these considerations, one might expect that vowel identification would be less accurate in hearing-impaired subjects than in normally hearing subjects, and that vowel identification would worsen progressively with decreasing frequency selectivity. There are at least some data to support this idea. Van Tasell *et al.* (1987) measured confusions among seven synthetic steady-state vowels for ten normally hearing subjects and three subjects with cochlear hearing loss. Confusions were greater for the impaired than for the normal subjects. They also used some of the vowels as forward maskers; the threshold of a brief sinusoidal signal was measured at each harmonic frequency. These vowel masking patterns (VMPs) can be used to infer the internal representation of the vowels including the effects of suppression. The VMPs of the impaired subjects showed poorer preservation of the vowels' formant structure than did the VMPs of the normal subjects. Vowel identification accuracy appeared to be related mainly to the positions of peaks in the VMPs rather than to the levels of peaks or between-peak characteristics.

Turner and Henn (1989) also compared vowel identification with measures of frequency selectivity for two normally hearing subjects and three subjects with cochlear losses. For each of several frequencies of a sinusoidal signal, they measured the signal threshold in forward masking for a sinusoidal masker of variable frequency but fixed level of 95 dB SPL. These 'input filter patterns' (Turner *et al.* 1987) were used to calculate the internal representations or excitation patterns of the vowel spectra (again, including the effects of suppression). They suggested that, the more similar the excitation patterns of two vowels, the more

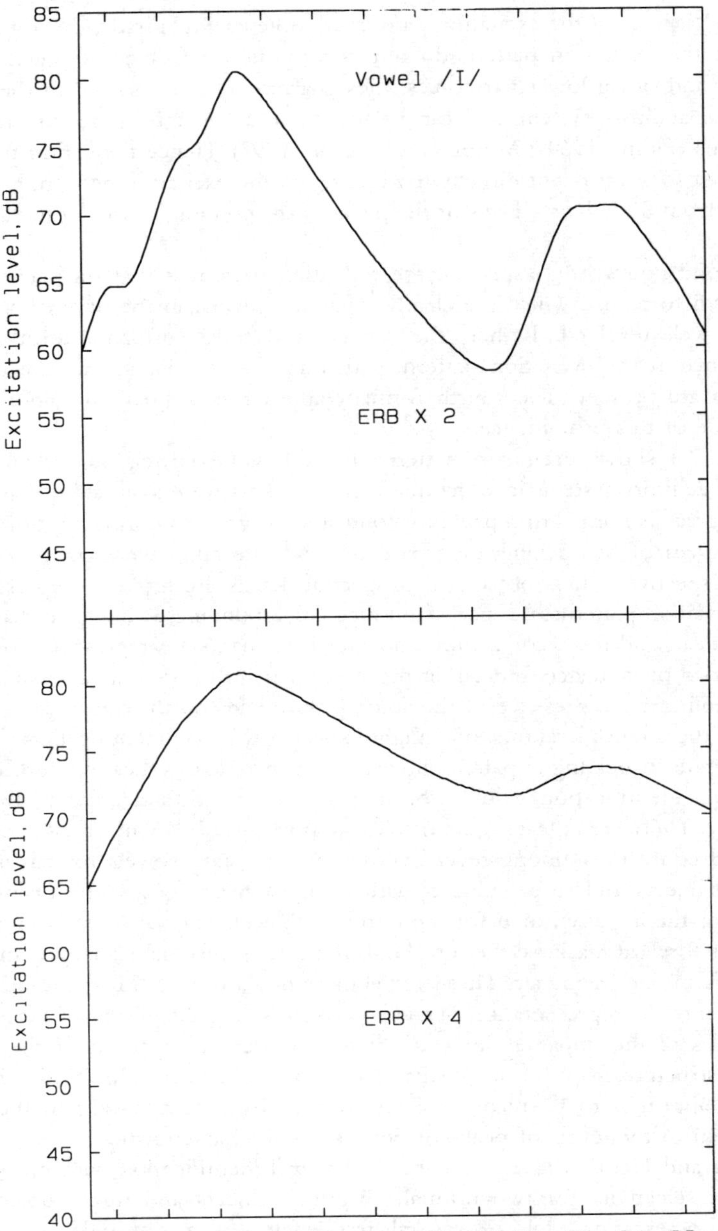

Fig. 7.4. The excitation pattern for the same vowel as in Figure 7.3, but calculated for impaired ears with auditory filters two times broader than normal (top panel) or four times broader than normal (bottom panel).

often they would be confused. This suggestion received some support when the measure of similarity was based on the entire shape of the inferred excitation patterns. However, it received stronger support when they used a measure that emphasized the similarities of spectral peak locations.

Although these experiments support the idea that reduced frequency selectivity can adversely affect vowel identification, everyday experience and studies using natural speech indicate that vowel identification by subjects with moderate cochlear hearing loss is often rather good. This may happen for at least two reasons. Firstly, the spectral differences between vowels are often very large, so that frequency selectivity has to be grossly impaired to prevent the differences being detected. Secondly, naturally produced vowels contain temporal cues (such as duration), as well as spectral cues, and these cues may be used to compensate for the effects of reduced frequency selectivity.

The use of simulations to assess the importance of psychoacoustic factors in speech perception

Another approach to assessing the importance of suprathreshold discrimination abilities for speech perception is to simulate the effect of one specific aspect of hearing impairment by processing the stimuli in a way that mimics the effect of this aspect. The processed stimuli are then used in tests with normally hearing subjects. Provided the simulation is accurate, this makes it possible to study the effect of that aspect in isolation. This general strategy has been used to study the importance of three psychoacoustical factors: loudness recruitment, frequency selectivity, and temporal resolution.

Loudness recruitment

The effects of loudness recruitment can be simulated by splitting the signal into a number of frequency bands and applying dynamic range expansion in each band before recombining the bands. Effectively, this simulation does the opposite of what happens in a normal cochlea, where stimuli are filtered along the basilar membrane, and fast-acting compression is applied at each CF (see chapter 1). The goal of the simulation is to process the level of the stimulus in each band, on a moment-by-moment basis, so as to create loudness sensations in a normal ear that would resemble those produced in an impaired ear with recruitment.

Villchur (1974) used a three-band system to process speech so as to simulate the effects of recruitment associated with severe hearing loss. The stimulus in each band was processed using a fast-acting expander. Subjects with unilateral hearing impairments judged processed stimuli presented to their normal ear to sound 'similar' or 'very similar' to unprocessed stimuli presented to their impaired ear. The intelligibility of the processed speech was not measured in formal tests. However, Villchur concluded that recruitment is a sufficient cause for loss of intelligibility in cases of severe hearing loss.

In a later study (Villchur 1977) he used a 16-channel system, with computer-controlled attenuators to achieve the dynamic range expansion. A severe sloping hearing loss was simulated. The intelligibility of speech in quiet at a level of 94 dB was adversely affected by the processing, both for isolated words and for sentences. The intelligibility of words and sentences in white noise was also adversely affected by the processing, the percent correct decreasing from about 69% to 50%. An even greater effect was found for speech in speech-shaped noise.

Duchnowski (1989) used digital signal processing to implement a 14-band system. The gain in each band was adjusted dynamically to reproduce the elevated absolute thresholds and abnormal loudness growth associated with cochlear hearing impairment. In one experiment, the processing was adjusted to simulate the hearing losses of the subjects tested by Zurek and Delhorne (1987); these subjects had mild-to-moderate hearing losses. The test stimuli were consonant-vowel (CV) syllables, presented in quiet and in various levels of speech-shaped noise. Generally, the pattern of results obtained using the simulation with normally hearing subjects matched the pattern obtained for the impaired subjects of Zurek and Delhorne. Thus, for these subjects, the threshold elevation and associated loudness recruitment appear sufficient to account for their difficulties in understanding speech.

In a second experiment, the hearing loss of subjects with more severe losses was simulated. When a flat frequency-gain characteristic was used, the pattern of results from the impaired subjects closely matched the results from the normal subjects listening to the processed stimuli. However, when high-frequency emphasis was employed, the impaired subjects generally performed more poorly than their normal counterparts listening to processed stimuli. This suggests that some factor other than threshold elevation and loudness recruitment contributed to the speech perceptual problems of the hearing-impaired subjects.

Moore and Glasberg (1993) simulated threshold elevation and loudness recruitment by splitting the input signal into 13 frequency bands, and processing the envelope in each band so as to create loudness sensations in a normal ear that would resemble those produced in an impaired ear with recruitment. In essence, the processing of the envelope for a given filter involved raising the envelope to a power N. Complete loudness recruitment was simulated, assuming that loudness reaches its 'normal' value at 100 dB SPL. If the envelope in a given frequency band is raised to the power N, then the level (in dB) of the processed stimulus in that band, L_P, is a linear function of the level of the unprocessed stimulus, L_U, with slope N:

$$L_P = NL_U + K, \qquad \text{Eq. 7.3}$$

where K is a constant. The overall levels were scaled so that $L_U = L_P$ when L_P = 100 dB. Hence $K = (1 - N)100$ and

$$L_P = NL_U - (N - 1)100 \qquad \text{Eq. 7.4}$$

For example, if N = 2, a value of L_U of 75 dB gives a value of L_P of 50 dB, and a value of L_U of 50 dB gives a value of L_P of 0 dB. A value of N of 2 simulates the type of recruitment typically found in cases of moderate to severe cochlear loss, where, for example, a 50-dB range of stimulus levels gives the same range of loudness as a 100-dB range of stimulus levels in a normal ear (Moore *et al.* 1985a); see chapter 3. After processing the envelope in each band in this way, the bands were recombined. All tests were performed using subjects with normal hearing.

The following processing conditions were used:

(1) Unprocessed (the control condition, R1).
(2) Uniform processing across bands with N = 2. This simulates a flat moderate hearing loss (threshold ≈ 50 dB HL) (condition R2).
(3) Uniform processing across bands with N = 3. This simulates a flat severe hearing loss (threshold ≈ 67 dB HL) (condition R3).
(4) Processing with more envelope expansion at high frequencies, to simulate a hearing loss increasing with frequency. The value of N was 1.5 for frequencies up to 1.0 kHz. The power was then increased smoothly to 3 as frequency increased to 4 kHz, and remained at 3 above 4 kHz (condition RX).

Moore and Glasberg also assessed whether there are deleterious effects of recruitment after the attenuative component of a hearing loss has been corrected as far as possible by linear amplification, as would be used in a conventional hearing aid. To do this, they ran a set of conditions in which the stimuli in conditions (2)-(4) were subjected to the frequency-dependent gain recommended by the NAL revised procedure (Byrne and Dillon 1986; see chapter 8 for more details). This gain is appropriate for speech presented at a moderate conversational level of about 65 dB SPL. This gave three more conditions, R2+, R3+ and RX+.

For speech in quiet, the simulation produced, as expected, a reduction in the ability to understand low-level speech. The level of speech required for 50% intelligibility was 16 dB SPL in condition R1, 64 dB in condition R2, 79 dB in condition R3, and 53 dB in condition RX. However, speech at sufficiently high levels was highly intelligible in all conditions. Also, linear amplification according to the NAL prescription reduced the 50% intelligibility points to less than 50 dB SPL for all conditions, and gave high intelligibility for speech at normal conversational levels. Thus, linear amplification was rather effective in improving the intelligibility of speech in quiet, although it did not allow speech to be both intelligible and comfortable over a wide range of sound levels; speech with input levels above about 70 dB SPL was judged to be unpleasantly loud in the conditions involving linear amplification.

For speech presented at a fixed input level of 65 dB SPL, against a background of a single competing talker, simulation of hearing loss produced substantial decrements in performance. This is illustrated in Figure 7.5 for the case where the background speech had a level of 71 dB SPL. Performance was almost perfect for condition R1, but not for the conditions simulating threshold elevation and loudness recruitment. The speech-to-background ratios in conditions R2 and RX had to be 11–13 dB higher than in condition R1 to achieve similar levels of performance. Linear amplification according to the NAL prescription improved performance markedly for the conditions simulating flat losses, but was

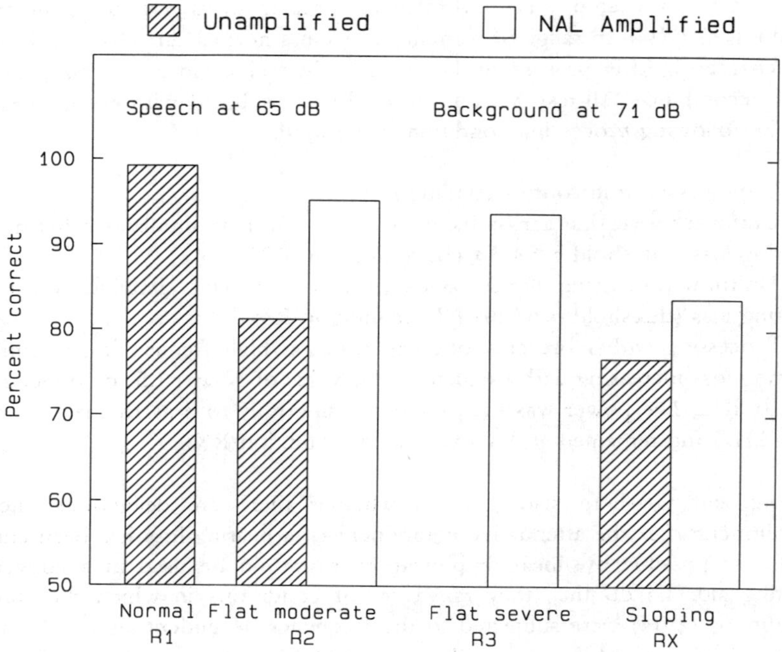

Fig. 7.5. Comparison of percent correct scores for the different conditions of Moore and Glasberg (1993), for a speech-to-background ratio of −6 dB. No score is shown for condition R3, since the target speech was inaudible for that condition.

less effective for the condition simulating a sloping loss. Performance in this condition remained well below that in the control condition, even after linear amplification.

In a second study, Moore *et al.* (1995) used similar processing conditions (R1, R2, R3 and RX), but the speech was presented in a background of speech-shaped noise instead of a single competing talker. The input level of the speech was fixed at 65 dB SPL, while the level of the background noise varied from 65 to 74 dB SPL. The speech in condition R3 was inaudible. For conditions R2 and RX, the speech-to-noise ratios had to be up to 6 dB higher than in the control condition (R1, unprocessed stimuli) to achieve similar levels of performance. When linear amplification according to the NAL prescription was applied before the simulation, performance improved markedly for conditions R2 and RX, and did not differ significantly from that for R1. For condition R3, performance with simulated NAL amplification remained below that for condition R1; the decrement in performance was equivalent to about a 1-dB change in speech-to-noise ratio.

The results obtained using speech-shaped noise differ in two ways from the results obtained using a single talker as the interfering sound: firstly, the deleterious effects of the simulations were generally smaller with speech-shaped noise;

secondly, linear amplification according to the NAL formula restored performance to normal for two of the three conditions tested (R2+ and RX+) using speech-shaped noise, whereas it did not when a single competing talker was used. In the remaining condition (R3+) the degradation in performance was significant, but was equivalent to a change of only 1 dB in speech-to-noise ratio.

The differences between the two sets of results can be understood in the following way. Normally hearing people can take advantage of spectral and temporal dips in a background of a single competing talker. Hence the speech-to-background ratio required to achieve a given level of performance is markedly lower than when the background is speech-shaped noise. However, 'dip listening' requires a wide dynamic range. Consider as an example, a situation where the target speech has a level 10 dB lower than that of the interfering speech, and where the overall level is such that the interfering speech is loud, but not uncomfortably so. The overall loudness is determined mainly by the levels of peaks in the interfering speech. In any given frequency band, the target speech may contain useful information at a level 40 dB below the peak level of the interfering speech (since for one voice the range of levels is about 30 dB — see the section on the AI). Such information may be audible during brief pauses in the interfering speech. Ideally, then, brief sounds should be audible and discriminable when their levels are 40 dB below the highest comfortable levels.

Loudness recruitment, either real or simulated, reduces the available dynamic range. If the level of the speech is set so that the more intense parts of the speech are comfortably loud, the weaker parts may be inaudible. Hence, people with recruitment cannot exploit 'dip listening' as effectively as normally hearing people. When a background of speech-shaped noise is used, 'dip listening' is of much less importance, since the noise does not contain dips of sufficient magnitude or duration. Hence speech intelligibility depends more on the higher-level portions of the speech and these are less affected by reduced dynamic range. Furthermore, linear amplification, which ensures that the higher level portions of speech are clearly audible, is effective in compensating for the simulated recruitment, except when the hearing loss is severe (condition R3).

In one respect, the results of the simulations differ from those obtained using subjects who have 'real' cochlear hearing loss. When threshold elevation and loudness recruitment are simulated using normally hearing subjects, performance is markedly better when the interfering sound is a single talker than when it is speech-shaped noise. However, people with cochlear hearing loss often show little or no difference in intelligibility for these two backgrounds (Duquesnoy and Plomp 1983; Festen and Plomp 1990; Moore *et al.* 1991). This suggests that some factor other than recruitment contributes to the reduced ability of hearing-impaired people to 'listen in the dips'. A likely factor is reduced frequency selectivity, which may have especially strong effects on the ability to listen in spectral dips of the interfering sound (Baer and Moore 1994).

In summary, the results of the simulations indicate that the reduced dynamic range associated with loudness recruitment can lead to difficulty in understanding speech in background sounds. When the background sound is a steady noise, the difficulty can be effectively compensated by linear amplification of the type commonly used in hearing aids, except when the loss is severe. When the background sound is fluctuating, as for a single talker, the deleterious effects of the reduced dynamic range are greater and are not fully compensated by linear amplification.

Simulation of reduced frequency selectivity

To simulate reduced frequency selectivity, the basic idea has been to smear or broaden the spectra of test signals, so that the excitation pattern produced in a normal ear resembles (albeit crudely in many of the simulations) the pattern that would be produced in an impaired ear using unprocessed signals. It should be noted that such spectral smearing does not simulate all of the effects of reduced frequency selectivity. Specifically, the time patterns at the outputs of the auditory filters are affected by reduced frequency selectivity in a way that is not reproduced by the simulations. Instead, the simulations alter the time patterns of the stimuli in a complex way that is a by-product of the specific processing used. Essentially, the simulation may be regarded as mimicking the consequences of reduced frequency selectivity in terms of place coding in the auditory system, but not in terms of time coding.

Several different techniques have been used to perform the spectral smearing. Smearing using analogue processing has generally been performed by filtering the signal into bands and multiplying each band by a bandpass noise (Villchur 1977; Summers and Al-Dabbagh 1982; Summers 1991). The width of the bandpass noise determines the degree of spectral smearing. In some studies, an independent bandpass noise was used for each band, the width of the bands increasing with centre frequency to simulate the way that the auditory filter bandwidth increases with centre frequency (see chapter 2). The results of these studies have shown that speech intelligibility declines as smearing bandwidth is increased. However, a serious problem with this approach is that the multiplication with random noise introduces spurious amplitude fluctuations that are uncorrelated with the speech signal.

In more recent studies, digital signal processing techniques have been used. Generally, short segments of the signal are transformed into spectra using a short-term Fast Fourier Transform (FFT). Modifications are then made in the spectral domain, always involving some operation on the power spectra, and the modified spectra are transformed back into time signals using an inverse FFT. This is repeated for a series of overlapping segments, and the resulting processed segments are added together. Hence, this is referred to as the overlap-add method (Allen 1977). The method has been used in several studies (Celmer and Bienvenue 1987; Howard-Jones and Summers 1992; ter Keurs *et al.* 1992; Baer and Moore 1993, 1994). The details of the processing have differed markedly across studies, especially in terms of how the power spectra have been modified and in terms of the degree of overlap of individual processed segments.

Ter Keurs *et al.* (1992) smeared the spectral *envelope* of each segment while leaving its fine structure unchanged. The envelope was first calculated from the power spectrum. It was then projected onto a log frequency scale and convolved with a Gaussian function to perform the smearing. They smeared the spectrum of speech and noise separately and then added the speech and noise together. The SRT in noise increased once the smearing bandwidth was increased beyond about 1/3 octave. Vowel identification was affected more than consonant identification.

In a second study (ter Keurs *et al.* 1993) they compared the effects of the smearing using either speech-shaped noise or a single talker as the background sound. For both types of masker, SRTs increased when the smearing bandwidth was increased. For unsmeared speech, SRTs were 5–7 dB lower when the background was a single talker than when it was speech-shaped noise. This difference decreased as the smearing bandwidth was increased. Hence, the effect of the spectral smearing on SRTs was greater for the speech masker than for the noise masker.

Baer and Moore (1993) measured the intelligibility of speech in quiet and in speech-shaped noise using the overlap–add method to perform spectral smearing. The magnitude spectrum itself was smeared (in contrast to the studies of ter Keurs *et al.*, which involved smearing of the spectral envelope, preserving spectral fine structure), but the phase spectrum was preserved. Normally hearing subjects listened to sentence material that had been processed to simulate varying degrees of loss of frequency selectivity. When speech in noise was used, the speech was mixed with the noise prior to processing. The procedure for simulating impaired frequency selectivity used a realistic form of spectral smearing, based on measured characteristics of auditory filters in hearing-impaired subjects. It was based on a procedure that was previously validated using non-speech signals (Moore *et al.* 1992a). The stimuli were processed so that the excitation pattern produced in a normal ear, calculated over a short period of time, would resemble that found with unprocessed stimuli in an impaired ear.

Several different types of smearing were used, simulating specific degrees of broadening and asymmetry of the auditory filter. Sentences in quiet and in speech-shaped noise were smeared and presented to normally hearing listeners in intelligibility tests. Some of the results are illustrated in Figure 7.6. The intelligibility of speech in quiet (the three left-most bars in Figure 7.6) was hardly affected by spectral smearing, even for smearing that simulated auditory filters six times broader than normal. However, this may partly reflect a ceiling effect, as scores were close to perfect in all conditions. The intelligibility of speech in noise was adversely affected by the smearing, especially for large degrees of smearing and at a low speech-to-noise ratio (–3 dB; see the three right-most bars in Figure 7.6). Simulation of asymmetrical broadening of the lower side of the auditory filter had a greater effect than simulation of asymmetrical broadening of the upper side, suggesting that upward spread of masking may be particularly important.

In a second study, Baer and Moore (1994) used a single competing talker as the background, instead of speech-shaped noise. The results were similar in form to those found using speech-shaped noise. Specifically, performance worsened with increasing smearing, and the worsening was greater at the more adverse speech-to-background ratio. The results agreed with those of ter Keurs *et al.* (1993) in

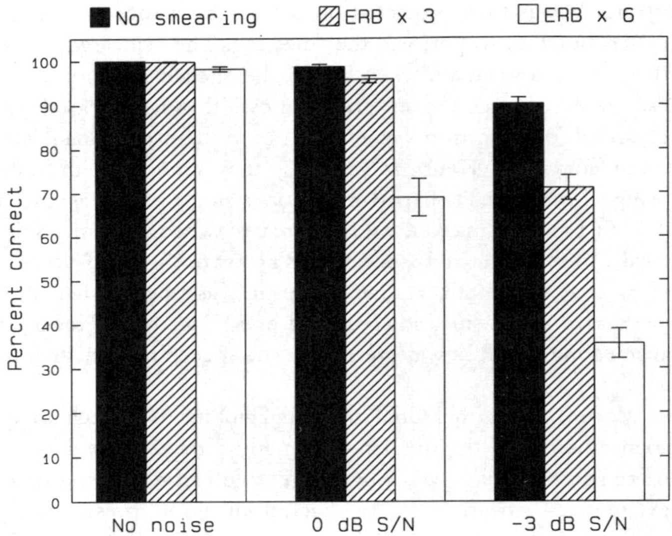

Fig. 7.6. Results of Baer and Moore (1993) showing the percentage of key words correct for three amounts of spectral smearing and three different amounts of background noise. The three amounts of smearing were: no smearing (solid bars); simulation of auditory filters with bandwidths three times greater than normal (diagonally shaded bars); and simulation of auditory filters with bandwidths six times greater than normal (open bars). Error bars indicate +/− one standard error.

showing that the deleterious effects of spectral smearing were greater for a speech masker than for a noise masker. Hence, the difference in masking produced by speech and noise maskers was less for spectrally smeared than for unprocessed stimuli. This is consistent with the finding noted earlier, that for normally hearing subjects SRTs are lower when the background is speech than when it is noise, while for hearing-impaired subjects the difference is smaller or absent.

In summary, the results of experiments on spectral smearing suggest that reduced frequency selectivity does contribute significantly to the difficulties experienced by people with cochlear damage in understanding speech in the presence of background sounds.

Simulation of reduced temporal resolution

In chapter 4 temporal resolution was described in terms of a four-stage model consisting of an array of bandpass filters (the auditory filters) each followed by a compressive nonlinearity, a sliding temporal integrator and a decision device. It was argued that cochlear damage can affect the first two stages, the filters and the nonlinearity, but that it usually did not affect the last two. Cochlear damage results in a broadening of the auditory filters and a reduction in the compressive nonlinearity. The end result is that temporal resolution is reduced only for certain specific stimuli, namely those with slowly fluctuating envelopes. In some situations, temporal resolution may be poor simply because of the low sensation level of the stimuli for people with cochlear damage.

The simulation of loudness recruitment described above effectively includes these effects; specifically, it models the effects of reduced sensation level and reduced compressive nonlinearity. Indeed, as described in chapter 4, simulation of loudness recruitment in this way results in poorer detection of temporal gaps in narrow bands of noise. One might question, therefore, whether it is appropriate to go any further in simulating the effects of abnormalities in temporal processing. However, some researchers have taken the approach of simulating the effects of reduced temporal resolution 'directly' by temporal smearing analogous to the spectral smearing used to simulate reduced frequency selectivity. Such work can be valuable because it provides a way of estimating the relative importance for speech intelligibility of temporal modulations at different rates.

Drullman *et al.* (1994) carried out a study of the effects of temporal envelope smearing on speech intelligibility. The study was not designed specifically as a simulation of reduced temporal resolution, but in effect the processing was equivalent to such a simulation. They split the input signal into a number of frequency bands covering the range 100–6400 Hz. The bands had widths of 0.25, 0.5 or 1 octave. The narrowest bandwidth corresponds roughly with the ERBs of normal auditory filters, while the wider bandwidths correspond roughly with the auditory filter bandwidths that might occur in people with moderate-to-severe cochlear losses. The amplitude envelope for each band was lowpass filtered with various cutoff frequencies. As the cutoff frequency was reduced, the envelope became more and more smeared in the time domain, simulating loss of temporal resolution. For all filtering bandwidths (0.25, 0.5 or 1 octave), the SRT of sentences in speech-shaped noise was almost unaffected by lowpass filtering the envelopes with cut-off frequencies of 64, 32 or 16 Hz; the SRT was elevated by only about 1 dB relative to that for a control condition with no envelope filtering. However, lowpass filtering with cutoff frequencies of 8 or 4 Hz produced mean elevations in SRT of 2.4 and 5.6 dB relative to the control condition. These results indicate that modulation of the envelopes of the filtered bands at rates of 16 Hz and above is relatively unimportant for speech intelligibility. Since most people with cochlear damage can easily detect modulation at rates up to 16 Hz (see, for example, Figure 4.7), this suggests that reduced temporal resolution is not a factor limiting speech intelligibility for most cases of cochlear damage.

Hou and Pavlovic (1994) carried out a study that was aimed at directly simulating the effects of reduced temporal resolution in the auditory system. They first filtered the speech into 23 bands using simulated auditory filters with bandwidths corresponding to those found in normal ears. They then smeared the temporal envelope in each band using a sliding temporal integrator similar to that described in chapter 4 for the model of temporal resolution (Moore *et al.* 1988; Plack and Moore 1990). When the equivalent rectangular duration (ERD) of the smearing integrator was less than the value of 8–9 ms found for the temporal integrator in the normal auditory system (see chapter 4), the smearing had no effect on the intelligibility of nonsense syllables in quiet. When the smearing ERD was longer, small but significant decreases in intelligibility occurred. However, even for a smearing ERD as large as 30 ms, the decrease in intelligibility was only 5–10%.

The results of Hou and Pavlovic indicate that temporal smearing can produce reduced intelligibility of nonsense syllables in quiet. They argued that reduced temporal resolution in the impaired auditory system was probably as detrimental to speech recognition as reduced frequency selectivity. However, it remains unclear whether temporal smearing is an appropriate way to model reduced temporal resolution in hearing-impaired subjects. The temporal smearing of Hou and Pavlovic would lead to reduced temporal resolution for all types of stimuli, whereas, as described in chapter 4, reduced temporal resolution in people with cochlear damage occurs only for stimuli at low SLs or with slowly fluctuating envelopes. In any case, the ERD of the temporal integrator measured for hearing-impaired subjects is not usually markedly greater than normal (Plack and Moore 1991).

Conclusions

People with mild or moderate cochlear losses can usually understand speech reasonably well when they are in a quiet room with only one person talking. However, they have difficulty when more than one person is talking at once, or when background noise or reverberation are present. People with severe or profound losses usually have difficulty even when listening to a single talker in a quiet room, and they generally have severe problems when background noise is present. The elevation of the SRT in noise, relative to the value for normally hearing subjects, is greater when the background sound is fluctuating (e.g. a single talker) than when it is a steady noise. This probably happens because people with cochlear damage are less able than normally hearing people to take advantage of temporal and spectral dips in fluctuating background sounds. People with cochlear damage are also less able than normally hearing people to exploit spatial separation between the target and interfering sounds.

The speech understanding difficulties of people with mild cochlear losses can be accounted for primarily in terms of audibility. With suitable linear amplification, such people can usually understand speech as well as normally hearing people. However, for people with moderate-to-severe cochlear losses, suprathreshold discrimination abilities also need to be taken into account. Although audibility is still of primary importance, it does not fully account for the difficulties experienced by such people.

It has proved difficult to determine the relative importance of different psychoacoustic factors that might affect speech intelligibility. However, evidence from a range of studies, including correlational studies, studies of the use of specific speech cues, and simulations, all indicate that reduced frequency selectivity plays a significant role. There is also evidence, mainly from simulations, that loudness recruitment is a significant factor. However, the most important aspect of loudness recruitment appears to be reduced dynamic range, rather than distorted loudness relationships.

8. Limitations and potentials of hearing aids

Introduction

Hearing aids have been used for many years to alleviate problems associated with cochlear damage. However, hearing-impaired people frequently complain that their hearing aids are of limited benefit. They find that the aids are sometimes useful in helping them to hear weak sounds, but that the aids do not help very much, if at all, when background noise is present. It seems clear that hearing aids are not like eye glasses. A well-fitted pair of eye glasses can give a clear visual percept if the visual problem is caused by poor focus of the image on the retina. Hearing aids do not restore hearing to normal. They can partially compensate for the loss of sensitivity produced by cochlear damage, but they do not compensate for the supra-threshold changes in perception caused, for example, by reduced frequency selectivity. This chapter reviews the capabilities and limitations of current hearing aids, and considers some ways in which hearing aids may be improved in the future.

The use of linear amplification to restore audibility

The primary goal of most hearing aids is relatively simple, namely to restore audibility via frequency-selective amplification. Many hearing aids operate essentially as linear amplifiers; over most of their operating range they apply a gain that is independent of level. For example, an aid may amplify by 20 dB at 1 kHz, and that same gain is applied regardless of the input level. A 1-kHz sinusoid with an input level of 40 dB SPL would be amplified to a level of 60 dB SPL, while an input level of 80 dB SPL would be amplified to 100 dB SPL. In practice, most hearing aids incorporate some means for limiting the maximum output, and if the limiter comes into operation the aid behaves in a non-linear manner. However, for convenience, aids which are normally used over the linear part of their operating range will still be referred to as linear.

It became apparent very soon after hearing aids first came into use that it was not practical to use linear amplification to compensate fully for the loss of audibility caused by cochlear damage. The major factor preventing this was loudness recruitment and the associated reduced dynamic range. Say, for example, a person had a cochlear hearing loss of 60 dB at all frequencies. The highest comfortable level (HCL) for such a person would typically be around 90–100 dB HL. If the person had a hearing aid that fully compensated for the loss of audibility, the aid would apply a gain of 60 dB at all frequencies. However, that would mean that any sound with a level above about 40 dB HL would be amplified to a level exceeding the HCL. In practice, many sounds encountered in everyday life would become unpleasantly loud.

As mentioned above, most hearing aids incorporate a way of limiting the maximum output of a hearing aid, so as to avoid discomfort to the user. In early hearing aids, and in many current hearing aids, this is achieved by electronic peak clipping in the output stage of the aid. The voltage is prevented from exceeding a certain absolute value (either positive of negative), which results in the larger peaks in the electrical signal being clipped or flattened off. Such clipping introduces unpleasant-sounding distortion, and in practice, most users of hearing aids set the volume control to avoid clipping in everyday listening situations. Even when aids include output limiting, it has been found to be impractical to compensate fully for loss of audibility. Rather, various prescriptive rules have been developed that can be used to derive an appropriate frequency-gain characteristic from the pattern of hearing loss as a function of frequency (Lybarger 1978; McCandless and Lyregard 1983; Byrne and Dillon 1986). Sometimes, suprathreshold measures such as the uncomfortable loudness level (ULL) or most comfortable level (MCL) are also taken into account. Invariably, such rules prescribe less gain than the hearing loss at a given frequency. Typically, the rules prescribe a gain that is between one-third and one-half of the hearing loss. For example, if the hearing loss is 60 dB at 1 kHz, then the prescribed gain is between 20 and 30 dB.

The goal of most of these rules is to select a frequency-gain characteristic that will amplify speech so as to improve intelligibility, while avoiding making speech uncomfortably loud. One rule that is quite widely used is the NAL(R) formula devised at the National Acoustics Laboratories of Australia (Byrne and Dillon 1986). The rule works solely on the basis of the pure-tone audiogram. It was derived by dividing speech into a number of contiguous 1/3-octave bands or one-octave bands covering the range 250 to 6 kHz, and working out what gain would be required in each band to amplify the speech in that band to the MCL, assuming that the speech was at a normal conversational level (typically about 65 dB SPL overall when the talker and listener are separated by about one metre). It should be noted that the user of a hearing aid is free to adjust the overall gain via the volume control on the aid. Hence, the main point of prescriptive rules, including NAL(R), is to select an appropriate shape for the frequency-gain characteristic. However, the NAL(R) formula prescribes a gain that is intended to correspond to the average gain actually used.

Although the various prescriptive rules do lead to different frequency-gain characteristics for a given hearing-impaired person, it has proved surprisingly difficult to demonstrate differences between the rules in terms of resulting speech recognition scores; for a review see Humes (1991). In any case, it should be realised that the goal of amplifying all bands of speech to the MCL could only be realised in practice for one specific speaker talking at one specific level. The long-term average spectrum of speech can vary markedly from one speaker to another. Also, the average shape of the speech spectrum for a given talker varies with vocal effort; a higher vocal effort leads to relatively more high-frequency emphasis. Thus, at best, a prescriptive rule can give a frequency-gain characteristic that will be appropriate for 'typical' listening situations encountered by the user. In practice, it is often necessary to do some 'fine tuning' of a hearing aid around the frequency-gain characteristic recommended by a given rule.

There are several factors that limit the usefulness of linear amplification in hearing aids. Firstly, it is often difficult or impossible to select an aid, or adjust an aid, so that its frequency-gain characteristic exactly matches the recommended one. A common problem is inadequate gain at high frequencies relative to low or medium frequencies. This is a particular problem when fitting people with hearing losses that increase rapidly at high frequencies. Nowadays, it has become relatively common to check the real-ear gain of hearing aids using a probe-tube microphone whose tip is placed inside the ear canal, close to the eardrum. This can reveal 'errors' in fitting which can then sometimes be reduced by modifications to the aid or to the 'plumbing', for example by changing the tubing leading from a behind-the-ear aid to the earmould. However, even after such modifications, the obtained frequency-gain characteristic may differ substantially from the one recommended by a prescriptive rule.

A second problem with linear amplification is connected with the gain selected by the user (i.e. the volume control setting) in everyday listening situations. There is evidence that the selected gain is often small, and certainly smaller than recommended by rules such as NAL(R) (Leijon 1989). In many cases, the gain is probably insufficient to ensure audibility of speech at normal conversational levels over a wide frequency range. Low gains are probably selected because the user wishes to avoid unpleasantly loud sounds, or to avoid the distortion associated with peak clipping. In my laboratory we have found that, under conditions where subjects are sure that they will not be exposed to any unexpected loud or unpleasant sounds, they will elect to use rather high gains, sometimes twice a great as those recommended by the NAL(R) formula. This can lead to better intelligibility than when lower gains are used. However, people do not use such high gains in everyday life. One may conclude that, in practice, the gain provided by linear hearing aids is usually less than would be required to provide optimum speech intelligibility.

A third problem with linear hearing aids is that users often find it necessary to adjust the volume control to deal with different listening situations. The overall level of speech and other sounds can vary considerably from one situation to another (Pearsons *et al.* 1976), and people with cochlear damage do not have sufficient dynamic range to deal with this. However, adjustment of the volume control can be difficult, especially for elderly people who may have limited manual dexterity, and placing a hand near the aid changes the acoustical conditions and may induce feedback (see below for details). This situation has been somewhat improved by the introduction of hearing aids with remote control of volume, although such aids are not in widespread use. Even with remote control, the need to adjust the volume control frequently is irksome.

On the positive side, linear hearing aids can have beneficial effects other than restoring audibility. Consider, as an example, a person with a 'flat' hearing loss. Most prescriptive rules would recommend a gain that increased with frequency up to about 1 kHz, and flattened off above that. The variation in gain with frequency is partly introduced to allow for the fact that the long-term average spectrum of speech typically slopes downwards for frequencies above about 500 Hz. The reduced gain below 1 kHz has the beneficial effect of reducing upward spread of masking (the masking of medium and high frequencies by lower frequencies). This is important since many environmental sounds (e.g. car noise) have most of their energy at low frequencies, and since many hearing-impaired people are particularly susceptible to the upward spread of masking (see chapter 2).

Some general problems with hearing aids

This section briefly discusses some problems that are inherent to most hearing aids, whether linear or not.

Feedback

Feedback occurs when the sound generated by a hearing aid leaks back to the microphone of the aid and sets up a self-sustaining oscillation. It is usually heard as a 'whistling' sound. It occurs when the gain from the microphone to the hearing aid receiver (the part that generates the sound) is greater than the acoustical attenuation in the feedback path from the receiver to the microphone. Feedback is usually unpleasant to listen to, and it may be accompanied by considerable distortion. In practice, feedback often limits the amount of gain that can be used in a hearing aid, especially at high frequencies. Sometimes, the user of an aid does not hear feedback (for example, when it occurs at a high frequency where the audiometric loss may be severe), but becomes embarassed about wearing the aid because they are aware that others can hear the feedback.

Feedback can be reduced in a number of ways. One way is to improve the seal of the aid or earmould to the ear canal, so that less sound leaks from the receiver to the microphone. This can be done by making a better-fitting aid or mould, or by smearing the ear canal with a substance like petroleum jelly before inserting the aid. A second way is to increase the distance between the microphone and the receiver. Generally, feedback is a greater problem with in-the-ear aids than with behind-the-ear aids. Feedback can be reduced considerably if the microphone is some distance from the receiver, as is possible, for example, with chest-worn aids. However, if the microphone is not worn on the head, sound localization may be markedly impaired (see chapter 6). A third way of reducing feedback is by smoothing the frequency response of the aid. Feedback usually occurs at one specific frequency where there is a peak in the frequency-gain characteristic, or in the response of the transmission path from the ear canal to the microphone, or both. If the frequency-gain characteristic is smoothed, then the overall gain can often be increased before feedback starts again. The frequency response can be smoothed either by electronic filtering or by modifications to the earmould and tubing, for example by the use of acoustic resistors.

There is one commercial hearing aid, the 'Danavox DFS Genius' which achieves feedback reduction in a very different way, using digital signal processing. It adds a small amount of white noise to the amplified microphone signal, and uses this to estimate the characteristics of the feedback path from the receiver to the microphone. It then constructs a digital filter which partially cancels the feedback signal. This system typically allows an increase in high-frequency gain of about 10 dB before feedback occurs. A drawback of the system is that the added white noise may be audible and have disturbing effects. The noise is typically added at a level 12 to 18 dB below the level of the speech signal, and its level changes as the speech level changes. However, this aid is mainly intended for people with severe or profound losses, who typically have a very small dynamic range. For these people, the added noise is usually barely audible, but the 10-dB extra gain can be very beneficial in improving audibility.

Peakiness of frequency response

The frequency response of a hearing aid on a real ear often shows two or three distinct peaks caused by resonances in the acoustical delivery system. This is especially true for behind-the-ear aids. It is usually possible to reduce these peaks, smoothing the overall frequency response, by suitable modifications to the tubing and/or by the use of acoustic resistors (dampers) (Libby 1981; Killion 1982). It is now widely accepted that the frequency response should be smoothed in this way as far as possible. While one study showed no significant differences in judged clarity and pleasantness between hearing aids with unsmoothed and smoothed responses (Cox and Gilmore 1986), most other studies have shown that hearing aids with smoothed frequency responses are preferred (Libby 1981; Mertz 1982; Dillon and Macrae 1984). For a review see Bornstein and Randolph (1983).

In any case, there are at least three benefits of smoothing the frequency response other than effects of sound quality. Firstly, smoothing the response can reduce acoustic feedback, as described above. Secondly, smoothing the response can reduce the distortion that often occurs at frequencies around peaks in the response. Finally, smoothing the response can allow a greater proportion of the speech spectrum to be above threshold before the uncomfortable loudness level is reached.

In spite of these good reasons for smoothing the frequency response, in clinical practice measures to smooth the frequency response are often not taken. This happens either because of ignorance or laziness on the part of the hearing-aid dispenser, or from the mistaken belief of the dispenser that there is no benefit in smoothing the response. It is to be hoped that this state of affairs will improve in the coming years, especially with the increasing use of real-ear probe tube measurement systems.

It should be noted that the acoustical delivery system can be important in other ways. The overall response of an aid at the eardrum can be markedly altered by changes in the tubing or by venting (introducing a small hole in the earmould). For example, the gain at high frequencies can be increased by 6–10 dB by using tubing whose bore increases progressively from the receiver to the inside end of the earmould (Libby 1982). It is unfortunate that many dispensers of hearing aids do not make full use of the opportunities that this provides for extending the effective frequency range of a hearing aid and for tailoring the frequency response to match a target.

The occlusion effect

People who wear hearing aids often complain that their own voice sounds unnatural, being excessively loud and 'hollow' sounding. This is sometimes called the 'occlusion effect'. The effect occurs when an earmould is worn that blocks the entrance to the ear canal. The sound of the person's own voice is transmitted through the bones of the head into the ear canal (meatus). The transmission occurs mainly through the flexible (cartilaginous) outer part of the ear canal. When the ear canal is blocked, the sound cannot escape, and the resulting sound pressure at the eardrum is markedly higher than would occur for an unblocked ear. Killion *et al.* (1988), using a probe tube microphone, showed that sound levels exceeding 90 dB SPL could occur for certain speech sounds such as /a/ as in 'car'.

The traditional way of alleviating the occlusion effect is to vent the earmould, by drilling a small hole through it. However, this can lead to acoustic feedback. Indeed, feedback often limits the size of the vent that can be used, so that the occlusion effect remains a significant problem. This is especially so in cases of near-normal low-frequency hearing with moderate or severe hearing loss at high frequencies, as is common in elderly people. The large vent that would be required to alleviate the occlusion effect would prevent the aid from providing adequate gain at high frequencies.

Recently, a new solution to this problem has emerged, based on some observations by Zwislocki (1953). He showed that the transmission of bone-conducted sound into the ear canal was much less when an earplug was inserted deeply into the ear canal than when it was inserted only into the flexible outer part. The inner part of the ear canal is composed of rigid bone, which accounts for the reduced transmission. Zwislocki's observations have been confirmed by Killion *et al.* (1988) who showed that the sound level in the ear canal produced by a person's own voice could be reduced by as much as 20 dB at low frequencies by using a deeply seated earplug or earmould, as compared to a shallow one.

In the case of hearing aids, the occlusion effect can be markedly reduced either by using an aid that is fitted deeply inside the ear canal (all-in-the-ear devices), or by using an earmould that extends deeply into the ear canal. This means that a 'deep' ear impression has to be taken, which is difficult and may require special techniques. However, users of hearing aids which fit deeply inside the ear canal do report that their own voices sound much more natural.

A completely different solution to this problem is offered by the 'Earlens' system currently being developed by the ReSound Corporation in the USA. A small but powerful magnet is embedded in a flexible plastic disc, the Earlens, which is somewhat smaller than a contact lens and is made to fit on the eardrum of the user. The eardrum is sprayed with mineral oil and the Earlens is placed on the eardrum by a medically qualified person; it adheres to the eardrum by surface tension and can remain in place indefinitely if a small amount of mineral oil is sprayed into the ear about once a week. The sound picked up by a microphone is amplified, filtered and compressed (if desired) and is then fed to a coil. The current passing through the coil creates a magnetic field that causes the magnet in the Earlens to move, which in turn moves the eardrum, creating a sensation of sound. The coil can be worn around the neck, or placed closer to the Earlens, for example, in the ear canal.

With this system, the ear canal remains open, so the occlusion effect simply does not occur. Hence, the user's own voice sounds natural. Other advantages of this system are that feedback is not a problem, and the sound quality is good because the frequency response is smooth and distortion is low. However, the system is only suitable for people with mild to moderate hearing losses; its gain is limited, especially at high frequencies.

The use of compression to compensate for reduced dynamic range

Linear amplification does not provide an effective way of dealing with the reduced dynamic range of people with cochlear hearing loss; with linear amplification it is not possible to restore audibility of weak sounds without intense sounds being over-amplified and becoming uncomfortably loud. It was suggested many years ago that this problem could be alleviated by the use of automatic gain control (AGC) (Steinberg and Gardner 1937). With AGC, it is possible to amplify weak sounds more than stronger ones, with the result that the wide dynamic range of the input signal is compressed into a smaller dynamic range at the output. Hence AGC systems are also called 'compressors'. Although this idea sounds simple, in practice there are many ways of implementing AGC, and there is still no clear consensus as to the 'best' method, if there is such a thing. There is also considerable controversy about the efficacy of AGC systems. To understand why things are not so simple, it is helpful first to consider some of the basic characteristics of AGC systems.

Basic characteristics of AGC systems

An AGC amplifier is an amplifier whose gain (output divided by input) is controlled by a feedback voltage. The voltage is derived either from the input to the amplifier or from its output. Essentially, the gain is reduced as the input level is increased. Most AGC amplifiers act as linear amplifiers for inputs below a certain level. Over the range where the amplifier is linear, the output is directly proportional to the input. If the output level in decibels is plotted as a function of the input level in decibels, the result is a straight line with a slope of one. Once the input level exceeds a certain value, the gain is reduced, and the slope of the line becomes less than one. This is illustrated by the input–output function in Figure 8.1. The compression

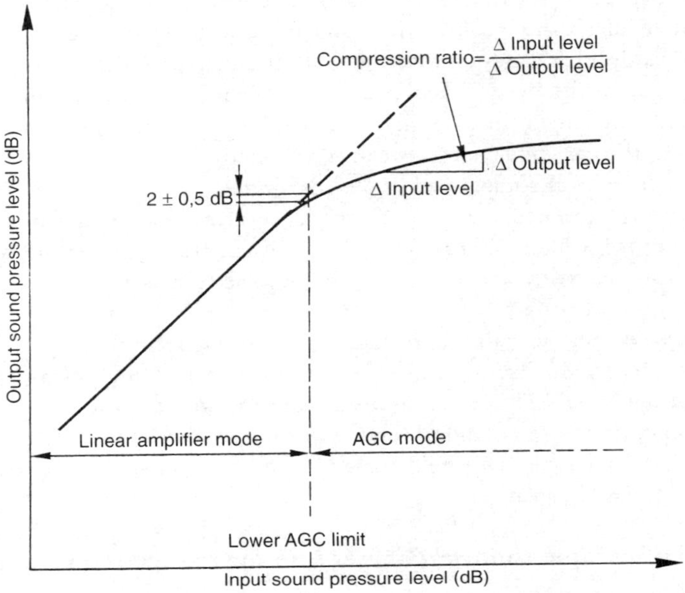

Fig. 8.1. An input–output function for an automatic gain control (AGC) system. The output in decibels is plotted as a function of the input in decibels.

threshold is defined as the input level at which the gain is reduced by two decibels, relative to the gain that would be produced by linear amplification.

The 'amount' of compression is specified by the compression ratio, which is the change in input level (in decibels) required to achieve a one-decibel change in output level (once the compression threshold is exceeded); the compression ratio is equal to the reciprocal of the slope of the input–output function in the range where the AGC is operating. For example, a compression ratio of three would mean that the output would grow by one decibel for each three decibels increase in input level.

AGC amplifiers vary in how fast they react to changes in input sound level. Typically, the speed of response is measured by using as an input a sound whose level changes abruptly between two values, normally 55 dB SPL and 80 dB SPL. When the sound level abruptly increases, the gain decreases, but this takes time to occur. Hence the output of the amplifier shows an initial 'spike' or 'overshoot', followed by a decline to a steady value. This is illustrated in Figure 8.2. The time taken for the output to get within two decibels of its steady value is called the attack time, and is labelled t_a in Figure 8.2. When the sound level abruptly decreases, the gain increases, but again this takes time to occur. Hence the output of the amplifier shows an initial dip, followed by an increase to a steady value. The time taken for the output to increase to within two decibels of its steady value is called the recovery time or release time, and is labelled t_r in Figure 8.2.

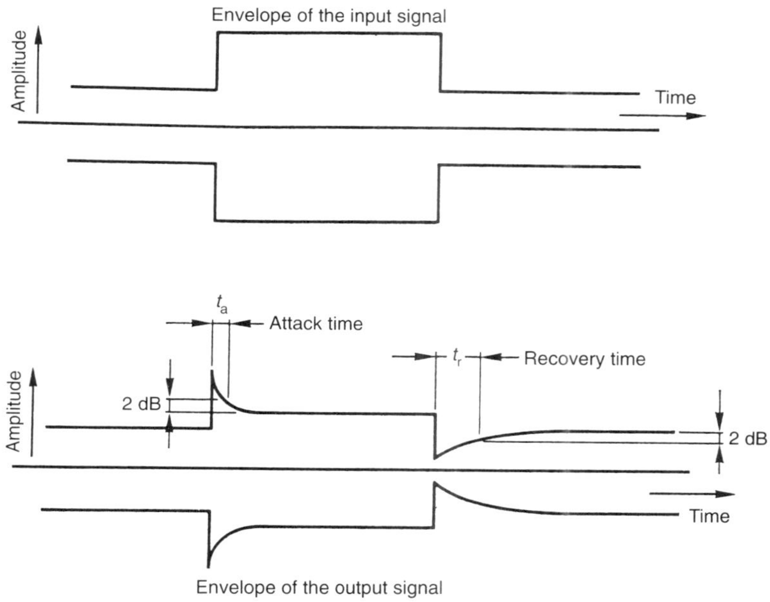

Fig. 8.2. Illustration of the temporal response of an AGC system. The envelope of the input signal is shown at the top. The envelope of the response of the system is shown at the bottom.

Varieties of AGC systems

AGC systems have been designed in many different forms, mostly on the basis of different rationales or design goals. For reviews see Moore (1990) and Hickson (1994). This section briefly decribes some of the different types.

Some systems are intended to adjust the gain automatically for different listening situations. Essentially, they are intended to relieve the user of the need to adjust the volume control to deal with these situations. Usually, such systems change their gain slowly with changes in sound level; this is achieved by making t_r, or t_r and t_a, relatively long (usually t_r is a few hundred milliseconds). These systems are often referred to as 'automatic volume control' (AVC). Although it is generally accepted that AVC can be useful, relatively few commercial hearing aids incorporate AVC. Some reasons for this are discussed below.

AGC is often used primarily to limit the maximum output of hearing aids, to prevent discomfort and/or circuit overload at high input sound levels. The compression ratio is usually very large and the compression threshold is usually relatively high. Such systems are known as 'compression limiters'. Compression limiters usually have a small value of t_a (1–10 ms) so as to respond rapidly to sudden increases in sound level. The recovery time, t_r, is also usually fairly small (20–100 ms). The function of compression limiters is similar to that of the peak clippers described earlier. However, peak clipping causes unpleasant-sounding distortion whereas the effects of compression limiting are not so noticeable. Hence compression limiters are quite widely used in hearing aids.

An alternative type of compressor, with lower compression ratios and lower compression thresholds, has been used in hearing aids in attempts to make the hearing-impaired person's perception of loudness more like that of a normal listener and to ensure that the weaker consonant sounds of speech will be audible without the more intense sounds (e.g. vowels) becoming uncomfortably loud. Such compressors usually have short time constants (typically 20–100 ms) and are often referred to as 'syllabic compressors', since the gain changes over times comparable to the durations of individual syllables.

Several authors (Villchur 1973; Mangold and Leijon 1979; Laurence *et al.* 1983) have proposed that syllabic compression should be applied separately in two or more frequency bands. There are at least two reasons why this might be beneficial. First, the amount of hearing loss, and usually the amount of recruitment, often varies markedly with frequency; typically, hearing loss and recruitment are both greater at high frequencies than at low. Hence, the amount of compression needed varies with frequency, and this requires that compression be applied independently in more than one band. A second reason is that relatively weak high-frequency components in speech (e.g. k, p, t), which can be important for intelligibility, are often accompanied by, or follow rapidly after, relatively intense low-frequency components. The use of fast-acting AGC in two or more separate bands can ensure that these weak high-frequency components are always audible.

Another rationale for the use of multi-band compression, as opposed to single-band (broad-band) compression is to reduce the effects of interfering sounds (Ono *et al.* 1983; van Dijkhuizen *et al.* 1991; Rankovic *et al.* 1992). Consider a hypothetical situation where a hearing-impaired person is trying to understand speech in the presence of an intense narrowband noise. A broad-band AGC system would reduce its gain in response to the intense noise, thereby reducing the audibility of the speech. A multi-band AGC system would reduce the gain only in the frequency region of the noise, reducing the masking effect and loudness of the noise without affecting the audibility of the parts of the speech spectrum remote from the frequency of the noise. Van Dijkhuizen *et al.* (1991) have argued that the gain in such systems should change slowly with time (i.e. t_a and t_r should be large, at least several hundred milliseconds).

Several commercial hearing aids incorporate a crude form of multi-band AGC based on this rationale. Usually, they have only two bands, and the gain in the low-frequency band is reduced when the input level exceeds a certain value. These aids, which are sometimes misleadingly called 'automatic signal processing' (ASP) aids, are based on the assumption that most intense environmental sounds have their energy concentrated at low frequencies. Reduction of low-frequency gain can, in principle, reduce the upward spread of masking from this noise. Evaluations of such aids have given mixed results. Where benefits have been found, they can probably be attributed at least partly to the fact that the ASP circuit reduces distortion that would otherwise be present at the output of the aids for high input sound levels (van Tasell and Crain 1992).

Research on the efficacy of multi-band compression

Research on the efficacy of multi-band compression has given somewhat conflicting results. The conflict arises partly from differences in the way that the compression systems have been implemented (based on different rationales, as described above) and partly on differences in methods of evaluation. Individual differences between the subjects used may also have played a role. Plomp (1988) has argued that fast-acting compression in multi-channel systems has deleterious effects, because it reduces spectral contrasts and it reduces the temporal modulation of the speech signal, which may carry useful information. He argued that slow-acting AGC (long attack and recovery times) should be more effective. However, his arguments apply mainly to systems using a large number of bands and large amounts of compression. Villchur (1989) has presented counter arguments to those of Plomp (1988), and has pointed out that in practice the amount of compression used is generally considerably less than that assumed by Plomp in his arguments.

Comprehensive reviews of results using multi-channel compression have been provided by Braida *et al.* (1982) and by Hickson (1994). Hickson surveyed 21 studies of multi-channel compression and noted that ten of the studies provided evidence for benefits of the compression. Some general trends can be discerned from the results:

(1) For speech in quiet, benefits of compression have often been found, in a variety of systems, when the speech materials used have covered a wide range of levels, as occurs in everyday life (Villchur 1973; Lippmann *et al.* 1981; Laurence *et al.* 1983; Moore *et al.* 1985c, 1991, 1992b; Moore and Glasberg 1986a, 1988a; Moore 1987a). When the speech material has been presented at one reasonably high level, and when the speech material has been carefully equalized in level during the recording process (as was the case in many studies), compression does not show benefits over linear amplification (Lippmann *et al.* 1981).

(2) For speech in background noise, benefits of fast-acting compression have sometimes (but not always) been found for systems with a small number of bands (channels) (Villchur 1973; Laurence *et al.* 1983; Moore *et al.* 1985c, 1991, 1992b; Moore and Glasberg 1986a, 1988a; Moore 1987a; Ringdahl *et al.* 1990). Benefits have not usually been found for systems with a large number of bands (Lippmann *et al.* 1981; Bustamante and Braida 1987). Adequate compensation for recruitment can probably be achieved with a small number of bands, say, two or three. There may be a disadvantage in using a large number of bands, since this tends to reduce spectral contrasts in complex stimuli. In a multi-band compression system with many bands, the differences in level between peaks and dips in the spectrum of the input are reduced. If the impaired ear has reduced frequency selectivity, as is often the case (see chapter 2), then the reduction in spectral contrast compounds the difficulties experienced in picking out the spectral features of complex sounds. To avoid this problem, the bands in a compression system should have bandwidths which are broad in comparison to the auditory filters of the impaired listener. In

practice, this means that only a few bands should be used, probably no more than three.

(3) The extent of the benefit of compression for the understanding of speech in noise depends upon how the frequency-gain characteristic was chosen for the control condition using linear amplification. Under laboratory conditions using speech in noise with carefully controlled levels and fixed spectra, it may be possible to use linear amplification to make the speech audible and comfortable over a wide frequency range. Under these conditions there may be little benefit of compression. However, if the linear condition is set up so that speech and/or environmental sounds with reasonably high input levels are not amplified to unpleasantly loud levels, then lower overall gains must be used. Under these conditions, benefits of compression may become apparent, because the compression allows more amplification for weaker sounds while not amplifying intense sounds excessively.

(4) Most (but not all) of the studies showing benefits of compression for listening to speech in noise have used aids that the subjects could wear in their everyday lives. This is important, since if a person has had a hearing impairment for many years, it may take some time for them to learn to use the new cues provided by a compression system (Gatehouse 1992).

The 'Cambridge' system

This section describes a system of automatic gain control which has been developed and improved in a series of studies in my laboratory. The original design was worked out by the late Roger F. Laurence, and the early studies were done in collaboration with him (Laurence *et al.* 1983; Moore *et al.* 1985c; Moore and Glasberg 1986a). However, what is described here is mainly the most recent implementation of the design. It is based on a consideration of the characteristics both of speech and of the impaired auditory system. The basic problem that we set out to solve was: how can the wide dynamic range of speech be 'squeezed' into the smaller dynamic range of the impaired auditory system so as to maximise intelligibility and listening comfort?

The wide dynamic range of speech arises in two ways. Firstly, in everyday situations the overall level of speech may vary over a 35 dB range (Pearsons *et al.* 1976). I refer to this as the long-term dynamic range. Secondly, the levels of individual speech sounds can vary over a range of at least 30 dB (Levitt 1982), even when the average level of the speech is held constant. I refer to this as the short-term dynamic range. Dealing with these two sources of wide dynamic range requires two separate forms of AGC. These are considered in the next two sections.

Compensating for variations in the overall level of speech

As described earlier, variations in the overall level of speech are sometimes dealt with using slow-acting automatic volume control (AVC) systems. However, conventional AVC systems involve a compromise between conflicting requirements. For speech with a fixed average level, the level may fluctuate markedly from moment to moment, and may drop to very low values during brief pauses in the speech. If the gain of an aid changes significantly during the speech itself, or during the pauses in the speech, then 'breathing' or 'pumping' noises may be heard which are objectionable to the user. These effects are particularly marked when moderate levels of background noise are present, as is often the case in everyday situations. In addition, the temporal envelope of the speech may be distorted by the changes in gain. To avoid these problems, the gain should change relatively slowly as a function of time, i.e. t_a and t_r should be long.

On the other hand, it is important to protect the user from sudden intense sounds, such as a door slamming or a cup being dropped. This requires the gain to change much more rapidly. This problem is usually dealt with by having an AVC system with a fast attack time (t_a in the range 1–10 ms), and a longer recovery time (t_r in the range 300–2000 ms). The fast attack time provides protection against sudden increases in sound level, but such a system has the disadvantage that the gain of the aid drops to a low value immediately after an intense transient; the aid effectively goes 'dead' for a while. A further problem is that a recovery time of a few hundred ms is not sufficiently long to prevent breathing sounds from being heard.

We (Moore and Glasberg 1988a; Moore *et al.* 1991) have developed an AVC system which provides a better solution to these problems. This system, referred to as 'dual front-end AGC', is illustrated in Figure 8.3. The signal picked up by the microphone (1) is fed to an AGC amplifier (2) whose gain is determined by a control voltage. There are two control voltage generators (3 and 4). Both of these act in such a way that the amplifier (2) behaves as a 'compression limiter'; it

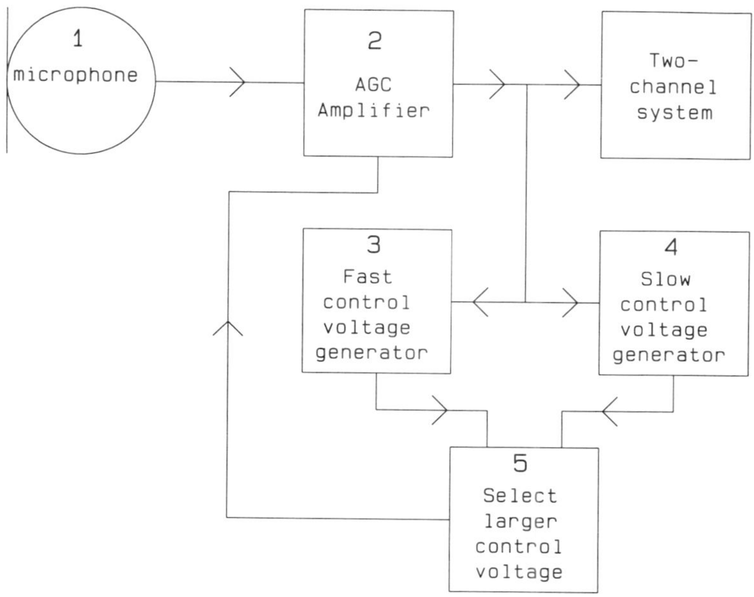

Fig. 8.3. A block diagram of the dual-front-end AGC system.

amplifies without compression for input levels up to a certain compression threshold, and has effectively an infinite compression ratio for levels above that. One of the control voltage generators (4) has a lower compression threshold (about 63 dB SPL) than the other one, and it changes only slowly in response to changes in sound level; in our early work it had an attack time of roughly a few hundred ms and a recovery time of several seconds. Normally, the operation of the AGC amplifier is determined by this slow-acting control voltage. The effect is that the gain changes slowly as the listening situation changes, in a way which is almost unnoticed by the user and which avoids audible breathing noises.

The fast-acting control voltage generator (3) has a compression threshold about 7 dB higher than that of the slower control voltage generator. It has an attack time of a few ms and a recovery time of about 100 ms. Normally it has little effect on the operation of the AGC amplifier. However, if an intense sound suddenly occurs, the fast-acting control voltage increases rapidly. When it exceeds the control voltage generated by (4), it is selected by circuit (5) to control the gain of the amplifier. The gain is rapidly reduced, thus protecting the user from over-amplification of the intense sound. However, the fast-acting control voltage decreases rapidly following the cessation of the intense sound, and control returns to the slow-acting control voltage. If the intense sound is brief, it does not significantly change the value of the slow-acting control voltage. Thus, following an intense transient, the gain returns to the original value determined by the overall level of the speech. In this way, intense transients are selectively attenuated, but the overall gain for the speech is held almost constant, except for a very brief period following the transient. Note that, although the transient is attenuated, it remains clearly audible, and can be identified, for example as a door slamming or cup being dropped.

We have conducted a series of experiments to optimize the time constants of the dual front-end AGC system (Moore *et al.* 1991; Moore 1993). In the initial experiments, the dual front-end AGC was implemented as a laboratory prototype. Later experiments have made use of a chest-worn prototype. The laboratory experiments showed that the optimum value of the recovery time of the fast component is about 80–150 ms and the optimum value of the attack time of the slow component is about 150–325 ms. Using these values, we were able to show significant benefits of the dual front-end AGC system. In situations where intense transient sounds (such as a door slamming or glass being tapped) were present, and there was either no background sound or continuous speech-shaped noise as a background, the dual front-end AGC gave significantly better speech intelligibility than linear amplification.

One significant problem with the dual front-end AGC was encountered in the laboratory experiments. The gain of the front-end AGC system was sometimes reduced as a result of the wearer of the aid talking. With the very long recovery time of the slow component, weak speech following soon after the wearer had been talking was sometimes inaudible. This problem was dealt with by making two changes in the design of the front-end AGC. Firstly, the input signal was subjected to high-frequency emphasis prior to generation of the slow-acting control signal. This reduced the contribution of the subject's own voice to the control signal.

Secondly, the recovery of the slow component was itself given two components: a hold-off time during which the gain did not change at all, and a recovery time following the end of the hold-off time. During pauses in speech shorter than the hold-off time, the gain did not change.

To assess the optimum values of the hold-off time and the recovery time, a field trial was conducted using a chest-worn prototype aid. Various values of the hold-off time and recovery times could be selected by the user via switches on the aid. Six subjects, all of whom had moderate sensorineural hearing loss, were asked to try out different combinations of the hold-off time and recovery time in different listening situations in everyday life, and to keep a diary noting which settings they preferred. The preferred hold-off time was either 0.375 seconds or 0.75 seconds, with most subjects preferring 0.75 seconds. The choice of recovery times varied more widely across subjects, but most were happy with a recovery time of 0.42 seconds. Note that the combined value of the hold-off and recovery times of about 1.2 seconds is much shorter than the original recovery time of several seconds, but the new system is still successful in avoiding audible pumping sounds.

Overall, the results indicate that the dual front-end AGC does achieve its design goals: it allows speech to be understood over a wide range of sound levels without any need to adjust the controls of the aid; it selectively reduces the gain for intense transients without affecting the long-term gain for speech; and it changes the gain in such a way that breathing and pumping noises are not audible. The reactions of users in the field trial were highly favourable.

Compensating for variations in the levels of individual speech sounds

Even when speech is presented at a constant average level, individual acoustic elements within the speech may vary over a range of at least 30 dB (Levitt 1982); see chapter 7. This short-term range may exceed the dynamic range available to the listener, especially at high frequencies, where the range of sound levels over which sounds are both clearly heard and comfortably loud may be as small as 10 dB, or even less. To deal with this problem it is necessary to use fast-acting AGC; the gain has to change rapidly from one speech sound to the next, so that weak sounds can be amplified more than intense sounds.

Moore and Glasberg (1988a) showed that if the dual front-end AGC was combined with a two-band system, then it was not necessary to apply fast acting compression in both bands; compression only in the upper band was sufficient. This probably happened because, when the overall level of speech was held at its optimum value by the front-end AGC, their hearing-impaired subjects had sufficient dynamic range at low frequencies not to require additional compression. However, this may not be true of all hearing-impaired persons, especially those with large hearing losses at low frequencies. Moore and Glasberg found that the two-channel system with fast-acting compression in the high-frequency band gave lower SRTs for speech in speech-shaped noise than a two-channel system in which the fast-acting compression was by-passed. In other words, the fast-acting compression led to improved speech intelligibility in noise.

It should be noted that the fast-acting compression used in this system was of the compression-limiting type. It remains unclear whether this is the 'best' form of compression to use. Compression with a smaller compression ratio and a lower compression threshold, such as used in the study of Moore *et al.* (1992b) may be more appropriate. However, when the overall level of the speech is held constant, the results of these two forms of compression are not greatly different (Stone and Moore 1992b).

Any form of fast-acting AGC inevitably distorts the temporal envelope of speech. Thus, the amount of compression applied in this way should be the minimum necessary to ensure audibility. In systems without a front-end AGC *all* of the compression is done using fast-acting (channel) AGC. In our system, less channel compression is needed, since the front-end AGC compensates for variations in the overall level of speech. Thus, our system gives less distortion of the temporal envelope of the speech. By using a front-end AGC, we ensure that the compression limiting operates only on speech peaks above a certain level relative to the mean level (in a given channel). For example, the limiting may be set to occur for peaks more than 4 dB above the mean level, meaning that compression occurs over a range of about 8 dB. The remaining 22 dB of short-term dynamic range (from 4 dB above the mean to 18 dB below it) is amplified linearly. If a front-end AGC were not used, the limiting would operate over a variable part of the short-term dynamic range of the speech depending on the overall input level of the speech. For speech with a high overall input level, limiting would occur over the whole short-term dynamic range of the speech, and this would almost certainly impair intelligibility (Bustamante and Braida 1987).

General conclusions about compression

It appears that compression can be beneficial in two ways. Firstly, it can allow speech in quiet to be understood over a wide range of sound levels without adjustment of the volume control and without the speech ever becoming uncomfortably loud. This can be achieved either by using a slow-acting front-end AGC (Moore *et al.* 1991) or by using multi-channel syllabic compression (Moore *et al.* 1992b). Secondly, it can improve the intelligibility of speech in background noise. This only seems to occur when fast-acting compression is used in a small number of bands and when the gain in the control condition with linear amplification is chosen realistically (to reflect the gain that would be usable in everyday life). The improvement is generally small, amounting to a 1–3 dB reduction in the SRT in noise, but it is nevertheless worthwhile. There is some reason to believe that larger benefits might be obtained with a background sound of a single talker as opposed to the speech-shaped noise that has been used in many studies (Moore *et al.* 1995).

There is little evidence to support the idea that the benefits of compression accrue from restoring the perception of loudness to 'normal'. Indeed, if fast-acting compression is set up to do this, hearing aid users complain that everything sounds too 'noisy'. In practice, the aids must be set up so as to 'under-compensate' for the loudness recruitment. Compression sufficient to restore loudness perception to 'normal' appears to have deleterious effects on speech intelligibility and is not liked by users (Moore *et al.* 1992c; Plomp 1994). It seems likely that the benefits of compression arise mainly from the fact that compression increases audibility while avoiding discomfort from loud sounds.

Attempts to improve speech intelligibility using spectral enhancement

Based on the evidence reviewed in chapter 7, it seems likely that impaired frequency selectivity is at least partly responsible for the reduced ability of people with cochlear hearing loss to understand speech in noise, although this causal link has not been universally accepted (Havens and Geisler 1991). Linear amplification and multi-band compression do not compensate for the effects of reduced frequency selectivity, although high-frequency emphasis can partially alleviate upward spread of masking. This section considers some forms of signal processing that attempt to compensate for reduced frequency selectivity. Such signal-processing is not yet available in wearable hearing aids, but it may become available within the next few years as digital-signal-processing (DSP) chips become more powerful while consuming less current.

One mechanism by which impaired frequency selectivity could affect the identification of speech in noise involves the perception of spectral shape. Broader auditory filters produce a more highly smoothed representation of the spectrum (the excitation pattern) than normal auditory filters (see Figures 7.3 and 7.4). If spectral features are not sufficiently prominent, they may be smoothed to such an extent that they become imperceptible. Adding a noise background to speech fills in the valleys between the spectral peaks and thus reduces their prominence, exacerbating the problem of perceiving them for people with broadened auditory filters.

A second possible effect of reduced frequency selectivity on speech perception in noise is connected with the temporal patterns at the outputs of individual auditory filters. The perceived frequency of a given formant and/or the fundamental frequency of voicing may be partly determined by the time pattern at the outputs of the auditory filters tuned close to the formant frequency (Young and Sachs 1979; Rosen and Fourcin 1986). Background noise disturbs this time pattern, which may lead to reduced accuracy in determining these frequencies. This effect would be greater in people with reduced frequency selectivity, since broader filters generally pass more background noise.

If reduced frequency selectivity impairs speech perception, then enhancement of spectral contrasts (magnifying the differences between peaks and dips in the spectrum) might improve it for the hearing-impaired person. Either of the two mechanisms outlined above, one based on degradation of spectral shape and the other on degradation of temporal patterns, provides a rationale for performing spectral enhancement. If spectral features are smoothed by an impaired auditory system, then preprocessing the signal to enhance spectral contrasts can produce an excitation pattern that more nearly resembles the excitation pattern evoked by an unprocessed signal in a normal auditory system. If temporal patterns are disturbed by the noise passing through a broadened auditory filter, then enhancing those portions of the spectrum where the signal-to-noise ratio is highest (the peaks) and supressing those portions where it is lowest (the valleys) should minimize this effect.

Several authors have described attempts to improve speech intelligibility for the hearing impaired by enhancement of spectral features. Boers (1980) processed a set of sentences so as to increase the level differences between peaks and valleys in the spectrum. Noise was added after the processing, and the effects of the processing were assessed by measuring the speech-to-noise ratio required for 50% of the words to be understood. Overall, the processing reduced intelligibility, although two impaired listeners did show a slight improvement with the processed signals. Even if it had systematically improved intelligibility, this kind of processing would not be feasible with naturally occurring signals; with these the speech would already be contaminated with noise, and the processing would have to operate on the speech-plus-noise.

Summerfield *et al.* (1985) synthesised 'whispered' speech sounds, and investigated the effect of narrowing the bandwidths of the formants used in synthesis. Narrowing these bandwidths led to both sharper spectral peaks and greater peak-to-valley ratios. However, it had only small effects on speech intelligibility; identification of consonants at the end of syllables tended to be slightly better for both normal and impaired listeners when the formant bandwidths were half their nominal normal values. Speech intelligibility in noise was not tested.

Simpson *et al.* (1990) described a method of digital signal processing of speech in noise so as to increase differences in level between peaks and valleys in the spectrum. The processing involved manipulation of the short-term spectrum of the speech in noise. Sampled segments of the signal were windowed, smoothed, spectrally enhanced, and then resynthesized using the overlap-add technique (Allen 1977). The steps in the processing are illustrated in Figure 8.4. A 12.8-ms segment of the speech in noise was weighted with a 12.8-ms Hamming window. This had the effect of tapering the amplitude of the segment towards zero at the edges of the segment. The segment was padded with zeros at the start and zeros at the end; this was done to allow for the fact that the duration of the segment can be increased when the spectrum is manipulated. A 256-point fast Fourier transform (FFT) of the windowed segment was calculated, giving the magnitude and phase at 128 frequencies. The phase values were stored and subsequent operations were carried out only on the magnitude spectrum.

To avoid enhancing spectral details that would be undetectable even for a normal ear, the magnitude spectrum was transformed to an auditory excitation pattern, using a procedure similar to that described in chapter 2. This involved calculating the output of an array of simulated auditory filters in response to the magnitude spectrum. As a result of this calculation, the original 128 magnitude values were replaced with 128 new values, representing a smoothed version of the original spectrum. The smoothing tended to remove minor irregularities in the spectrum, but to preserve peaks corresponding to major spectral prominences in the speech.

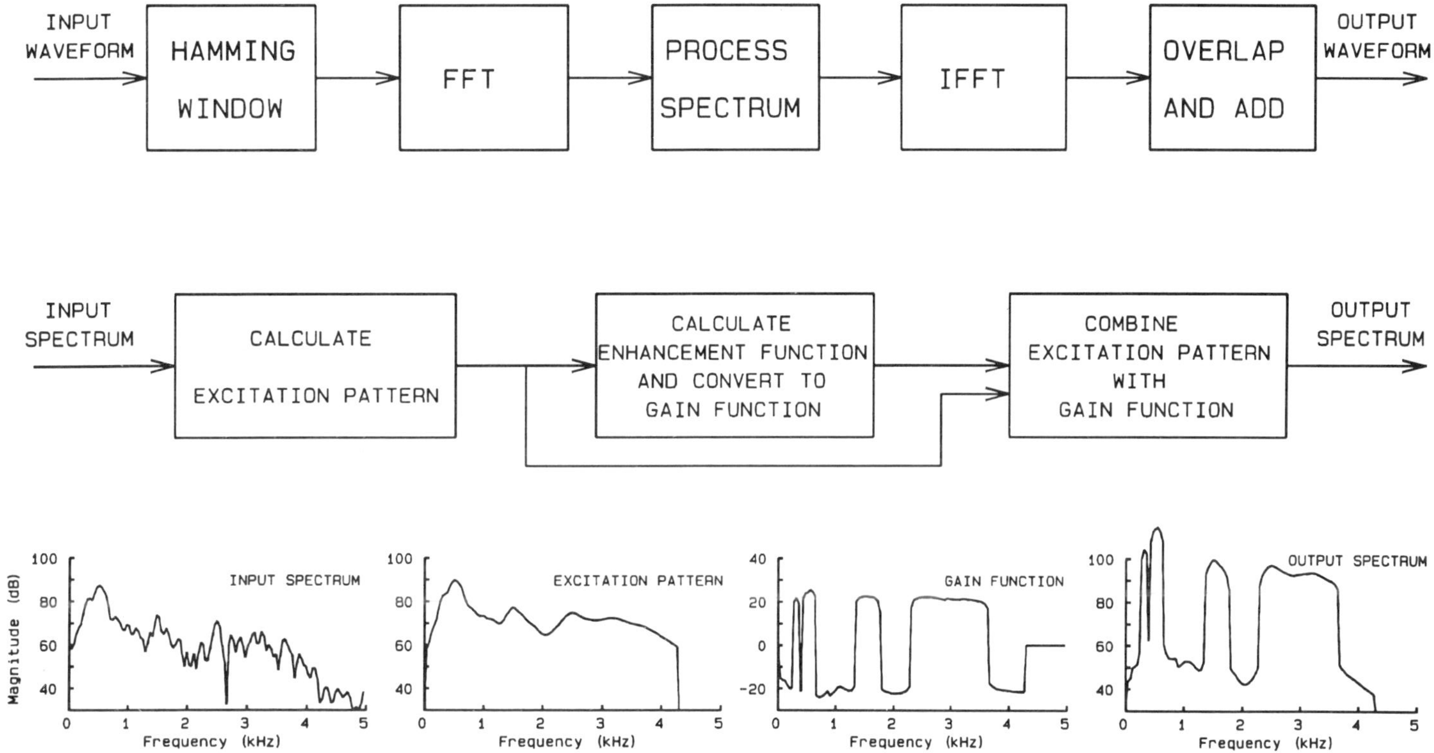

Fig. 8.4. Schematic diagram of the sequence of stages involved in the spectral enhancement processing of Simpson *et al.* (1990). The top row shows all stages of the processing. The middle row shows the stage "process spectrum" in more detail. The bottom row shows an example of the spectral processing for a particular segment.

The next stage was to enhance contrast in the excitation pattern. An enhancement function was derived from the excitation pattern using a difference-of-Gaussians (DoG) function. This function is the sum of a positive Gaussian and a negative Gaussian that has twice the width of the positive Gaussian. The width of the DoG function increased with increasing centre frequency according to the ERB scale described in chapter 2; the idea here was to enhance spectral features on a frequency scale that was relevant to the operation of the normal auditory system.

The DoG function was centred on the frequency of each of the 128 magnitude values of the excitation pattern in turn. For a given centre frequency of the DoG function, the value of the excitation pattern at each frequency (in linear power units) was multiplied by the value of the DoG function at that same frequency, and the products obtained in this way were summed. The magnitude value of the excitation pattern at that centre frequency was then replaced by that sum.

The enhancement function derived in this way was then used to modify the excitation pattern. At centre frequencies where the enhancement function was positive, the excitation pattern was increased in magnitude, and at centre frequencies where the enhancement function was negative, the excitation pattern was decreased in magnitude.

The magnitude values from the enhanced excitation pattern, expressed in linear amplitude units, were then combined with the original phase values and an inverse FFT was used to produce a 25.6-ms segment of spectrally enhanced speech in noise. This process was repeated, and the resultant overlapping segments were summed to give a complete processed waveform. In summary, the processing had the effect of enhancing spectral contrast in the magnitude spectrum while preserving the phase spectrum.

Simpson *et al.* (1990) measured the intelligibility of the speech in speech-shaped noise using subjects with moderate cochlear hearing loss. The results showed small but reasonably consistent improvements in speech intelligibility for the processed speech, typically of 6–7%.

Stone and Moore (1992a) described a speech-processing system similar to that used by Simpson *et al.* (1990), but one that was simpler, and based on analogue electronics running in real time, using a 16-channel band-pass filter bank. Each channel generated an 'activity function' that was proportional to the magnitude of the signal envelope in that channel, averaged over a short period of time. A positively weighted activity function from the nth channel was combined with negatively weighted functions from channels $n-2$, $n-1$, $n+1$, and $n+2$, giving a correction signal used to control the gain of the band-pass signal in the nth channel. Recombining the band-pass signals resulted in a signal with enhanced spectral contrast. Two different experiments were described, the first using the activity function as described, and the second using a non-linear transform of the activity function. In both experiments several different weighting patterns were used in calculating the correction signal. The intelligibility of speech in speech-shaped noise processed by the system was measured for subjects with moderate sensorineural hearing loss. In both experiments no improvement in intelligibility was found. However, subjective ratings of the stimuli used in the second experiment indicated that some subjects judged the processed stimuli to have both higher quality and higher intelligibility than unprocessed stimuli.

Bunnell (1990) described a method of digital signal processing to enhance spectral contrasts. Contrasts were enhanced mainly at middle frequencies, leaving high and low frequencies relatively unaffected. Unlike the processing used by Simpson *et al.* (1990) and by Stone and Moore (1992a), the enhancement was performed on a spectral envelope that was calculated with a linear frequency scale rather than a scale reflecting auditory frequency selectivity. Small improvements were found in the identification of stop consonants (p, t, k, b, d, g) presented in quiet to subjects with sloping hearing losses. No measurements of the intelligibility of speech in noise were reported.

Baer *et al.* (1993) carried out an experiment similar to that of Simpson *et al.* (1990), but the amount of enhancement and the bandwidth (in ERBs) of the enhancement processing were systematically varied. Large amounts of enhancement produced decreases in the intelligibility of speech in noise. Performance for moderate degrees of enhancement was generally similar to that for the control condition. This rather disappointing result may have occurred because subjects did not have sufficient experience with the processed speech.

In a second experiment, subjects judged the relative quality and intelligibility of speech in noise processed using a subset of the conditions of the first experiment. Generally, processing with a moderate degree of enhancement was preferred over the control condition, for both quality and intelligibility. Subjects varied in their preferences for high degrees of enhancement.

A third experiment used a modified processing algorithm, with a moderate degree of spectral enhancement, and examined the effects of combining the enhancement with broadband fast-acting compression. The intelligibility of speech in noise improved with practice, and, after a small amount of practice, scores for the condition combining enhancement with a moderate degree of compression were found to be significantly higher than for the control condition.

A problem with most of the experiments described so far on spectral enhancement is that the measure used, the percent correct of words identified, may not have been suitable for revealing all of the effects of the processing. Specifically, the measure probably did not tap the dimension of 'ease of listening', which can be especially important in everyday situations involving decision making and selective attention. Also, because of the limited speech materials available, it was not possible to give much practice in the different processing conditions.

In a fourth experiment, Baer *et al.* addressed these problems by assessing performance using a sentence verification test (SVT) that measured both intelligibility and response times. The SVT can be administered repeatedly, and it includes a measure of response time which is probably related to ease of listening. They evaluated a subset of conditions from the third experiment. The results are illustrated in Figure 8.5. They showed highly significant benefits of the processing, revealed by increases in percent correct and decreases in response times. Spectral enhancement alone was superior to the control condition, and enhancement combined with compression was superior to enhancement alone. When expressed

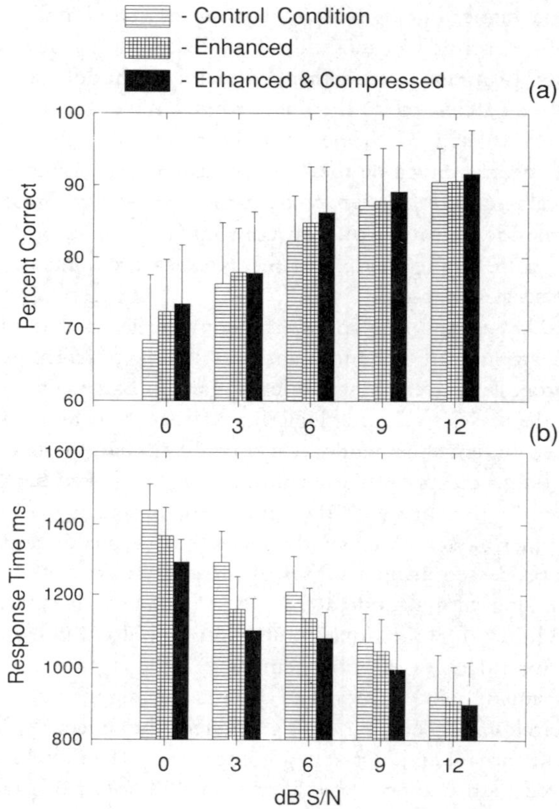

Fig. 8.5. Results of Baer *et al.* (1993) for three conditions: a control condition, a condition using spectral enhancement, and a condition combining spectral enhancement with a moderate degree of compression. Results are shown for several speech-to-noise ratios. The upper panel (a) shows intelligibility scores, and the lower panel (b) shows response times.

in terms of equivalent changes in signal-to-masker ratio, the benefits were about twice as great for the response time measures as for the identification scores, and they were also statistically more robust for the response time measures. This suggests that the major benefits of the processing may be in terms of increased ease of listening rather than in intelligibility. The overall effect of spectral enhancement combined with compression was equivalent to an improvement of speech-to-noise ratio by 4.2 dB.

In summary, studies of the effects of spectral enhancement have given mixed results. Some studies have shown no benefit, while others have shown modest benefits. However, the benefits can show up both in increased intelligibility of speech in noise (percent correct) and in decreased response times. The latter may reflect greater 'ease of listening'. It should be noted that none of the studies on spectral enhancement has used wearable aids. Thus subjects did not have extensive experience listening to the processed stimuli. It seems likely that such experience may be necessary to allow the full benefits of the processing to be measured (Gatehouse 1992).

Methods of improving the speech-to-noise ratio

Directional microphones

One of the few ways of achieving a true improvement in speech-to-noise ratio is to use a directional microphone. Such a microphone is more sensitive to sounds coming from certain directions than to sounds coming from other directions. In the case of a hearing aid microphone, it is assumed that the user will normally face towards the desired sound source, so the microphone is designed to be more sensitive to sounds coming from the front than to sounds coming from the sides or back. In practice the directional pattern is affected by placement of the microphone close to the head, and the direction of maximum sensitivity is displaced somewhat away from straight ahead. The directivity of a microphone is a measure of the sensitivity to sounds from the desired direction relative to the sensitivity to sounds from other directions. In principle, a higher directivity gives a greater improvement in speech-to-noise ratio whenever the noise comes from one or more directions other than the desired direction. However, the beneficial effects of directional microphones are reduced in reverberant rooms, since, in such rooms, some of the interfering sound comes from the frontal direction.

Simple directional microphones have been used in hearing aids for many years. Their directivity has not generally been very high, but they have been found to give worthwhile improvements in the ability to understand speech in noise. In a situation where the speech comes from in front (0° azimuth) and interfering sounds are used at various azimuths, the SRT in noise can be reduced by 2–3 dB compared to what is obtained with omni-directional microphones or unaided listening (Nielsen and Ludvigsen 1978; Laurence *et al.* 1983; Hawkins and Yacullo 1984; Leeuw and Dreschler 1991). This is equivalent to improvements of intelligibility between 20 and 45% in difficult listening situations. Directional microphones can also improve the ability to localize sounds (Leeuw and Dreschler 1991).

Soede *et al.* (1993a,b) have developed and evaluated two microphone arrays with improved directionality. The arrays consist of five microphones which can be mounted either along the front of a pair of spectacles (broadside array) or along the side (endfire array). The microphone signals are combined in such a way as to give high directivity. The arrays were evaluated using 30 normally hearing subjects and 45 hearing-impaired subjects listening to speech coming from the frontal direction. Independent speech-shaped noises were emitted from eight loudspeakers positioned on each side of the subject, and below and above the subject. Initial tests were conducted using one ear only (the other ear being plugged). The results showed that SRTs in noise were substantially decreased (improved) relative to unaided listening or listening with an omni-directional microphone. Both the broadside array and the endfire array led to reductions in SRT averaging about 7 dB.

Subsequent tests using hearing-impaired subjects listening with two endfire arrays showed that SRTs were typically about 2 dB lower for binaural than for monaural listening. This is comparable to the diotic advantage usually found for listening to speech in noise, as described in chapter 6. It can be concluded that this system is very effective in improving the ability to understand speech in background noise. Additional physical measurements indicated that the arrays were also effective in reverberant environments, and would decrease the interfering effects of the reverberation. One drawback with the arrays is their physical size (14 cm for the broadside array and 10 cm for the endfire array), which is necessary to achieve high directionality. However, it is to be hoped that users will accept the large size given the substantial advantages in intelligibility that can be achieved.

Adaptive beamforming

Several researchers have studied systems known as adaptive beamformers (Griffiths and Jim 1982). In principle, such systems resemble directional microphone systems, but they differ from these in two important ways. Firstly, adaptive beamformers use only a small number of microphones, typically two, and these do not have to be widely spaced. Hence the microphone array can be quite compact. Secondly, they adapt to the characteristics of the interfering sounds, so as to remove as much of the interference as possible. Generally, the goal is to preserve sounds coming from in front while removing sounds coming from other directions as much as possible.

The operation of a simple beamformer is illustrated in Figure 8.6. In this example, two microphones are used. One is the primary microphone, which picks up a mixture of the desired signal, usually speech (S), and the background interference (N1). The second microphone, the reference microphone, is intended to pick up mainly the interference. This can be achieved, for example, by using a microphone which responds to sounds from all directions except the frontal direction. Alternatively, a reference signal can be derived from two omnidirectional microphones, equally distant from the desired signal, by subtracting their outputs. The reference signal, which contains a somewhat different version of the noise (N2), is passed through a digital filter whose amplitude and phase response can be adjusted. The output of this filter is subtracted from the primary signal. The basic idea is to adjust the characteristics of the digital filter so as to cancel as much as possible of the interference in the primary signal. This is done using an adaptive procedure that minimises the resultant output. The quantity that is minimised is usually the power at the output, although this is probably not the best criterion from a perceptual point of view.

Evaluations of such systems have shown that they can give substantial improvements (20 dB or more) in speech-to-background ratio provided that the listening room is not too reverberant (Peterson *et al.* 1987; Schwander and Levitt 1987; Weiss 1987; Greenberg and Zurek 1992). However, under reverberant conditions, they do not work

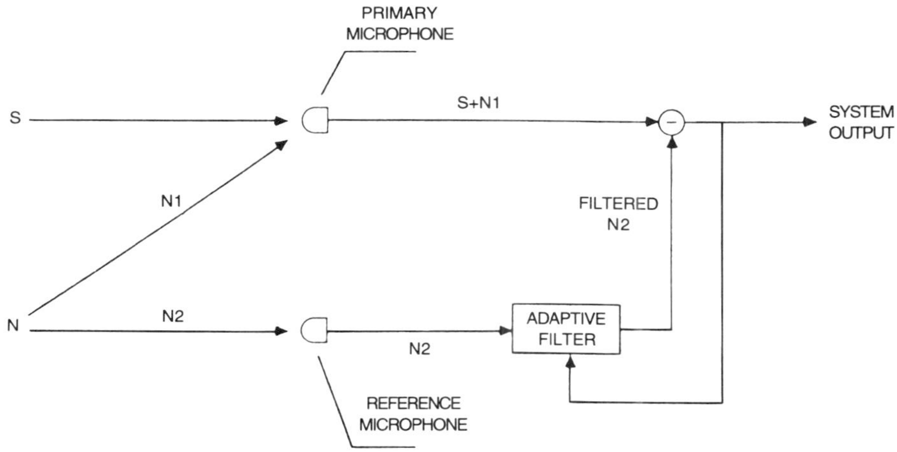

Fig. 8.6. A block diagram of a simple adaptive beamformer. Redrawn from Weiss (1987).

well. Kompis and Dillier (1994) investigated the effect of combining directional microphones with an adaptive beamformer. They reported that the combination gave better intelligibility of speech in noise than either approach alone for sounds in an 'office' sized room with moderate reverberation (reverberation time = 0.4 s).

One significant problem with adaptive beamformers should be noted. The adaptation of the digital filter takes a certain time to occur. The more accurate the required cancellation of the interference, the longer is the response time. The changing response of the adaptive filter can have audible and disturbing effects, especially during head movements of the user.

Binaural processing algorithms

Kollmeier and his co-workers have described several methods of processing sounds that are based on the use of binaural cues to enhance speech-to-background ratios (Kollmeier *et al.* 1993; Kollmeier and Koch 1994). An example of one of their processing schemes is illustrated in Figure 8.7. The scheme is based on the overlap-add method described earlier. It is assumed that the user of the system would wear microphones mounted in or close to their ear canals. For research purposes, sounds are picked up using microphones mounted in the ear canals of a dummy head, so the microphone signals contain the cues for localization that would occur in the ear canals of a normal listener (see chapter 6). Short segments of the sampled sound in each channel are Fourier transformed to give magnitude and phase spectra at the two ears. The magnitude spectra are converted to logarithic (dB) form. For each frequency component, the interaural level and phase differences are computed and compared with those of the 'reference' interaural level and phase differences that occur for a sound from the 'target' direction. Usually, the target direction is straight ahead, and the reference interaural level and phase differences are close to zero. The deviation between actual and reference values serves as the input to a weighting function, *g*, which applies no attenuation if the deviation is small and applies an attenuation up to 20 dB if the deviation is large. To reduce processing artifacts, the function *g* is smoothed by averaging over time and frequency. The smoothed function is used to control the gain in both channels at a given frequency. After weighting, a time signal is constructed from the magnitude and phase spectrum by inverse Fourier transformation, and the resulting processed time segments are overlapped and added. The overall effect of the processing is that sounds from the target direction are preserved, while sounds from other directions are attenuated.

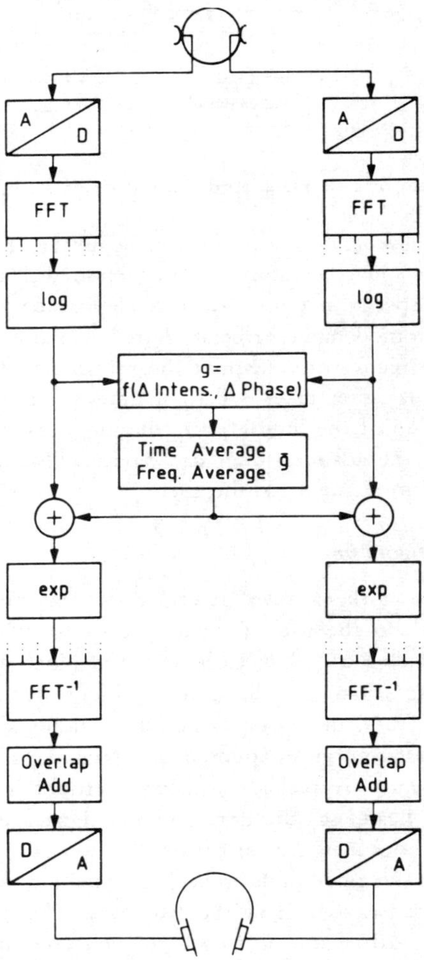

Fig. 8.7. A block diagram of the binaural processing algorithm used by Kollmeier *et al.* (1993).

Evaluations of this system (Kollmeier *et al.* 1993) showed that it could give significant improvements in the intelligibility of speech in a 'cocktail party' situation (with several interfering speakers at various angles), provided that there was no reverberation; the improvements were roughly equivalent to those produced by a 5-dB change in speech-to-background ratio. However, the performance of the algorithm worsened when reverberation was present.

Kollmeier *et al.* (1993) also evaluated a scheme for reducing reverberation. This was similar to the scheme illustrated in Figure 8.7, except that it involved calculation of the short-term cross correlation between the two channels. The direct sound from the target is highly correlated between the two channels, whereas the reverberation is less correlated. The algorithm essentially enhanced spectral components that were well correlated and attenuated components that were poorly correlated. Subjective rankings of this algorithm improved, relative to those for a control condition, with increasing reverberation. Formal intelligibility measurements were not reported.

Kollmeier and Koch (1994) described a binaural noise suppression algorithm based on the construction of a two-dimensional representation of the signal in each channel. One dimension is centre frequency and the other is modulation frequency, representing the spectrum of the amplitude fluctuations at each frequency. As in the algorithm illustrated in Figure 8.7, a weighting function is constructed for each centre frequency, based on a comparison of the two channels. However, in this case the modulation spectra of the two channels are compared and used to compute the weighting function. The algorithm was evaluated using normally hearing subjects. It was found to give small but consistent improvments in the intelligibility of speech in the presence of speech-shaped noise or competing talkers, even at adverse speech-to-noise ratios or under conditions of reverberation. The improvements were equivalent to those produced by about a 2-dB increase in speech-to-background ratio. Under anechoic conditions, larger improvements could be achieved.

In summary, schemes based on binaural processing have the potential for improving the effective speech-to-background ratio for target speech sounds that come from straight ahead. However, the schemes are computationally intensive, and it may be some time before they can be evaluated using wearable hearing aids.

Concluding remarks on schemes to improve the speech-to-noise ratio

Of the schemes described above, directional microphones are the most practical and straightforward. The microphone arrays described by Soede and co-workers (Soede *et al.* 1993a,b) can be implemented without elaborate electronics. They produce a true improvement in speech-to-background ratio in both reverberant and non-reverberant environments and they do this without introducing processing artifacts. Furthermore, they do not introduce significant time delays. However, they are physically rather large, and this may limit their acceptability.

One other problem should be noted. While high directionality is useful in noisy situations, it can be a problem in other situations, since the user becomes effectively 'deaf' for certain directions. This makes it more difficult to detect voices coming from non-frontal directions and to detect environmental sounds such as approaching cars. This problem can be alleviated by allowing the directional characteristic to be selected by the user (as in some aids made by Phonak), or by making the microphone omnidirectional at low sound levels and directional at high sound levels (as in a recent aid made by Viennatone).

Schemes based on digital signal processing are computationally intensive and will require extensive development work before they can be implemented in wearable hearing aids. The schemes sometimes introduce processing artifacts, which may be audible and disturbing. Furthermore, they can introduce significant time delays. This may be a problem when the user is trying to combine visual information (lip-reading) with auditory information. The delay may also affect perception of the user's own voice, since their voice will often be heard both via bone conduction and via the aid. The interference of delayed and non-delayed sound can create disturbing echoes and colouration. Processing algorithms will need to be designed so as to minimise time delays, preferably keeping them below a few tens of milliseconds.

In spite of these difficulties, approaches based on digital signal processing show great promise and are clearly worth further development. Apart from its use in noise reduction, digital signal processing can also be used to provide compensation for loudness recruitment, and to tailor a frequency-gain characteristic precisely to suit an individual person (Suzuki and Sone 1994; Kollmeier and Hohmann 1995).

Signal-processing aids for severe and profound hearing loss

People with severe or profound hearing loss often get little or no benefit from conventional hearing aids. They usually have very small dynamic ranges so extreme compression may be required to make speech audible without it being uncomfortably loud. In people with profound losses, residual hearing may be limited to a small frequency range, say up to 1000 Hz. Even when speech is made audible, as far as possible, the residual auditory capacities, such as frequency and temporal resolution, may be very poor (Faulkner *et al.* 1990a,b), so the ability to understand speech, in quiet or in noise, is greatly diminished in comparison to normally hearing people.

One approach to designing more effective hearing aids for such people is based on the concept of extraction and presentation of speech features. The basic idea is to extract simple features or patterns from speech, such as the fundamental frequency of the speech, and to present those features in a simplified form that is matched to the auditory abilities of the user. The extracted features may be designed specifically to be used in conjunction with lip-reading. For example, the presence or absence of voicing (vibration of the vocal folds) is difficult or impossible to determine by looking at the face of the talker, but it conveys important linguistic information. By supplementing lip-reading with an auditory signal that signals the presence or absence of voicing, speech understanding may be improved. The improvement can be larger if information about the fundamental frequency (f0) of the voice is also conveyed (Rosen *et al.* 1981).

Faulkner *et al.* (1992) described an evaluation of an aid based on this principle, called the SiVo (Sinusoidal Voice) aid. The aid detects when voicing occurs and extracts the f0 of the speaker's voice on a period-by-period basis. A sinusoid is synthesized whose period is equal to that of the extracted f0 and this synthesised signal is presented to the user. Optionally, the frequency of the synthesised sinusoid can be shifted downwards. This is useful in cases where the speaker has a voice with a high average f0 (for example a child); shifting f0 downwards can have the effect of making the sinusoid more audible and of increasing the discriminability of changes in f0, which convey intonation and linguistic structure (see chapter 7). The synthesized sinsuoid is generated with an output level that is independent of the input level of the speech; rather it is set to the user's most comfortable listening level for the specific frequency being generated. This ensures that the signal is always audible and comfortable. One rationale for synthesizing a sinusoid rather than a complex periodic signal is that, for people with profound hearing loss, frequency discrimination is sometimes better for sinusoids than it is for complex tones.

Faulkner *et al.* evaluated the SiVo aid by comparing it with 'conventional' hearing aids with AGC and an extended low-frequency output (to make optimal use of the residual hearing of the subjects), using an audio-visual consonant recognition task. Out of eleven profoundly hearing-impaired subjects, four scored more highly with the SiVo aid, five performed better with the conventional aids and two achieved similar scores for the two types of aids.

In a second study, they evaluated a more complex laboratory prototype version of the SiVo aid, that presented more speech features. The amplitude envelope of the whole speech signal was represented by amplitude modulation of the output sinusoid, with appropriate compression so as to map the amplitude fluctuations into the user's available dynamic range. The presence of noise-like speech sounds (e.g. s, sh, p, t, k) was signalled by low-frequency noise. This compound speech-pattern aid was demonstrated to give better consonant identification than the simple SiVo aid. Of five subjects tested with this aid, three showed better speech recognition than with a 'conventional' aid and two showed similar performance for the speech-pattern aid and the conventional aid. The better performance for the speech-pattern aid was obtained both for consonant identification and for the tracking of connected discourse.

Overall, these results seem promising, and they are likely to be improved further by new algorithms that increase the robustness of the pattern-extraction processes, so that they work well in noise and reverberant conditions (Walliker and Howard 1990). Speech-pattern hearing aids may prove to be a useful alternative to conventional aids or to cochlear implants (see below) for those with profound hearing loss.

Cochlear implants

Cochlear implants represent a form of treatment for total or near total deafness arising from damage to the cochlea. Usually, such deafness is associated with loss of function of the outer and inner hair cells, but the auditory nerve survives to some extent. The treatment involves the implantation of electrodes so as to stimulate the surviving neurones electrically. This results in sensations of sound.

It is beyond the scope of this book to give more than a cursory overview of this topic. For reviews see Clark *et al.* (1990) and Tyler (1993). Briefly, the systems currently in use have two major parts. One part is external to the patient. It consists of a microphone to pick up the sound, and a processor (that may be analogue or digital) that analyses the sound and derives from it signals appropriate for delivery to the individual electrodes. These signals are transmitted through the skin to the implanted part of the system. This consists of a receiver of the transmitted signals, and a device which assigns each electrical signal to its appropriate electrode. The electrodes are usually implanted within the cochlea, by insertion through the round window (see Figure 1.1).

The majority of cochlear implants currently being implanted are multi-channel devices, using several electrodes, although some devices have only one channel. The multi-channel devices attempt to exploit the tonotopic or 'place' organization of the cochlea. The electrodes are distributed as far as possible along the length of the cochlea and each is intended to stimulate neurones with a limited range of CFs (here, CF is used to refer to the frequency that would best excite a given neurone if the cochlea were not damaged). In practice, it is difficult to insert the electrode array very deeply into the cochlea, so the electrodes mainly lie close to neurones with medium and high CFs. Also, the electrical current from a given electrode or electrode pair tends to spread out within the cochlea, so the stimulation is not confined to neurones with a small range of CFs.

Information is transmitted in a cochlear implant in two basic ways: in terms of which electrode is active or of the distribution of current across electrodes ('place' coding); and in terms of the amplitude and time pattern of stimulation on individual electrodes ('temporal' coding). Changes in the place of stimulation generally give rise to changes in perceived timbre; stimulation at the basal end gives a 'sharp' timbre while stimulation towards the apical end gives a more mellow or bass-like timbre. Changes in the rate of stimulation on a single electrode can give rise to changes in perceived pitch, if the rate is below a few hundred Hertz.

Many different coding 'strategies' have been used in cochlear implants. Some strategies are based on the extraction of certain speech features, an approach similar to that used with the SiVo aid described above. For example, the 'Nucleus' device (Clark *et al.* 1987) extracts f0 and the frequencies of the first three formants. The value of f0 is signalled by the rate of electrical pulses, while the formant frequencies are signalled by which electrodes are stimulated. The device also detects the presence of frication and signals this by an irregular pulse pattern on electrodes towards the base of the cochlea.

Other devices filter the signal into frequency bands; the output from each band is used to derive a signal which stimulates a specific electrode. In one coding strategy, called compressed analogue (CA), the input waveform is first compressed, then filtered, and the resulting analogue waveforms are applied directly to the electrodes (Eddington 1983). In another strategy, the envelopes of the outputs of the filters are used to control the amplitudes of brief electrical pulses that are delivered at a constant high rate (typically about 800 pulses per second). The pulses are interleaved on the different electrodes, hence the name 'continuous interleaved sampling' (CIS) (Wilson *et al.* 1991). The interleaving is done to reduce interactions of electrical fields between electrodes, so as to improve the specificity of place coding.

Recently, Nucleus have introduced a new sound processor called the Spectral Maxima Sound Processor (SMSP) (McDermott *et al.* 1992). The processor incorporates 16 (digital) bandpass filters with centre frequencies spaced from 250 to 5400 Hz. Every 4 ms, the six filters with the largest outputs are selected and six corresponding electrodes are stimulated by current pulses whose amplitudes are determined by the respective filter outputs.

Results obtained using cochlear implants vary widely across patients even for a single type of implant. However, it is remarkable that for each of the different types of implants described above, some patients have achieved good levels of speech understanding without lip-reading. Almost all patients find that the quality of their lives has been improved by the implants. It is difficult to determine which system is the 'best'. Current evidence suggests that CIS gives better speech intelligibility than CA (Wilson *et al.* 1991), and the new SMSP Nucleus processor gives better speech intelligibility than the earlier processor based on feature extraction (McKay and McDermott 1993).

When cochlear implants were first introduced, they were restricted to people with total or near-total hearing loss. However, the results have been sufficiently good that their use has been extended to people with a small amount of residual hearing. An important area for future research is to devise criteria to decide on the most important treatment for a specific person with a profound hearing loss; should they be given a 'conventional' aid (with AGC), a speech-pattern aid, or a cochlear implant?

Some concluding remarks

Hearing aids have improved considerably in recent years. Aids are available with low distortion and with smooth wideband frequency responses. Many aids, and especially the newer programmable aids, have a high degree of flexibility in shaping their frequency-gain characteristic. In principle it is usually possible to tailor the frequency response of a linear aid to suit an individual patient. Hearing aids are also available that offer reasonably effective compensation for loudness recruitment. In practice, many hearing-impaired people are still being fitted with hearing aids that have significant distortion, that have an irregular frequency response with an inappropriate shape, and that do not offer effective compensation for loudness recruitment.

Even the best possible current hearing aids do not restore hearing to normal; especially when listening to speech in noise or competing speech, hearing-impaired subjects listening through hearing aids perform more poorly than normally hearing people. This situation may be improved in the future through the use of directional microphones and through the use of digital signal processing to enhance spectral contrast and/or to improve speech-to-background ratios. Digital hearing aids also offer the possibility of very precise frequency response shaping and compensation for loudness recruitment. People with severe or profound hearing losses may benefit from future developments in speech-pattern hearing aids and cochlear implants.

References

Allen, J. B. (1977). Short term spectral analysis, synthesis and modification by discrete Fourier transform. *IEEE Trans. Acoust. Speech Sig. Proc.*, **25,** 235–238.

Allen, J. B., and Jeng, P. S. (1990). Loudness growth in 1/2-octave bands (LGOB); a procedure for the assessment of loudness. *J. Acoust. Soc. Am.*, **88,** 745–753.

American Standards Association (1960). *Acoustical Terminology SI, 1-1960 American Standards Association, New York.*

Aniansson, G. (1974). Methods for assessing high-frequency hearing loss in everyday situations. *Acta Otolaryngol.*, Suppl. **320**, 1–50.

Arehart, K. H. (1994). Effects of harmonic content on complex-tone fundamental-frequency discrimination in hearing-impaired listeners. *J. Acoust. Soc. Am.*, **95**, 3574–3585.

Arthur, R. M., Pfeiffer, R. R., and Suga, N. (1971). Properties of 'two-tone inhibition' in primary auditory neurones. *J. Physiol.*, **212**, 593–609.

Attneave, F., and Olson, R. K. (1971). Pitch as a medium: A new approach to psychophysical scaling. *Am. J. Psychol.*, **84**, 147–166.

Bachem, A. (1950). Tone height and tone chroma as two different pitch qualities. *Acta Psychol.*, **7**, 80–88.

Bacon, S. P., and Gleitman, R. M. (1992). Modulation detection in subjects with relatively flat hearing losses. *J. Speech Hear. Res.*, **35**, 642–653.

Bacon, S. P., and Viemeister, N. F. (1985). Temporal modulation transfer functions in normal-hearing and hearing-impaired subjects. *Audiology*, **24**, 117–134.

Baer, T., and Moore, B. C. J. (1993). Effects of spectral smearing on the intelligibility of sentences in the presence of noise. *J. Acoust. Soc. Am.*, **94**, 1229–1241.

Baer, T., and Moore, B. C. J. (1994). Effects of spectral smearing on the intelligibility of sentences in the presence of interfering speech. *J. Acoust. Soc. Am.*, **95**, 2277–2280.

Baer, T., Moore, B. C. J., and Gatehouse, S. (1993). Spectral contrast enhancement of speech in noise for listeners with sensorineural hearing impairment: effects on intelligibility, quality and response times. *J. Rehab. Res. Devel.*, **30**, 49–72.

Bernstein, R. S., and Raab, D. H. (1990). The effects of bandwidth on the detectability of narrow- and wideband signals. *J. Acoust. Soc. Am.*, **88**, 2115–2125.

Blauert, J. (1983). *Spatial Hearing.* MIT Press, Cambridge, Mass.

Boers, P. M. (1980). Formant enhancement of speech for listeners with sensorineural hearing loss. *IPO Ann. Prog. Rep.*, **15**, 21–28.

Bonding, P. (1979a). Critical bandwidth in loudness summation in sensorineural hearing loss. *Brit. J. Audiol.*, **13**, 23–30.

Bonding, P. (1979b). Frequency selectivity and speech discrimination in sensorineural hearing loss. *Scand. Audiol.*, **8**, 205–216.

Bonding, P., and Elberling, C. (1980). Loudness summation across frequency under masking and in sensorineural hearing loss. *Audiology*, **19**, 57–74.

Bornstein, S. P., and Randolph, K. J. (1983). Research on smooth, wideband frequency responses: Current status and unresolved issues. *Hear. Inst.*, **34**, 12–16.

Braida, L. D., Durlach, N. I., De Gennaro, S. V., Peterson, P. M., and Bustamante, D. K. (1982). Review of recent research on multiband amplitude compression for the hearing impaired. In *The Vanderbilt Hearing-Aid Report*, (ed. G. A. Studebaker and F. H. Bess), pp. 133–140. Monographs in Contemporary Audiology, Upper Darby, Pennsylvania.

Bronkhurst, A. W., and Plomp, R. (1988). The effect of head-induced interaural time and level differences on speech intelligibility in noise. *J. Acoust. Soc. Am.*, **83**, 1508–1516.

Bronkhurst, A. W., and Plomp, R. (1989). Binaural speech intelligibility in noise for hearing-impaired listeners. *J. Acoust. Soc. Am.*, **86**, 1374–1383.

Bunnell, H. T. (1990). On enhancement of spectral contrast in speech for hearing-impaired listeners. *J. Acoust. Soc. Am.*, **88**, 2546–2556.

Burkhard, M. D., and Sachs, R. M. (1975). Anthropometric manikin for acoustic research. *J. Acoust. Soc. Am.*, **58**, 214–222.

Burns, E. M., and Turner, C. (1986). Pure-tone pitch anomalies. II. Pitch-intensity effects and diplacusis in impaired ears. *J. Acoust. Soc. Am.*, **79**, 1530–1540.

Bustamante, D. K., and Braida, L. D. (1987). Multiband compression limiting for hearing-impaired listeners. *J. Rehab. Res. Dev.*, **24**, 149–160.

Buunen, T. J. F., Festen, J. M., Bilsen, F. A., and van den Brink, G. (1974). Phase effects in a three-component signal. *J. Acoust. Soc. Am.*, **55**, 297–303.

Buus, S., and Florentine, M. (1985). Gap detection in normal and impaired listeners: the effect of level and frequency. In *Time Resolution in Auditory Systems*, (ed. A. Michelsen), pp. 159–179. Springer-Verlag, New York.

Buus, S., Florentine, M., and Redden, R. B. (1982a). The SISI test: A review. Part I. *Audiology*, **21**, 273–293.

Buus, S., Florentine, M., and Redden, R. B. (1982b). The SISI test: A review. Part II. *Audiology*, **21**, 365–385.

Buus, S., Schorer, E., Florentine, M., and Zwicker, E. (1986). Decision rules in detection of simple and complex tones. *J. Acoust. Soc. Am.*, **80**, 1646–1657.

Byrne, D. (1986). Effects of bandwidth and stimulus type on most comfortable loudness levels of hearing-impaired listeners. *J. Acoust. Soc. Am.*, **80**, 484–492.

Byrne, D., and Dillon, H. (1986). The National Acoustic Laboratories' (NAL) new procedure for selecting the gain and frequency response of a hearing aid. *Ear Hear.*, **7**, 257–265.

Carlyon, R. P., Buus, S., and Florentine, M. (1990). Temporal integration of trains of tone pulses by normal and by cochlearly impaired listeners. *J. Acoust. Soc. Am.*, **87**, 260–268.

Carney, A. E., and Nelson, D. A. (1983). An analysis of psychophysical tuning curves in normal and pathological ears. *J. Acoust. Soc. Am.*, **73**, 268–278.

Celmer, R. D., and Bienvenue, G. R. (1987). Critical bands in the perception of speech signals by normal and sensorineural hearing loss listeners. In *The Psychophysics of Speech Perception*, (ed. M. E. H. Schouten), pp. 473–480. Nijhoff, Dordrecht, Netherlands.

Chistovich, L. A. (1957). Frequency characteristics of masking effect. *Biophys.*, **2**, 743–755.

Chung, D. Y. (1981). Masking, temporal integration, and sensorineural hearing loss. *J. Speech Hear. Res.*, **24**, 514–520.

Clark, G. M., Tong, Y. C., and Patrick, J. F. (1990). *Cochlear Prostheses.* Churchill Livingstone, Edinburgh.

Clark, G. M. *et al.* (1987). *The University of Melbourne-Nucleus Multi-electrode Cochlear Implant.* Karger, Basel.

Cokely, C. G., and Humes, L. E. (1993). Two experiments on the temporal boundaries for the nonlinear additivity of masking. *J. Acoust. Soc. Am.*, **94**, 2553–2559.

Colburn, H. S., and Trahiotis, C. (1992). Effects of noise on binaural hearing. In *Noise-Induced Hearing Loss*, (ed. A. Dancer, D. Henderson, R. Salvi and R. Hamernik), pp. 293–302. Mosby, St. Louis.

Cox, R. M., and Gilmore, C. (1986). Damping and the hearing aid frequency response: Effects on speech clarity and preferred listening level. *J. Speech Hear. Res.*, **29**, 357–365.

Davis, A., Haggard, M., and Bell, I. (1990). Magnitude of diotic summation in speech-in-noise tasks: performance region and appropriate baseline. *Brit. J. Audiol.*, **24**, 11–16.

Davis, A. C., and Haggard, M. P. (1982). Some implications of audiological measures in the population for binaural aiding strategies. *Scand. Audiol.*, Suppl. **15**.

Davis, H. (1962). Advances in the neurophysiology and neuroanatomy of the cochlea. *J. Acoust. Soc. Am.*, **34**, 1377–1385.

de Filippo, C. L., and Snell, K. B. (1986). Detection of a temporal gap in low-frequency narrow-band signals by normal hearing and hearing-impaired listeners. *J. Acoust. Soc. Am.*, **80**, 1354–1358.

de Mare, G. (1948). Investigations into the functions of the auditory apparatus in perception deafness. *Acta Otolaryngol.*, **Suppl. 74**, 107–116.

Delgutte, B. (1988). Physiological mechanisms of masking. In *Basic Issues in Hearing*, (ed. H. Duifhuis, J. W. Horst and H. P. Wit), pp. 204–214. Academic Press, London.

Delgutte, B. (1990). Physiological mechanisms of psychophysical masking: Observations from auditory-nerve fibers. *J. Acoust. Soc. Am.*, **87**, 791–809.

Dillon, H., and Macrae, J. (1984). *Derivation of Design Specifications for Hearing Aids (NAL report Number 102).* Australian Government Publishing Service, Canberra.

Dix, M., Hallpike, C., and Hood, J. (1948). Observations upon the loudness recruitment phonemenon with especial reference to the differential diagnosis of disorders of the internal ear and VIIIth nerve. *J. Laryngol. Otol*, **62**, 671–686.

Dreschler, W. A., and Plomp, R. (1980). Relations between psychophysical data and speech perception for hearing-impaired subjects. I. *J. Acoust. Soc. Am.*, **68**, 1608–1615.

Dreschler, W. A., and Plomp, R. (1985). Relations between psychophysical data and speech perception for hearing-impaired subjects. II. *J. Acoust. Soc. Am.*, **78**, 1261–1270.

Drullman, R., Festen, J. M., and Plomp, R. (1994). Effect of temporal envelope smearing on speech reception. *J. Acoust. Soc. Am.*, **95**, 1053–1064.

Dubno, J. R., and Dirks, D. D. (1989). Auditory filter characteristics and consonant recognition for hearing-impaired listeners. *J. Acoust. Soc. Am.*, **85**, 1666–1675.

Dubno, J. R., and Schaefer, A. B. (1992). Comparison of frequency selectivity and consonant recognition among hearing-impaired and masked normal-hearing listeners. *J. Acoust. Soc. Am.*, **91**, 2110–2121.

Duchnowski, P. (1989). Simulation of sensorineural hearing impairment. M.S. Thesis, MIT, Cambridge, MA.

Dugal, R., Braida, L. D., and Durlach, N. I. (1978). Implications of previous research for the selection of frequency-gain characteristics. In *Acoustical Factors Affecting Hearing Aid Performance*, (ed. G. A. Studebaker and I. Hochberg), pp. 379–403. University Park Press, Baltimore.

Duifhuis, H. (1973). Consequences of peripheral frequency selectivity for nonsimultaneous masking. *J. Acoust. Soc. Am.*, **54**, 1471–1488.

Duquesnoy, A. J. (1983). Effect of a single interfering noise or speech source on the binaural sentence intelligibility of aged persons. *J. Acoust. Soc. Am.*, **74**, 739–743.

Duquesnoy, A. J., and Plomp, R. (1983). The effect of a hearing aid on the speech-reception threshold of hearing-impaired listeners in quiet and in noise. *J. Acoust. Soc. Am.*, **73**, 2166–2173.

Durlach, N. I., Thompson, C. L., and Colburn, H. S. (1981). Binaural interaction in impaired listeners. *Audiology*, **20**, 181–211.

Dye, R. H., and Hafter, E. R. (1984). The effects of intensity on the detection of interaural differences of time in high-frequency trains of clicks. *J. Acoust. Soc. Am.*, **75**, 1593–1598.

Eddington, D. K. (1983). Speech recognition in deaf subjects with multichannel intracochlear electrodes. *Ann. New York Acad. Sci.*, **405**, 241–258.

Eddins, D. A., Hall, J. W., and Grose, J. H. (1992). Detection of temporal gaps as a function of frequency region and absolute noise bandwidth. *J. Acoust. Soc. Am.*, **91**, 1069–1077.

Egan, J. P., and Hake, H. W. (1950). On the masking pattern of a simple auditory stimulus. *J. Acoust. Soc. Am.*, **22**, 622–630.

Elliott, L. L. (1975). Temporal and masking phenomena in persons with sensorineural hearing loss. *Audiology* **14**, 336–353.

Evans, E. F. (1975). The sharpening of frequency selectivity in the normal and abnormal cochlea. *Audiology*, **14**, 419–442.

Evans, E. F., and Harrison, R. V. (1976). Correlation between outer hair cell damage and deterioration of cochlear nerve tuning properties in the guinea pig. *J. Physiol.*, **252**, 43–44p.

Exner, S. (1876). Zur Lehre von den Gehörsempfindungen. *Pflügers Archiv*, **13**, 228–253.

Fabry, D. A., and van Tasell, D. J. (1986). Masked and filtered simulation of hearing loss: Effects on consonant recognition. *J. Speech Hear. Res.*, **29**, 170–178.

Fastl, H. (1976a). Masking patterns of subcritical versus critical band maskers at 8.5 kHz. *Acustica*, **34**, 167–171.

Fastl, H. (1976b). Temporal masking effects: I. Broad band noise masker. *Acustica*, **35**, 287–302.

Faulkner, A., Ball, V., Rosen, S., Moore, B. C. J., and Fourcin, A. J. (1992). Speech pattern hearing aids for the profoundly hearing impaired: Speech perception and auditory abilities. *J. Acoust. Soc. Am.*, **91**, 2136–2155.

Faulkner, A., Fourcin, A. J., and Moore, B. C. J. (1990a). Psychoacoustic aspects of speech pattern coding for the deaf. *Acta Otolaryngol. Suppl.*, **469**, 172–180.

Faulkner, A., Rosen, S., and Moore, B. C. J. (1990b). Residual frequency selectivity in the profoundly hearing-impaired listener. *Brit. J. Audiol.*, **24**, 381–392.

Feddersen, W. E., Sandel, T. T., Teas, D. C., and Jeffress, L. A. (1957). Localization of high-frequency tones. *J. Acoust. Soc. Am.*, **29**, 988–991.

Festen, J. M., and Plomp, R. (1983). Relations between auditory functions in impaired hearing. *J. Acoust. Soc. Am.*, **73**, 652–662.

Festen, J. M., and Plomp, R. (1990). Effects of fluctuating noise and interfering speech on the speech-reception threshold for impaired and normal hearing. *J. Acoust. Soc. Am.*, **88**, 1725–1736.

Fitzgibbons, P. J. (1983). Temporal gap detection in noise as a function of frequency, bandwidth and level. *J. Acoust. Soc. Am.*, **74**, 67–72.

Fitzgibbons, P. J., and Gordon-Salant, S. (1987). Minimum stimulus levels for temporal gap resolution in listeners with sensorineural hearing loss. *J. Acoust. Soc. Am.*, **81**, 1542–1545.

Fitzgibbons, P. J., and Wightman, F. L. (1982). Gap detection in normal and hearing-impaired listeners. *J. Acoust. Soc. Am.*, **72**, 761–765.

Flanagan, J. L., and Saslow, M. G. (1958). Pitch discrimination for synthetic vowels. *J. Acoust. Soc. Am.*, **30**, 435–442.

Fletcher, H. (1940). Auditory patterns. *Rev. Mod. Phys.*, **12**, 47–65.

Fletcher, H. (1952). The perception of sounds by deafened persons. *J. Acoust. Soc. Am.*, **24**, 490–497.

Fletcher, H., and Munson, W. A. (1933). Loudness, its definition, measurement and calculation. *J. Acoust. Soc. Am.*, **5**, 82–108.

Fletcher, H., and Munson, W. A. (1937). Relation between loudness and masking. *J. Acoust. Soc. Am.*, **9**, 1–10.

Florentine, M., and Buus, S. (1981). An excitation-pattern model for intensity discrimination. *J. Acoust. Soc. Am.*, **70**, 1646–1654.

Florentine, M., and Buus, S. (1984). Temporal gap detection in sensorineural and simulated hearing impairment. *J. Speech Hear. Res.*, **27**, 449–455.

Florentine, M., Buus, S., Scharf, B., and Zwicker, E. (1980). Frequency selectivity in normally-hearing and hearing-impaired observers. *J. Speech Hear. Res.*, **23**, 643–669.

Florentine, M., Fastl, H., and Buus, S. (1988). Temporal integration in normal hearing, cochlear impairment, and impairment simulated by masking. *J. Acoust. Soc. Am.*, **84**, 195–203.

Florentine, M., and Houtsma, A. J. M. (1983). Tuning curves and pitch matches in a listener with a unilateral, low-frequency hearing loss. *J. Acoust. Soc. Am.*, **73**, 961–965.

Florentine, M., Reed, C. M., Rabinowitz, W. M., Braida, L. D., Durlach, N. I., and Buus, S. (1993). Intensity perception. XIV. Intensity discrimination in listeners with sensorineural hearing loss. *J. Acoust. Soc. Am.*, **94**, 2575–2586.

Florentine, M., and Zwicker, E. (1979). A model of loudness summation applied to noise-induced hearing loss. *Hear. Res.*, **1**, 121–132.

Formby, C. (1982). Differential sensitivity to tonal frequency and to the rate of amplitude modulation of broad-band noise by hearing-impaired listeners. Ph.D. Thesis, Washington University, St. Louis.

Fowler, E. P. (1936). A method for the early detection of otosclerosis. *Arch. Otolaryngol.*, **24**, 731–741.

French, N. R., and Steinberg, J. C. (1947). Factors governing the intelligibility of speech sounds. *J. Acoust. Soc. Am.*, **19**, 90–119.

Freyman, R. L., and Nelson, D. A. (1986). Frequency discrimination as a function of tonal duration and excitation-pattern slopes in normal and hearing-impaired listeners. *J. Acoust. Soc. Am.*, **79**, 1034–1044.

Freyman, R. L., and Nelson, D. A. (1987). Frequency discrimination of short- versus long-duration tones by normal and hearing-impaired listeners. *J. Speech Hear. Res.*, **30**, 28–36.

Freyman, R. L., and Nelson, D. A. (1991). Frequency discrimination as a function of signal frequency and level in normal-hearing and hearing-impaired listeners. *J. Speech Hear. Res.*, **34**, 1371–1386.

Gabriel, K. J., Koehnke, J., and Colburn, H. S. (1992). Frequency dependence of binaural performance in listeners with impaired binaural hearing. *J. Acoust. Soc. Am.*, **91**, 336–347.

Gaeth, J., and Norris, T. (1965). Diplacusis in unilateral high frequency hearing losses. *J. Speech Hear. Res.*, **8**, 63–75.

Garner, W. R., and Miller, G. A. (1947). The masked threshold of pure tones as a function of duration. *J. Exp. Psychol.*, **37**, 293–303.

Gatehouse, S. (1992). The time course and magnitude of perceptual acclimatization to frequency responses: Evidence from monaural fitting of hearing aids. *J. Acoust. Soc. Am.*, **92**, 1258–1268.

Gatehouse, S., and Haggard, M. P. (1987). The effects of air-bone gap and presentation level on word identification. *Ear Hear.*, **8**, 140–146.

Gengel, R. W. (1973). Temporal effects on frequency discrimination by hearing-impaired listeners. *J. Acoust. Soc. Am.*, **54**, 11–15.

Gengel, R. W., and Watson, C. S. (1971). Temporal integration: I. Clinical implications of a laboratory study. II. Additional data from hearing-impaired subjects. *J. Speech. Hear. Disord.*, **36**, 213–224.

Glasberg, B. R., and Moore, B. C. J. (1986). Auditory filter shapes in subjects with unilateral and bilateral cochlear impairments. *J. Acoust. Soc. Am.*, **79**, 1020–1033.

Glasberg, B. R., and Moore, B. C. J. (1989). Psychoacoustic abilities of subjects with unilateral and bilateral cochlear impairments and their relationship to the ability to understand speech. *Scand. Audiol. Suppl.*, **32**, 1–25.

Glasberg, B. R., and Moore, B. C. J. (1990). Derivation of auditory filter shapes from notched-noise data. *Hear. Res.*, **47**, 103–138.

Glasberg, B. R., and Moore, B. C. J. (1992). Effects of envelope fluctuations on gap detection. *Hear. Res.*, **64**, 81–92.

Glasberg, B. R., Moore, B. C. J., and Bacon, S. P. (1987). Gap detection and masking in hearing-impaired and normal-hearing subjects. *J. Acoust. Soc. Am.*, **81**, 1546–1556.

Glasberg, B. R., Moore, B. C. J., and Nimmo-Smith, I. (1984). Comparison of auditory filter shapes derived with three different maskers. *J. Acoust. Soc. Am.*, **75**, 536–544.

Goldstein, J. L. (1973). An optimum processor theory for the central formation of the pitch of complex tones. *J. Acoust. Soc. Am.*, **54**, 1496–1516.

Goldstein, J. L., and Srulovicz, P. (1977). Auditory-nerve spike intervals as an adequate basis for aural frequency measurement. In *Psychophysics and Physiology of Hearing*, (ed. E. F. Evans and J. P. Wilson), pp. 337-346. Academic Press, London.

Goodman, A. (1965). Reference zero levels for pure-tone audiometer. *ASHA*, **7**, 262–263.

Grant, K. W. (1987). Frequency modulation detection by normally hearing and profoundly hearing-impaired listeners. *J. Speech Hear. Res.*, **30**, 558–563.

Grant, K. W., Ardell, L. H., Kuhl, P. K., and Sparks, D. W. (1985). The contributions of fundamental frequency, amplitude envelope, and voicing duration cues to speechreading in normal-hearing subjects. *J. Acoust. Soc. Am.*, **77**, 671–677.

Grantham, D. W. (1995). Spatial hearing and related phenomena. In *Handbook of Perception and Cognition, Vol. 6, Hearing* (ed. B. C. J. Moore), pp. 297–345. Academic, New York.

Green, D. M. (1973). Temporal acuity as a function of frequency. *J. Acoust. Soc. Am.*, **54**, 373–379.

Green, D. M. (1985). Temporal factors in psychoacoustics. In *Time Resolution in Auditory Systems*, (ed. A. Michelsen), pp. 122–140. Springer-Verlag, New York.

Green, D. M., and Forrest, T. G. (1988). Detection of amplitude modulation and gaps in noise. In *Basic Issues in Hearing*, (ed. H. Duifhuis, J. W. Horst and H. P. Wit), pp. 323–330. Academic Press, New York.

Greenberg, J. E., and Zurek, P. M. (1992). Evaluation of an adaptive beamforming method for hearing aids. *J. Acoust. Soc. Am.*, **91**, 1662–1676.

Greenwood, D. D. (1961a). Auditory masking and the critical band. *J. Acoust. Soc. Am.*, **33**, 484–501.

Greenwood, D. D. (1961b). Critical bandwidth and the frequency coordinates of the basilar membrane. *J. Acoust. Soc. Am.*, **33**, 1344–1356.

Greenwood, D. D. (1971). Aural combination tones and auditory masking. *J. Acoust. Soc. Am.*, **50**, 502–543.

Griffiths, L. J., and Jim, C. W. (1982). An alternative approach to linearly constrained adaptive beamforming. *IEEE Trans. Antennas Propag.*, AP-**30**, 27–34.

Hall, J. W., and Fernandes, M. A. (1983). Temporal integration, frequency resolution, and off-frequency listening in normal-hearing and cochlear-impaired listeners. *J. Acoust. Soc. Am.*, **74**, 1172–1177.

Hall, J. W., Haggard, M. P., and Fernandes, M. A. (1984a). Detection in noise by spectro-temporal pattern analysis. *J. Acoust. Soc. Am.*, **76**, 50–56.

Hall, J. W., Tyler, R. S., and Fernandes, M. A. (1984b). Factors influencing the masking level difference in cochlear hearing-impaired and normal-hearing listeners. *J. Speech Hear. Res.*, **27**, 145–154.

Hall, J. W., and Wood, E. J. (1984). Stimulus duration and frequency discrimination for normal-hearing and hearing-impaired subjects. *J. Speech Hear. Res.*, **27**, 252–256.

Hamilton, P. M. (1957). Noise masked thresholds as a function of tonal duration and masking noise bandwidth. *J. Acoust. Soc. Am.*, **29**, 506–511.

Handel, S. (1995). Timbre perception and auditory object identification. In *Handbook of Perception and Cognition, Vol. 6. Hearing, (ed. B. C. J. Moore),* pp. 425–461. Academic Press, Florida.

Harris, J. D. (1963). Loudness discrimination. *J. Speech. Hear. Disord.*, Monographs, Supplement **11**, 1–63.

Harrison, R. V., and Evans, E. F. (1979). Some aspects of temporal coding by single cochlear fibres from regions of cochlear hair cell degeneration in the guinea pig. *Arch. Otolaryngol.*, **224**, 71–78.

Häusler, R., Colburn, H. S., and Marr, E. (1983). Sound localization in subjects with impaired hearing. *Acta Otolaryngol.*, **Suppl. 400**, 1–62.

Havens, J. F., and Geisler, C. D. (1991). Speech recognition and frequency selectivity for hearing impaired listeners. In *Proceedings of the International Conference on Acoustics Speech and Signal Processing*, pp. 3629–3632. IEEE, New York.

Hawkins, D. B., and Wightman, F. L. (1980). Interaural time discrimination ability of listeners with sensori-neural hearing loss. *Audiol.*, **19**, 495–507.

Hawkins, D. B., and Yacullo, W. S. (1984). Signal-to-noise ratio advantage of binaural hearing aids and directional microphones under different levels of reverberation. *J. Speech. Hear. Disord.*, **49**, 278–286.

Hellbrück, J., and Moser, L. M. (1985). Hörgeräte Audiometrie: Ein computer-unterstütztes psychologisches Verfahren zur Hörgeräteanpassung. *Psychologische Beiträge*, **27**, 494–509.

Hellman, R. P. (1978). Dependence of loudness growth on skirts of excitation patterns. *J. Acoust. Soc. Am.*, **63**, 1114–1119.

Hellman, R. P. (1994). Relation between the growth of loudness and high-frequency excitation. *J. Acoust. Soc. Am.*, **96**, 2655–2663.

Hellman, R. P., and Meiselman, C. H. (1986). Is high-frequency hearing necessary for normal loudness growth at low frequencies? 12th ICA, Paper B11-5.

Hellman, R. P., and Meiselman, C. H. (1990). Loudness relations for individuals and groups in normal and impaired hearing. *J. Acoust. Soc. Am.*, **88**, 2596–2606.

Hellman, R. P., and Meiselman, C. H. (1993). Rate of loudness growth for pure tones in normal and impaired hearing. *J. Acoust. Soc. Am.*, **93**, 966–975.

Hellman, R. P., Scharf, B., Teghtsoonian, M., and Teghtsoonian, R. (1987). On the relation between the growth of loudness and the discrimination of intensity for pure tones. *J. Acoust. Soc. Am.*, **82**, 448–453.

Henning, G. B. (1967). A model for auditory discrimination and detection. *J. Acoust. Soc. Am.*, **42**, 1325–1334.

Henning, G. B. (1974). Detectability of interaural delay in high-frequency complex waveforms. *J. Acoust. Soc. Am.*, **55**, 84–90.

Hickson, L. M. H. (1994). Compression amplification in hearing aids. *Am. J. Audiol*, **3**, 51–65.

Hirsh, I. J. (1948). Influence of interaural phase on interaural summation and inhibition. *J. Acoust. Soc. Am.*, **20**, 536–544.

Hoekstra, A. (1979). Frequency discrimination and frequency analysis in hearing, Ph.D. Thesis, Institute of Audiology, University Hospital, Groningen, Netherlands.

Hoekstra, A., and Ritsma, R. J. (1977). Perceptive hearing loss and frequency selectivity. In *Psychophysics and Physiology of Hearing*, (ed. E. F. Evans and J. P. Wilson), pp. 263–271. Academic Press, London.

Hood, J. D. (1984). Speech discrimination in bilateral and unilateral loss due to Ménière's disease. *Brit. J. Audiol.*, **18**, 173–78.

Horst, J. W. (1987). Frequency discrimination of complex signals, frequency selectivity and speech perception in hearing-impaired subjects. *J. Acoust. Soc. Am.*, **82**, 874–885.

Hou, Z., and Pavlovic, C. V. (1994). Effects of temporal smearing on temporal resolution, frequency selectivity, and speech intelligibility. *J. Acoust. Soc. Am.*, **96**, 1325–1340.

Houtgast, T. (1972). Psychophysical evidence for lateral inhibition in hearing. *J. Acoust. Soc. Am.*, **51**, 1885–1894.

Houtgast, T. (1973). Psychophysical experiments on 'tuning curves' and 'two-tone inhibition'. *Acustica*, **29**, 168–179.

Houtgast, T. (1974). Lateral suppression in hearing, Ph.D. Thesis, Free University of Amsterdam.

Houtgast, T. (1977). Auditory-filter characteristics derived from direct-masking data and pulsation-threshold data with a rippled-noise masker. *J. Acoust. Soc. Am.*, **62**, 409–415.

Houtsma, A. J. M., and Smurzynski, J. (1990). Pitch identification and discrimination for complex tones with many harmonics. *J. Acoust. Soc. Am.*, **87**, 304–310.

Howard-Jones, P. A., and Summers, I. R. (1992). Temporal features in spectrally degraded speech. *Acoust. Lett.*, **15**, 159–163.

Hughes, J. W. (1946). The threshold of audition for short periods of stimulation. *Proc. Roy. Soc. B*, **133**, 486–490.

Humes, L. E. (1991). Prescribing gain characteristics of linear hearing aids. In *The Vanderbilt Hearing Aid Report II*, (ed. G. A. Studebaker, F. H. Bess and L. B. Beck), pp. 13–22. York Press, Parkton, Maryland.

Humes, L. E., Dirks, D. D., and Kincaid, G. E. (1987). Recognition of nonsense syllables by hearing-impaired listeners and by noise masked normal listeners. *J. Acoust. Soc. Am.*, **81**, 765–773.

Humes, L. E., and Roberts, L. (1990). Speech-recognition difficulties of the hearing-impaired elderly: The contributions of audibility. *J. Speech. Hear. Res.*, **33**, 726–735.

Hygge, S., Rönnberg, J., Larsby, B., and Arlinger, S. (1992). Normal-hearing and hearing-impaired subjects' ability to just follow conversation in competing speech, reversed speech, and noise backgrounds. *J. Speech Hear. Res.*, **35**, 208–215.

Jerger, J. (1962). The SISI test. *Int. Audiol.*, **1**, 246–247.

Jerger, J., Brown, D., and Smith, S. (1984). Effect of peripheral hearing loss on the MLD. *Arch. Otolaryngol.*, **110**, 290–296.

Jerger, J., Shedd, J., and Harford, E. (1959). On the detection of extremely small changes in sound intensity. *Arch. Otolaryngol.*, **69**, 200–211.

Jesteadt, W., Bilger, R. C., Green, D. M., and Patterson, J. H. (1976). Temporal acuity in listeners with sensorineural hearing loss. *J. Speech Hear. Res.*, **19**, 357–370.

Jesteadt, W., Wier, C. C., and Green, D. M. (1977a). Comparison of monaural and binaural discrimination of intensity and frequency. *J. Acoust. Soc. Am.*, **61**, 1599–1603.

Jesteadt, W., Wier, C. C., and Green, D. M. (1977b). Intensity discrimination as a function of frequency and sensation level. *J. Acoust. Soc. Am.*, **61**, 169–177.

Johnson-Davies, D., and Patterson, R. D. (1979). Psychophysical tuning curves: restricting the listening band to the signal region. *J. Acoust. Soc. Am.*, **65**, 675–770.

Kemp, D. T. (1978). Stimulated acoustic emissions from within the human auditory system. *J. Acoust. Soc. Am.*, **64**, 1386–1391.

Kendall, M. G., and Stuart, A. (1967). *The Advanced Theory of Statistics, Vol. II.* Griffin, London.

Khanna, S. M., and Leonard, D. G. B. (1982). Basilar membrane tuning in the cat cochlea. *Science*, **215**, 305–306.

Kiang, N. Y.-S., Watanabe, T., Thomas, E. C., and Clark, L. F. (1965). *Discharge Patterns of Single Fibers in the Cat's Auditory Nerve.* MIT Press, Cambridge, Mass.

Kiang, N. Y. S. (1968). A survey of recent developments in the study of auditory physiology. *Ann. Otol. Rhinol. Laryngol.*, **77**, 656–675.

Kiang, N. Y. S., Moxon, E. C., and Levine, R. A. (1970). Auditory nerve activity in cats with normal and abnormal cochleas. In *Sensorineural Hearing Loss*, (ed. G. E. W. Wolstenholme and J. J. Knight), pp. 241–268. Churchill, London.

Kidd, G., and Feth, L. L. (1982). Effects of masker duration in pure-tone forward masking. *J. Acoust. Soc. Am.*, **72**, 1384–1386.

Kiessling, J., Steffens, T., and Wagner, I. (1993). Untersuchungen zur praktischen Anwendbarkeit der Lautheitsskalierung. *Audiologische Akustik*, **4/93**, 100–115.

Killion, M. C. (1982). Transducers, earmolds and sound quality considerations. In *The Vanderbilt Hearing-Aid Report*, (ed. G. A. Studebaker and F. H. Bess), pp. 104–111. Monographs in Contemporary Audiology, Upper Darby, PA.

Killion, M. C., Wilber, L. A., and Gudmundsen, G. I. (1988). Zwislocki was right: A potential solution to the 'hollow voice' problem (the amplified occlusion effect) with deeply sealed earmolds. *Hear. Inst.*, **39**, 14–18.

Kinkel, M., and Kollmeier, B. (1992). Binaurales Hören bei Normalhörenden und Schwerhörigen.II. Analyse der Ergebnisse. *Audiologishe Akustik*, **1/92**, 22–33.

Kinkel, M., Kollmeier, B., and Holube, I. (1991). Binaurales Hören bei Normalhörenden und Schwerhörigen.I. Meßmethods und Meßergebnisse. *Audiologishe Akustik*, **6/91**, 192–201.

Klump, R. G., and Eady, H. R. (1956). Some measurements of interaural time difference thresholds. *J. Acoust. Soc. Am.*, **28**, 859–860.

Kohlrausch, A. (1988). Masking patterns of harmonic complex tone maskers and the role of the inner ear transfer function. In *Basic Issues in Hearing*, (ed. H. Duifhuis, J. W. Horst and H. P. Wit), pp. 339–346. Academic, London.

Kollmeier, B., and Hohmann, V. (1995). Loudness estimation and compensation employing a categorical scale. In *Advances in Hearing Research*, (ed. G. A. Manley, G. M. Klump, C. Köppl, H. Fastl and H. Oeckinghaus). World Scientific Publishers, Singapore (in press).

Kollmeier, B., and Koch, R. (1994). Speech enhancement based on physiological and psychoacoustical models of modulation perception and binaural interaction. *J. Acoust. Soc. Am.*, **95**, 1593–1602.

Kollmeier, B., Peissig, J., and Hohman, V. (1993). Binaural noise-reduction hearing aid scheme with real-time processing in the frequency domain. *Scand. Audiol.*, **Suppl. 38, 28-38**.

Kompis, M., and Dillier, N. (1994). Noise reduction for hearing aids:Combining directional microphones with an adaptive beamformer. *J. Acoust. Soc. Am.*, **96**, 1910–1913.

Kryter, K. D. (1962). Methods for the calculation and use of the Articulation Index. *J. Acoust. Soc. Am.*, **34**, 467–477.

Lamore, P. J. J., Verweij, C., and Brocaar, M. P. (1984). Reliability of auditory function tests in severely hearing-impaired and deaf subjects. *Audiology*, **23**, 453–466.

Laroche, C., Hétu, R., Quoc, H. T., Josserand, B., and Glasberg, B. R. (1992). Frequency selectivity in workers with noise-induced hearing loss. *Hear. Res.*, **64**, 61–72.

Laurence, R. F., Moore, B. C. J., and Glasberg, B. R. (1983). A comparison of behind-the-ear high-fidelity linear aids and two-channel compression hearing aids in the laboratory and in everyday life. *Brit. J. Audiol.*, **17**, 31–48.

Lee, L. W., and Humes, L. E. (1993). Evaluating a speech-reception threshold model for hearing-impaired listeners. *J. Acoust. Soc. Am.*, **93**, 2879–2885.

Leek, M. R., and Summers, V. (1993). Auditory filter shapes of normal-hearing and hearing-impaired listeners in continuous broadband noise. *J. Acoust. Soc. Am.*, **94**, 3127–3137.

Leeuw, A. R., and Dreschler, W. A. (1991). Advantages of directional hearing aid microphones related to room acoustics. *Audiology*, **30**, 330–344.

Leeuw, A. R., and Dreschler, W. A. (1994). Frequency-resolution measurements with notched noise for clinical purposes. *Ear Hear.*, **15**, 240–255.

Leijon, A. (1989). Optimization of hearing-aid gain and frequency response for cochlear hearing losses. Ph.D. Thesis, Chalmers University of Technology, Sweden.

Leonard, D. G. B., and Khanna, S. M. (1984). Histological evaluation of damage in cat cochleas used for measurement of basilar membrane mechanics. *J. Acoust. Soc. Am.*, **75**, 515–527.

Leshowitz, B., and Lindstrom, R. (1977). Measurement of nonlinearities in listeners with sensorineural hearing loss. In *Psychophysics and Physiology of Hearing*, (ed. E. F. Evans and J. P. Wilson), pp. 283–292. Academic Press, London.

Leshowitz, B., Linstrom, R., and Zurek, P. (1975). Psychophysical tuning curves in normal and impaired ears. *J. Acoust. Soc. Am.*, 58, **Suppl. 1, s71**.

Levitt, H. (1982). Speech discrimination ability in the hearing impaired: Spectrum considerations. In *The Vanderbilt Hearing-Aid Report*, (ed. G. A. Studebaker and F. H. Bess), pp. 32–43. Monographs in Contemporary Audiology, Upper Darby, PA.

Levitt, H., and Rabiner, L. R. (1967). Binaural release from masking for speech and gain in intelligibility. *J. Acoust. Soc. Am.*, **42**, 601–608.

Libby, E. R. (1981). Achieving a transparent, smooth, wideband hearing aid response. *Hear. Inst.*, **32**, 9–12.

Libby, E. R. (1982). In search of transparent hearing aid responses. In *The Vanderbilt Hearing Aid Report*, (ed. G. A. Studebaker and F. H. Bess), pp. 112–123. Monographs in Contemporary Audiology, Upper Darby, PA.

Liberman, M. C. (1978). Auditory-nerve response from cats raised in a low-noise chamber. *J. Acoust. Soc. Am.*, **63**, 442–455.

Liberman, M. C. (1982). The cochlear frequency map for the cat: Labeling auditory-nerve fibers of known characteristic frequency. *J. Acoust. Soc. Am.*, **72**, 1441–1449.

Liberman, M. C., and Dodds, L. W. (1984). Single neuron labeling and chronic cochlea pathology. III. Stereocilia damage and alterations in threshold tuning curves. *Hear. Res.*, **16**, 54–74.

Liberman, M. C., Dodds, L. W., and Learson, D. A. (1986). Structure-function correlation in noise-damaged ears: A light and electron-microscopic study. In *Basic and Applied Aspects of Noise-Induced Hearing Loss*, (ed. R. J. Salvi, D. Henderson, R. P. Hamernik and V. Colletti), pp. 163–176. Plenum, New York.

Licklider, J. C. R. (1948). The influence of interaural phase relations upon the masking of speech by white noise. *J. Acoust. Soc. Am.*, **20**, 150–159.

Licklider, J. C. R. (1956). Auditory frequency analysis. In *Information Theory*, (ed. C. Cherry), pp. 253–268. Academic, New York.

Lindsay, P. H., and Norman, D. A. (1972). *Human Information Processing*. Academic Press, New York.

Lippmann, R. P., Braida, L. D., and Durlach, N. I. (1981). Study of multi-channel amplitude compression and linear amplification for persons with sensorineural hearing loss. *J. Acoust. Soc. Am.*, **69**, 524–534.

Loeb, G. E., White, M. W., and Merzenich, M. M. (1983). Spatial cross correlation: A proposed mechanism for acoustic pitch perception. *Biol. Cybern.*, **47**, 149–163.

Lundeen, C., and Small, A. M. (1984). The influence of temporal cues on the strength of periodicity pitches. *J. Acoust. Soc. Am.*, **75**, 1578–1587.

Lüscher, E., and Zwislocki, J. J. (1949). A simple method for indirect determination of the recruitment phenomenon (difference limen in intensity in different types of deafness). *Acta Otolaryngol.*, **Suppl. 78**, 156-168.

Lutman, M. E. (1991). Degradations in frequency and temporal resolution with age and their impact on speech identification. *Acta Otolaryngol. (Stockh)*, **Suppl. 4**, 120-126.

Lybarger, S. F. (1978). Selective amplification—A review and evaluation. *J. Am. Audit. Soc*, **3**, 258–266.

Mangold, S., and Leijon, A. (1979). Programmable hearing aid with multi-channel compression. *Scand. Audiol.*, **8**, 121–126.

McCandless, G. A., and Lyregard, P. E. (1983). Prescription of gain/output (POGO) for hearing aids. *Hear. Inst.*, **34**, 16–21.

McDermott, H. J., McKay, C. M., and Vandali, A. E. (1992). A new portable soundprocessor for the University of Melbourne/Nucleus Limited multielectrode cochlear implant. *J. Acoust. Soc. Am.*, **91**, 3367–3371.

McKay, C. M., and McDermott, H. J. (1993). Perceptual performance of subjects with cochlear implants using the spectral maxima sound processor (SMSP) and the mini speech processor (MSP). *Ear Hear.*, **15**, 350–367.

Meddis, R., and Hewitt, M. (1991). Virtual pitch and phase sensitivity studied using a computer model of the auditory periphery: Pitch identification. *J. Acoust. Soc. Am.*, **89**, 2866–2882.

Mertz, P. (1982). Clinical applications of innovative earmold coupling systems. *Audecibel*, **31**, 24–26.

Miller, G. A. (1947). Sensitivity to changes in the intensity of white noise and its relation to masking and loudness. *J. Acoust. Soc. Am.*, **191**, 609–619.

Mills, A. W. (1958). On the minimum audible angle. *J. Acoust. Soc. Am.*, **30**, 237–246.

Mills, A. W. (1960). Lateralization of high-frequency tones. *J. Acoust. Soc. Am.*, **32**, 132–134.

Mills, A. W. (1972). Auditory localization. In *Foundations of Modern Auditory Theory Vol. II*, (ed. J. V. Tobias), pp. 303–348. Academic Press, New York.

Mills, J. H., and Schmeidt, R. A. (1983). Frequency selectivity: Physiological and psychophysical tuning curves and suppression. In *Hearing Research and Theory, Vol. 2,* (ed. J. V. Tobias and E. D. Schubert), pp. 233-336. Academic, New York.

Miskolczy-Fodor, F. (1960). Relation between loudness and duration of tonal pulses. III. Response in cases of abnormal loudness function. *J. Acoust. Soc. Am.*, **32**, 486–492.

Moore, B. C. J. (1973a). Frequency difference limens for short-duration tones. *J. Acoust. Soc. Am.*, **54**, 610–619.

Moore, B. C. J. (1973b). Some experiments relating to the perception of complex tones. *Q. J. Exp. Psych.*, **25**, 451–475.

Moore, B. C. J. (1974). Relation between the critical bandwidth and the frequency-difference limen. *J. Acoust. Soc. Am.*, **55**, 359.

Moore, B. C. J. (1976). Comparison of frequency DL's for pulsed tones and modulated tones. *Brit. J. Audiol.*, **10**, 17–20.

Moore, B. C. J. (1977). Effects of relative phase of the components on the pitch of three-component complex tones. In *Psychophysics and Physiology of Hearing*, (ed. E. F. Evans and J. P. Wilson), pp. 349–358. Academic Press, London.

Moore, B. C. J. (1978). Psychophysical tuning curves measured in simultaneous and forward masking. *J. Acoust. Soc. Am.*, **63**, 524–532.

Moore, B. C. J. (1980). Detection cues in forward masking. In *Psychophysical, Physiological and Behavioural Studies in Hearing*, (ed. G. van den Brink and F. A. Bilson), pp. 222–229. Delft University Press, Delft.

Moore, B. C. J. (1981). Interactions of masker bandwidth with signal duration and delay in forward masking. *J. Acoust. Soc. Am.*, **70**, 62–68.

Moore, B. C. J. (1982). *An Introduction to the Psychology of Hearing, 2nd Ed.* Academic Press, London.

Moore, B. C. J. (1987a). Design and evaluation of a two-channel compression hearing aid. *J. Rehab. Res. Dev.*, **24**, 181–192.

Moore, B. C. J. (1987b). Distribution of auditory-filter bandwidths at 2 kHz in young normal listeners. *J. Acoust. Soc. Am.*, **81**, 1633–1635.

Moore, B. C. J. (1988). Dynamic aspects of auditory masking. In *Auditory Function: Neurobiological Bases of Hearing*, (ed. G. Edelman, W. Gall and W. Cowan), pp. 585–607. Wiley, New York.

Moore, B. C. J. (1989). *An Introduction to the Psychology of Hearing, 3rd Ed.* Academic Press, London.

Moore, B. C. J. (1990). How much do we gain by gain control in hearing aids? *Acta Otolaryngol. Suppl.*, **469**, 250–256.

Moore, B. C. J. (1991). Characterization and simulation of impaired hearing: implications for hearing aid design. *Ear Hear.*, **12**, Suppl., 154S–161S.

Moore, B. C. J. (1993). Signal processing to compensate for reduced dynamic range. In *Recent Developments in Hearing Instrument Technology*, (ed. J. Beilin and G. R. Jensen), pp. 147–165. Danavox Foundation, Kolding, Denmark.

Moore, B. C. J. (1995). Frequency analysis and masking. In *Handbook of Perception and Cognition, Volume 6. Hearing*, (ed. B. C. J. Moore) pp. 161–205. Academic Press, Orlando, Florida.

Moore, B. C. J., and Glasberg, B. R. (1981). Auditory filter shapes derived in simultaneous and forward masking. *J. Acoust. Soc. Am.*, **70**, 1003–1014.

Moore, B. C. J., and Glasberg, B. R. (1982). Contralateral and ipsilateral cueing in forward masking. *J. Acoust. Soc. Am.*, **71**, 942–945.

Moore, B. C. J., and Glasberg, B. R. (1983a). Growth of forward masking for sinusoidal and noise maskers as a function of signal delay: implications for suppression in noise. *J. Acoust. Soc. Am.*, **73**, 1249–1259.

Moore, B. C. J., and Glasberg, B. R. (1983b). Masking patterns of synthetic vowels in simultaneous and forward masking. *J. Acoust. Soc. Am.*, **73**, 906–917.

Moore, B. C. J., and Glasberg, B. R. (1983c). Suggested formulae for calculating auditory-filter bandwidths and excitation patterns. *J. Acoust. Soc. Am.*, **74**, 750–753.

Moore, B. C. J., and Glasberg, B. R. (1985). The danger of using narrowband noise maskers to measure suppression. *J. Acoust. Soc. Am.*, **77**, 2137–2141.

Moore, B. C. J., and Glasberg, B. R. (1986a). A comparison of two-channel and single-channel compression hearing aids. *Audiol.*, **25**, 210–226.

Moore, B. C. J., and Glasberg, B. R. (1986b). Comparisons of frequency selectivity in simultaneous and forward masking for subjects with unilateral cochlear impairments. *J. Acoust. Soc. Am.*, **80**, 93–107.

Moore, B. C. J., and Glasberg, B. R. (1986c). The relationship between frequency selectivity and frequency discrimination for subjects with unilateral and bilateral cochlear impairments. In *Auditory Frequency Selectivity*, (ed. B. C. J. Moore and R. D. Patterson), pp. 407–414. Plenum, New York.

Moore, B. C. J., and Glasberg, B. R. (1986d). The role of frequency selectivity in the perception of loudness, pitch and time. In *Frequency Selectivity in Hearing*, (ed. B. C. J. Moore), pp. 251–308. Academic Press, London.

Moore, B. C. J., and Glasberg, B. R. (1987). Formulae describing frequency selectivity as a function of frequency and level and their use in calculating excitation patterns. *Hear. Res.*, **28**, 209–225.

Moore, B. C. J., and Glasberg, B. R. (1988a). A comparison of four methods of implementing automatic gain control (AGC) in hearing aids. *Brit. J. Audiol.*, **22**, 93–104.

Moore, B. C. J., and Glasberg, B. R. (1988b). Effects of the relative phase of the components on the pitch discrimination of complex tones by subjects with unilateral and bilateral cochlear impairments. In *Basic Issues in Hearing*, (ed. H. Duifhuis, H. Wit and J. Horst), pp. 421–430. Academic Press, London.

Moore, B. C. J., and Glasberg, B. R. (1988c). Gap detection with sinusoids and noise in normal, impaired and electrically stimulated ears. *J. Acoust. Soc. Am.*, **83**, 1093–1101.

Moore, B. C. J., and Glasberg, B. R. (1988d). Pitch perception and phase sensitivity for subjects with unilateral and bilateral cochlear hearing impairments. In *Clinical Audiology*, (ed. A. Quaranta), pp. 104-109. Laterza, Bari, Italy.

Moore, B. C. J., and Glasberg, B. R. (1989). Mechanisms underlying the frequency discrimination of pulsed tones and the detection of frequency modulation. *J. Acoust. Soc. Am.*, **86**, 1722–1732.

Moore, B. C. J., and Glasberg, B. R. (1990). Frequency selectivity in subjects with cochlear loss and its effects on pitch discrimination and phase sensitivity. In *Advances in Audiology*, (ed. F. Grandori, G. Cianfrone and D. T. Kemp), pp. 187–200. Karger, Basel.

Moore, B. C. J., and Glasberg, B. R. (1993). Simulation of the effects of loudness recruitment and threshold elevation on the intelligibility of speech in quiet and in a background of speech. *J. Acoust. Soc. Am.*, **94**, 2050–2062.

Moore, B. C. J., and Glasberg, B. R. (1995). A revision of Zwicker's loudness model. *Acustica*, (in press).

Moore, B. C. J., Glasberg, B. R., Donaldson, E., McPherson, T., and Plack, C. J. (1989). Detection of temporal gaps in sinusoids by normally hearing and hearing-impaired subjects. *J. Acoust. Soc. Am.*, **85**, 1266–1275.

Moore, B. C. J., Glasberg, B. R., Hess, R. F., and Birchall, J. P. (1985a). Effects of flanking noise bands on the rate of growth of loudness of tones in normal and recruiting ears. *J. Acoust. Soc. Am.*, **77**, 1505–1515.

Moore, B. C. J., Glasberg, B. R., and Peters, R. W. (1985b). Relative dominance of individual partials in determining the pitch of complex tones. *J. Acoust. Soc. Am.*, **77**, 1853–1860.

Moore, B. C. J., Glasberg, B. R., Plack, C. J., and Biswas, A. K. (1988). The shape of the ear's temporal window. *J. Acoust. Soc. Am.*, **83**, 1102–1116.

Moore, B. C. J., Glasberg, B. R., and Roberts, B. (1984a). Refining the measurement of psychophysical tuning curves. *J. Acoust. Soc. Am.*, **76**, 1057–1066.

Moore, B. C. J., Glasberg, B. R., and Shailer, M. J. (1984b). Frequency and intensity difference limens for harmonics within complex tones. *J. Acoust. Soc. Am.*, **75**, 550–561.

Moore, B. C. J., Glasberg, B. R., and Simpson, A. (1992a). Evaluation of a method of simulating reduced frequency selectivity. *J. Acoust. Soc. Am.*, **91**, 3402–3423.

Moore, B. C. J., Glasberg, B. R., and Stone, M. A. (1991). Optimization of a slow-acting automatic gain control system for use in hearing aids. *Brit. J. Audiol.*, **25**, 171–182.

Moore, B. C. J., Glasberg, B. R., and Vickers, D. A. (1995). Simulation of the effects of loudness recruitment on the intelligibility of speech in noise. *Brit. J. Audiol.*, (in press).

Moore, B. C. J., Johnson, J. S., Clark, T. M., and Pluvinage, V. (1992b). Evaluation of a dual-channel full dynamic range compression system for people with sensorineural hearing loss. *Ear Hear.*, **13**, 349–370.

Moore, B. C. J., Laurence, R. F., and Wright, D. (1985c). Improvements in speech intelligibility in quiet and in noise produced by two-channel compression hearing aids. *Brit. J. Audiol.*, **19**, 175–187.

Moore, B. C. J., Lynch, C., and Stone, M. A. (1992c). Effects of the fitting parameters of a two-channel compression system on the intelligibility of speech in quiet and in noise. *Brit. J. Audiol.*, **26**, 369–379.

Moore, B. C. J., and O'Loughlin, B. J. (1986). The use of nonsimultaneous masking to measure frequency selectivity and suppression. In *Frequency Selectivity in Hearing*, (ed. B. C. J. Moore), pp. 179–250. Academic Press, London.

Moore, B. C. J., and Ohgushi, K. (1993). Audibility of partials in inharmonic complex tones. *J. Acoust. Soc. Am.*, **93**, 452–461.

Moore, B. C. J., and Peters, R. W. (1992). Pitch discrimination and phase sensitivity in young and elderly subjects and its relationship to frequency selectivity. *J. Acoust. Soc. Am.*, **91**, 2881–2893.

Moore, B. C. J., Peters, R. W., and Glasberg, B. R. (1990). Auditory filter shapes at low center frequencies. *J. Acoust. Soc. Am.*, **88**, 132–140.

Moore, B. C. J., Peters, R. W., and Glasberg, B. R. (1993a). Detection of temporal gaps in sinusoids: Effects of frequency and level. *J. Acoust. Soc. Am.*, **93**, 1563–1570.

Moore, B. C. J., Peters, R. W., and Glasberg, B. R. (1993b). Effects of frequency on the detection of decrements and increments in sinusoids. *J. Acoust. Soc. Am.*, **94**, 3190–3198.

Moore, B. C. J., Poon, P. W. F., Bacon, S. P., and Glasberg, B. R. (1987). The temporal course of masking and the auditory filter shape. *J. Acoust. Soc. Am.*, **81**, 1873–1880.

Moore, B. C. J., and Rosen, S. M. (1979). Tune recognition with reduced pitch and interval information. *Q. J. Exp. Psychol.*, **31**, 229–240.

Moore, B. C. J., and Sek, A. (1994). Effects of carrier frequency and background noise on the detection of mixed modulation. *J. Acoust. Soc. Am.*, **96**, 741–751.

Moore, B. C. J., and Sek, A. (1995). Effects of carrier frequency, modulation rate and modulation waveform on the detection of modulation and the discrimination of modulation type (AM vs FM). *J. Acoust. Soc. Am.*, **97**, 2468–2478.

Moore, B. C. J., Shailer, M. J., Hall, J. W., and Schooneveldt, G. P. (1993c). Comodulation masking release in subjects with unilateral and bilateral cochlear hearing impairment. *J. Acoust. Soc. Am.*, **93**, 435–451.

Moore, B. C. J., Shailer, M. J., and Schooneveldt, G. P. (1992d). Temporal modulation transfer functions for band-limited noise in subjects with cochlear hearing loss. *Brit. J. Audiol.*, **26**, 229–237.

Murray, N., and Byrne, D. (1986). Performance of hearing-impaired and normal hearing listeners with various high-frequency cut-offs in hearing aids. *Aust. J. Audiol.*, **8**, 21–28.

Neff, D. L. (1985). Stimulus parameters governing confusion effects in forward masking. *J. Acoust. Soc. Am.*, **78**, 1966–1976.

Nelson, D. A. (1991). High-level psychophysical tuning curves: Forward masking in normal-hearing and hearing-impaired listeners. *J. Speech Hear. Res.*, **34**, 1233–1249.

Nielsen, H. B., and Ludvigsen, C. (1978). Effect of hearing aids with directional microphones in different acoustic environments. *Scand. Audiol.*, **7**, 217–224.

Nordlund, B. (1964). Directional Audiometry. *Acta Otolaryngol.*, **57**, 1–18.

O'Loughlin, B. J., and Moore, B. C. J. (1981a). Improving psychoacoustical tuning curves. *Hear. Res.*, **5**, 343–346.

O'Loughlin, B. J., and Moore, B. C. J. (1981b). Off-frequency listening: effects on psychoacoustical tuning curves obtained in simultaneous and forward masking. *J. Acoust. Soc. Am.*, **69**, 1119–1125.

Ohgushi, K., and Hatoh, T. (1991). Perception of the musical pitch of high frequency tones. In *Ninth International Symposium on Hearing: Auditory Physiology and Perception*, (ed. Y. Cazals, L. Demany and K. Horner), pp. 207–212. Pergamon, Oxford.

Ohm, G. S. (1843). Über die Definition des Tones, nebst daran geknüpfter Theorie der Sirene und ähnlicher tonbildender Vorrichtungen. *Annalen der Physik und Chemie*, **59**, 513–565.

Ono, H., Kanzaki, J., and Mizoi, K. (1983). Clinical results of hearing aid with noise-level-controlled selective amplification. *Audiology*, **22**, 494–515.

Oxenham, A. J., and Moore, B. C. J. (1994). Modeling the additivity of nonsimultaneous masking. *Hear. Res.*, **80**, 105–118.

Oxenham, A. J., and Moore, B. C. J. (1995). Additivity of masking in normally hearing and hearing-impaired subjects. *J. Acoust. Soc. Am.*, (in press).

Palmer, A. R. (1987). Physiology of the cochlear nerve and cochlear nucleus. In *Hearing*, (ed. M. P. Haggard and E. F. Evans), pp. 838-855. Churchill Livingstone, Edinburgh.

Palmer, A. R., and Russell, I. J. (1986). Phase-locking in the cochlear nerve of the guinea-pig and its relation to the receptor potential of inner hair-cells. *Hear. Res.*, **24**, 1–15.

Pascoe, D. P. (1978). An approach to hearing aid selection. *Hear. Inst.*, **29**, 12–16.

Patterson, R. D. (1973). The effects of relative phase and the number of components on residue pitch. *J. Acoust. Soc. Am.*, **53**, 1565–1572.

Patterson, R. D. (1974). Auditory filter shape. *J. Acoust. Soc. Am.*, **55**, 802–809.

Patterson, R. D. (1976). Auditory filter shapes derived with noise stimuli. *J. Acoust. Soc. Am.*, **59**, 640–654.

Patterson, R. D. (1987). A pulse ribbon model of peripheral auditory processing. In *Auditory Processing of Complex Sounds*, (ed. W. A. Yost and C. S. Watson), pp. 167-179. Erlbaum, New Jersey.

Patterson, R. D., and Henning, G. B. (1977). Stimulus variability and auditory filter shape. *J. Acoust. Soc. Am.*, **62**, 649–664.

Patterson, R. D., and Moore, B. C. J. (1986). Auditory filters and excitation patterns as representations of frequency resolution. In *Frequency Selectivity in Hearing*, (ed. B. C. J. Moore), pp. 123-177. Academic Press, London.

Patterson, R. D., and Nimmo-Smith, I. (1980). Off-frequency listening and auditory filter asymmetry. *J. Acoust. Soc. Am.*, **67**, 229–245.

Patterson, R. D., Nimmo-Smith, I., Weber, D. L., and Milroy, R. (1982). The deterioration of hearing with age: Frequency selectivity, the critical ratio, the audiogram, and speech threshold. *J. Acoust. Soc. Am.*, **72**, 1788–1803.

Patterson, R. D., and Wightman, F. L. (1976). Residue pitch as a function of component spacing. *J. Acoust. Soc. Am.*, **59**, 1450–1459.

Patuzzi, R., Sellick, P. M., and Johnstone, B. M. (1984). The modulation of the sensitivity of the mammalian cochlea by low-frequency tones. III. Basilar membrane motion. *Hear. Res.*, **13**, 19–27.

Patuzzi, R. B. (1992). Effects of noise on auditory nerve fiber response. In *Noise Induced Hearing Loss*, (ed. A. Dancer, D. Henderson, R. Salvi and R. Hamernik), pp. 45–59. Mosby Year Book, St. Louis.

Pavlovic, C. V. (1984). Use of the articulation index for assessing residual auditory function in listeners with sensorineural hearing impairment. *J. Acoust. Soc. Am.*, **75**, 1253–1258.

Pavlovic, C. V. (1987). Derivation of primary parameters and procedures for use in speech intelligibility predictions. *J. Acoust. Soc. Am.*, **82**, 413–422.

Pavlovic, C. V., Studebaker, G. A., and Sherbecoe, R. (1986). An articulation index based procedure for predicting the speech recognition performance of hearing-impaired individuals. *J. Acoust. Soc. Am.*, **80**, 50–57.

Pearsons, K. S., Bennett, R. L., and Fidell, S. (1976). *Speech Levels in Various Environments. Report No. 3281*. Bolt, Beranek and Newman, Cambridge, Massachussets.

Pedersen, C. B., and Elberling, C. (1973). Temporal integration of acoustic energy in patients with presbyacusis. *Acta Otolaryngol.*, **75**, 32–37.

Penner, M. J. (1972). Neural or energy summation in a Poisson counting model. *J. Math. Psych.*, **9**, 286–293.

Penner, M. J. (1978). A power law transformation resulting in a class of short-term integrators that produce time-intensity trades for noise bursts. *J. Acoust. Soc. Am.*, **63**, 195–201.

Penner, M. J. (1980a). The coding of intensity and the interaction of forward and backward masking. *J. Acoust. Soc. Am.*, **67**, 608–616.

Penner, M. J. (1980b). Two-tone forward masking patterns and tinnitus. *J. Speech Hear. Res.*, **23**, 779–786.

Penner, M. J., and Shiffrin, R. M. (1980). Nonlinearities in the coding of intensity within the context of a temporal summation model. *J. Acoust. Soc. Am.*, **67**, 617–627.

Peters, R. W., and Moore, B. C. J. (1992). Auditory filter shapes at low center frequencies in young and elderly hearing-impaired subjects. *J. Acoust. Soc. Am.*, **91**, 256–266.

Peters, R. W., Moore, B. C. J., and Glasberg, B. R. (1995). Effects of level and frequency on the detection of decrements and increments in sinusoids. *J. Acoust. Soc. Am.*, (in press).

Peterson, P. M., Durlach, N. I., Rabinowitz, W. M., and Zurek, P. M. (1987). Multimicrophone adaptive beamforming for interference reduction in hearing aids. *J. Rehab. Res. Devel.*, **24**, 103–110.

Phillips, D. P. (1987). Stimulus intensity and loudness recruitment: neural correlates. *J. Acoust. Soc. Am.*, **82**, 1–12.

Pick, G. F. (1980). Level dependence of psychophysical frequency resolution and auditory filter shape. *J. Acoust. Soc. Am.*, **68**, 1085–1095.

Pick, G. F., Evans, E. F., and Wilson, J. P. (1977). Frequency resolution in patients with hearing loss of cochlear origin. In *Psychophysics and Physiology of Hearing*, (ed. E. F. Evans and J. P. Wilson), pp. 273–281. Academic Press, London.

Pickles, J. O. (1986). The neurophysiological basis of frequency selectivity. In *Frequency Selectivity in Hearing*, (ed. B. C. J. Moore), pp. 51–121. Academic Press, London.

Pickles, J. O. (1988). *An Introduction to the Physiology of Hearing, 2nd Ed.* Academic Press, London.

Plack, C. J., and Moore, B. C. J. (1990). Temporal window shape as a function of frequency and level. *J. Acoust. Soc. Am.*, **87**, 2178–2187.

Plack, C. J., and Moore, B. C. J. (1991). Decrement detection in normal and impaired ears. *J. Acoust. Soc. Am.*, **90**, 3069–3076.

Plomp, R. (1964a). The ear as a frequency analyzer. *J. Acoust. Soc. Am.*, **36**, 1628–1636.

Plomp, R. (1964b). The rate of decay of auditory sensation. *J. Acoust. Soc. Am.*, **36**, 277–282.

Plomp, R. (1967). Pitch of complex tones. *J. Acoust. Soc. Am.*, **41**, 1526–1533.

Plomp, R. (1976). *Aspects of Tone Sensation.* Academic Press, London.

Plomp, R. (1978). Auditory handicap of hearing impairment and the limited benefit of hearing aids. *J. Acoust. Soc. Am.*, **63**, 533–549.

Plomp, R. (1986). A signal-to-noise ratio model for the speech-reception threshold of the hearing impaired. *J. Speech Hear. Res.*, **29**, 146–154.

Plomp, R. (1988). The negative effect of amplitude compression in multichannel hearing aids in the light of the modulation-transfer function. *J. Acoust. Soc. Am.*, **83**, 2322–2327.

Plomp, R. (1994). Noise, amplification, and compression: Considerations of three main issues in hearing aid design. *Ear Hear.*, **15**, 2–12.

Plomp, R., and Mimpen, A. M. (1979). Improving the reliability of testing the speech reception threshold for sentences. *Audiology*, **18**, 43–53.

Plomp, R., and Steeneken, H. J. M. (1973). Place dependence of timbre in reverberant sound fields. *Acustica*, **28**, 50–59.

Pluvinage, V. (1989). Clinical measurement of loudness growth. *Hear. Instr.*, **39**, 28–29,32.

Preminger, J., and Wiley, T. L. (1985). Frequency selectivity and consonant intelligibility in sensorineural hearing loss. *J. Speech Hear. Res.*, **28**, 197–206.

Quaranta, A., and Cervellera, G. (1974). Masking level differences in normal and pathological ears. *Audiology*, **13**, 428–431.

Rankovic, C. M., Freyman, R. L., and Zurek, P. M. (1992). Potential benefits of adaptive frequency-gain characteristics for speech reception in noise. *J. Acoust. Soc. Am.*, **91**, 354–362.

Rankovic, C. M., Viemeister, N. F., Fantini, D. A., Cheesman, M. F., and Uchiyama, C. L. (1988). The relation between loudness and intensity difference limens for tones in quiet and noise backgrounds. *J. Acoust. Soc. Am.*, **84**, 150–155.

Rayleigh, Lord. (1907). On our perception of sound direction. *Phil. Mag.*, **13**, 214–232.

Rhode, W. S. (1971). Observations of the vibration of the basilar membrane in squirrel monkeys using the Mössbauer technique. *J. Acoust. Soc. Am.*, **49**, 1218–1231.

Rhode, W. S. (1977). Some observations on two-tone interaction measured with the Mössbauer effect. In *Psychophysics and Physiology of Hearing*, (ed. E. F. Evans and J. P. Wilson), pp. 27–41. Academic Press, London.

Rhode, W. S., and Robles, L. (1974). Evidence from Mössbauer experiments for non-linear vibration in the cochlea. *J. Acoust. Soc. Am.*, **55**, 588–596.

Riesz, R. R. (1928). Differential intensity sensitivity of the ear for pure tones. *Physical Reviews*, **31**, 867–875.

Ringdahl, A., Eriksson-Mangold, M., Israelsson, B., Lindkvist, A., and Mangold, S. (1990). Clinical trials with a programmable hearing aid set for various listening environments. *Brit. J. Audiol.*, **24**, 235–242.

Risberg, A. (1974). The importance of prosodic elements for the lipreader. In *Visual and Audio-visual Perception of Speech*, (ed. H. B. Nielson and E. Klamp), pp. 153–164. Almquist and Wiksell, Stockholm.

Ritsma, R. J. (1962). Existence region of the tonal residue. I. *J. Acoust. Soc. Am.*, **34**, 1224–1229.

Ritsma, R. J. (1963). Existence region of the tonal residue. II. *J. Acoust. Soc. Am.*, **35**, 1241–1245.

Ritsma, R. J. (1967). Frequencies dominant in the perception of the pitch of complex sounds. *J. Acoust. Soc. Am.*, **42**, 191–198.

Ritsma, R. J. (1970). Periodicity detection. In *Frequency Analysis and Periodicity Detection in Hearing*, (ed. R. Plomp and G. F. Smoorenburg), pp. 250–263. Sijthoff, Leiden.

Robertson, D., and Manley, G. A. (1974). Manipulation of frequency analysis in the cochlear ganglion of the guinea pig. *J. Comp. Physiol.*, **91**, 363–375.

Robinson, D. W., and Dadson, R. S. (1956). A re-determination of the equal-loudness relations for pure tones. *Brit. J. Appl. Phys.*, **7**, 166–181.

Robles, L., Ruggero, M. A., and Rich, N. C. (1986). Basilar membrane mechanics at the base of the chinchilla cochlea. I. Input–output functions, tuning curves, and response phases. *J. Acoust. Soc. Am.*, **80**, 1364–1374.

Robles, L., Ruggero, M. A., and Rich, N. C. (1991). Two-tone distortion in the basilar membrane of the cochlea. *Nature*, **349**, 413–414.

Rose, J. E., Brugge, J. F., Anderson, D. J., and Hind, J. E. (1968). Patterns of activity in single auditory nerve fibres of the squirrel monkey. In *Hearing Mechanisms in Vertebrates*, (ed. A. V. S. de Reuck and J. Knight), pp. 144–157. Churchill, London.

Rosen, S. (1987). Phase and the hearing impaired. In *The Psychophysics of Speech Perception*, (ed. M. E. H.Schouten), pp. 481–488. Martinus Nijhoff, Dordrecht.

Rosen, S., and Fourcin, A. (1986). Frequency selectivity and the perception of speech. In *Frequency Selectivity in Hearing*, (ed. B. C. J. Moore), pp. 373–487. Academic Press, London.

Rosen, S. M., Fourcin, A. J., and Moore, B. C. J. (1981). Voice pitch as an aid to lipreading. *Nature*, **291**, 150–152.

Ruggero, M. A. (1992). Responses to sound of the basilar membrane of the mammalian cochlea. *Curr. Opin. Neurobiol.*, **2**, 449–456.

Ruggero, M. A., and Rich, N. C. (1987). Timing of spike initiation in cochlear afferents: Dependence on site of innervation. *J. Neurophysiol.*, **58**, 379–403.

Ruggero, M. A., and Rich, N. C. (1991). Furosemide alters organ of Corti mechanics: Evidence for feedback of outer hair cells upon the basilar membrane. *J. Neurosci.*, **11**, 1057–1067.

Ruggero, M. A., Rich, N. C., and Recio, A. (1993). Alteration of basilar membrane response to sound by acoustic overstimulation. In *Biophysics of Hair Cell Sensory Systems*, (ed. H. Duifhuis, J. W. Horst, P. van Dijk and S. M. van Netten), pp. 258–265. World Scientific, Singapore.

Ruggero, M. A., Robles, L., and Rich, N. C. (1992). Two-tone suppression in the basilar membrane of the cochlea: Mechanical basis of auditory-nerve rate suppression. *J. Neurophysiol.*, **68**, 1087–1099.

Ruggero, M. A., Robles, L., Rich, N. C., and Costalupes, J. A. (1986). Basilar membrane motion and spike initiation in the cochlear nerve. In *Auditory Frequency Selectivity* , (ed. B. C. J. Moore and R. D. Patterson), pp. 189–196. Plenum, New York.

Ryan, A. F., and Dallos, P. (1984). Physiology of the cochlea. In *Hearing Disorders*, (ed. J. L. Northern), pp. 253–266. Little Brown, Boston.

Sachs, M. B., and Abbas, P. J. (1974). Rate versus level functions for auditory-nerve fibers in cats:tone-burst stimuli. *J. Acoust. Soc. Am.*, **56**, 1835–1847.

Sachs, M. B., and Kiang, N. Y. S. (1968). Two-tone inhibition in auditory nerve fibers. *J. Acoust. Soc. Am.*, **43**, 1120–1128.

Salvi, R. J., and Arehole, S. (1985). Gap detection in chinchillas with temporary high-frequency hearing loss. *J. Acoust. Soc. Am.*, **77**, 1173–1177.

Scharf, B., and Hellman, R. P. (1966). A model of loudness summation applied to impaired ears. *J. Acoust. Soc. Am.*, **40**, 71–78.

Schlauch, R. S. (1994). Intensity resolution and loudness in high-pass noise. *J. Acoust. Soc. Am.*, **95**, 2171–2179.

Schlauch, R. S., and Wier, C. C. (1987). A method for relating loudness matching and intensity-discrimination data. *J. Speech Hear. Res.*, **30**, 13–20.

Schoeny, Z., and Carhart, R. (1971). Effects of unilateral Ménière's disease on masking level differences. *J. Acoust. Soc. Am.*, **50**, 1143–1150.

Schooneveldt, G. P., and Moore, B. C. J. (1989). Comodulation masking release (CMR) as a function of masker bandwidth, modulator bandwidth and signal duration. *J. Acoust. Soc. Am.*, **85**, 273–281.

Schouten, J. F. (1940). The residue and the mechanism of hearing. *Proc. Kon. Akad. Wetenschap.*, **43**, 991–999.

Schouten, J. F. (1970). The residue revisited. In *Frequency Analysis and Periodicity Detection in Hearing*, (ed. R. Plomp and G. F. Smoorenburg), pp. 41–54. Sijthoff, Lieden, The Netherlands.

Schouten, J. F., Ritsma, R. J., and Cardozo, B. L. (1962). Pitch of the residue. *J. Acoust. Soc. Am.*, **34**, 1418–1424.

Schroder, A. C., Viemeister, N. F., and Nelson, D. A. (1994). Intensity discrimination in normal-hearing and hearing-impaired listeners. *J. Acoust. Soc. Am.*, **96**, 2683–2693.

Schwander, T. J., and Levitt, H. (1987). Effect of two-microphone noise reduction on speech recognition by normal-hearing listeners. *J. Rehab. Res. Devel.*, **24**, 87–92.

Sek, A., and Moore, B. C. J. (1995). Frequency discrimination as a function of frequency, measured in several ways. *J. Acoust. Soc. Am.*, **97**, 2479–2486.

Sellick, P. M., Patuzzi, R., and Johnstone, B. M. (1982). Measurement of basilar membrane motion in the guinea pig using the Mössbauer technique. *J. Acoust. Soc. Am.*, **72**, 131–141.

Shackleton, T. M., and Carlyon, R. P. (1994). The role of resolved and unresolved harmonics in pitch perception and frequency modulation discrimination. *J. Acoust. Soc. Am.*, **95**, 3529–3540.

Shailer, M. J., and Moore, B. C. J. (1983). Gap detection as a function of frequency, bandwidth and level. *J. Acoust. Soc. Am.*, **74**, 467–473.

Shailer, M. J., and Moore, B. C. J. (1985). Detection of temporal gaps in band-limited noise: effects of variations in bandwidth and signal-to-masker ratio. *J. Acoust. Soc. Am.*, **77**, 635–639.

Shailer, M. J., and Moore, B. C. J. (1987). Gap detection and the auditory filter: phase effects using sinusoidal stimuli. *J. Acoust. Soc. Am.*, **81**, 1110–1117.

Shailer, M. J., Moore, B. C. J., Glasberg, B. R., Watson, N., and Harris, S. (1990). Auditory filter shapes at 8 and 10 kHz. *J. Acoust. Soc. Am.*, **88**, 141–148.

Shamma, S. A. (1985). Speech processing in the auditory system II: Lateral inhibition and the central processing of speech evoked activity in the auditory nerve. *J. Acoust. Soc. Am.*, **78**, 1622–1632.

Shannon, R. V. (1976). Two-tone unmasking and suppression in a forward masking situation. *J. Acoust. Soc. Am.*, **59**, 1460–1470.

Shaw, W. A., Newman, E. B., and Hirsh, I. J. (1947). The difference between monaural and binaural thresholds. *J. Exp. Psychol.*, **37**, 229–242.

Sher, A. E., and Owens, E. (1974). Consonant confusions associated with hearing loss above 2000 Hz. *J. Speech Hear. Res.*, **17**, 669–681.

Shower, E. G., and Biddulph, R. (1931). Differential pitch sensitivity of the ear. *J. Acoust. Soc. Am.*, 2, 275-287.

Siebert, W. M. (1970). Frequency discrimination in the auditory system: place or periodicity mechanisms. *Proc. IEEE*, **58**, 723–730.

Simon, H. J., and Yund, E. W. (1993). Frequency discrimination in listeners with sensorineural hearing loss. *Ear Hear.*, **14**, 190–199.

Simpson, A. M., Moore, B. C. J., and Glasberg, B. R. (1990). Spectral enhancement to improve the intelligibility of speech in noise for hearing-impaired listeners. *Acta Otolaryngol. Suppl.*, **469**, 101–107.

Slepecky, N., Hamernik, R., Henderson, D., and Coling, D. (1982). Correlation of audiometric data with changes in cochlear hair cell stereocilia resulting from impulse noise trauma. *Acta Otolaryngol.*, **93**, 329–340.

Small, A. M. (1959). Pure-tone masking. *J. Acoust. Soc. Am.*, **31**, 1619–1625.

Smoorenburg, G. F. (1972a). Audibility region of combination tones. *J. Acoust. Soc. Am.*, **52**, 603–614.

Smoorenburg, G. F. (1972b). Combination tones and their origin. *J. Acoust. Soc. Am.*, **52**, 615–632.

Smoorenburg, G. F. (1992). Speech reception in quiet and in noisy conditions by individuals with noise-induced hearing loss in relation to their tone audiogram. *J. Acoust. Soc. Am.*, **91**, 421–437.

Smoski, W. J., and Trahiotis, C. (1986). Discrimination of interaural temporal disparities by normal-hearing listeners and listeners with high-frequency sensorineural hearing loss. *J. Acoust. Soc. Am.*, **79**, 1541–1547.

Snell, K. B., Ison, J. R., and Frisina, D. R. (1994). The effects of signal frequency and absolute bandwidth on gap detection in noise. *J. Acoust. Soc. Am.*, **96**, 1458–1464.

Soede, W., Berkhout, A. J., and Bilsen, F. A. (1993a). Development of a directional hearing instrument based on array technology. *J. Acoust. Soc. Am.*, **94**, 785–798.

Soede, W., Bilsen, F. A., and Berkhout, A. J. (1993b). Assessment of a directional microphone array for hearing-impaired listeners. *J. Acoust. Soc. Am.*, **94**, 799–808.

Sommers, M. S., and Humes, L. E. (1993). Auditory filter shapes in normal-hearing, noise-masked normal, and elderly listeners. *J. Acoust. Soc. Am.*, **93**, 2903–2914.

Spiegel, M. F. (1981). Thresholds for tones in maskers of various bandwidths and for signals of various bandwidths as a function of signal frequency. *J. Acoust. Soc. Am.*, **69**, 791–795.

Spoendlin, H. (1970). Structural basis of peripheral frequency analysis. In *Frequency Analysis and Periodicity Detection in Hearing*, (ed. R. Plomp and G. F. Smoorenburg), pp. 2–40. Sijthoff, Leiden.

Srulovicz, P., and Goldstein, J. L. (1983). A central spectrum model: a synthesis of auditory-nerve timing and place cues in monaural communication of frequency spectrum. *J. Acoust. Soc. Am.*, **73**, 1266–1276.

Staffel, J. G., Hall, J. W., Grose, J. H., and Pillsbury, H. C. (1990). NoSo and NoSπ detection as a function of masker bandwidth in normal-hearing and cochlear-impaired listeners. *J. Acoust. Soc. Am.*, **87**, 1720–1727.

Steinberg, J. C., and Gardner, M. B. (1937). The dependency of hearing impairment on sound intensity. *J. Acoust. Soc. Am.*, **9**, 11–23.

Stelmachowicz, P. G., Jesteadt, W., Gorga, M. P., and Mott, J. (1985). Speech perception ability and psychophysical tuning curves in hearing-impaired listeners. *J. Acoust. Soc. Am.*, **77**, 621–627.

Stelmachowicz, P. G., Lewis, D. E., Larson, L. L., and Jesteadt, W. (1987). Growth of masking as a measure of response growth in hearing-impaired listeners. *J. Acoust. Soc. Am.*, **81**, 1881–1887.

Stern, R. M., and Trahiotis, C. (1995). Models of binaural interaction. In *Handbook of Perception and Cognition, Vol. 6, Hearing,* (ed. B. C. J. Moore), pp. 347–386. Academic Press, New York.

Stevens, S. S. (1957). On the psychophysical law. *Psychol. Rev.*, **64**, 153–181.

Stevens, S. S., and Newman, E. B. (1936). The localization of actual sources of sound. *Am. J. Psychol.*, **48**, 297–306.

Stillman, J. A., Zwislocki, J. J., Zhang, M., and Cefaratti, L. K. (1993). Intensity just-noticeable differences at equal-loudness levels in normal and pathological ears. *J. Acoust. Soc. Am.*, **93**, 425–434.

Stone, M. A., Glasberg, B. R., and Moore, B. C. J. (1992). Simplified measurement of impaired auditory filter shapes using the notched-noise method. *Brit. J. Audiol.*, **26**, 329–334.

Stone, M. A., and Moore, B. C. J. (1992a). Spectral feature enhancement for people with sensorineural hearing impairment: effects on speech intelligibility and quality. *J. Rehab. Res. Devel.*, **29**, 39–56.

Stone, M. A., and Moore, B. C. J. (1992b). Syllabic compression: Effective compression ratios for signals modulated at different rates. *Brit. J. Audiol.*, **26**, 351–361.

Summerfield, A. Q., Foster, J., Tyler, R. S., and Bailey, P. J. (1985). Influences of formant narrowing and auditory frequency selectivity on identification of place of articulation in stop consonants. *Speech Commun.*, **4**, 213–229.

Summers, I. R. (1991). Electronically simulated hearing loss and the perception of degraded speech. In *Bioinstrumentation and Biosensors*, (ed. D. L. Wise), pp. 589–610. Marcel Dekker, New York.

Summers, I. R., and Al-Dabbagh, A. D. (1982). Simulated loss of frequency selectivity and its effects on speech perception. *Acoust. Lett.*, **5**, 129–132.

Suzuki, Y., and Sone, T. (1994). Frequency characteristics of loudness perception: Principles and applications. In *Contributions to Psychological Acoustics*, (ed. A. Schick), pp. 193–221. Bibliotheks- und Informationssytem der Universitat Oldenburg, Oldenburg.

Tabachnick, B. G., and Fidell, L. S. (1983). *Using Multi-variate Statistics.* Harper and Row, New York.

ter Keurs, M., Festen, J. M., and Plomp, R. (1992). Effect of spectral envelope smearing on speech reception. I. *J. Acoust. Soc. Am.*, **91**, 2872–2880.

ter Keurs, M., Festen, J. M., and Plomp, R. (1993). Effect of spectral envelope smearing on speech reception.II. *J. Acoust. Soc. Am.*, **93**, 1547–1552.

Terhardt, E. (1974). Pitch, consonance, and harmony. *J. Acoust. Soc. Am.*, **55**, 1061–1069.

Thibodeau, L. M., and van Tasell, D. J. (1987). Tone detection and synthetic speech discrimination in band-reject noise by hearing-impaired listeners. *J. Acoust. Soc. Am.*, **82**, 864–873.

Thornton, A. R., and Abbas, P. J. (1980). Low-frequency hearing loss: perception of filtered speech, psychophysical tuning curves, and masking. *J. Acoust. Soc. Am.*, **67,** 638–643.

Tobias, J. V., and Zerlin, S. (1959). Lateralization threshold as a function of stimulus duration. *J. Acoust. Soc. Am.*, **31**, 1591– 1594.

Turner, C. W., Burns, E. M., and Nelson, D. A. (1983). Pure tone pitch perception and low-frequency hearing loss. *J. Acoust. Soc. Am.*, **73**, 966–975.

Turner, C. W., Fabry, D. A., Barrett, S., and Horwitz, A. R. (1992). Detection and recognition of stop consonants by normal-hearing and hearing-impaired listeners. *J. Speech Hear. Res.*, **35**, 942–949.

Turner, C. W., and Henn, C. C. (1989). The relation between vowel recognition and measures of frequency resolution. *J. Speech Hear. Res.*, **32**, 49–58.

Turner, C. W., Holte, L. A., and Relkin, E. R. (1987). Auditory filtering and the discrimination of spectral shapes by normal and hearing-impaired listeners. *J. Rehab. Res. Devel.*, **24**, 229–238.

Turner, C. W., and Robb, M. P. (1987). Audibility and recognition of stop consonants in normal and hearing-impaired subjects. *J. Acoust. Soc. Am.*, **81**, 1566–1573.

Turner, C. W., Zwislocki, J. J., and Filion, P. R. (1989). Intensity discrimination determined with two paradigms in normal and hearing-impaired subjects. *J. Acoust. Soc. Am.*, **86**, 109–115.

Tyler, R. S. (1986). Frequency resolution in hearing-impaired listeners. In *Frequency Selectivity in Hearing*, (ed. B. C. J. Moore), pp. 309–371. Academic Press, London.

Tyler, R. S. (1993). *Cochlear Implants: Audiological Foundations*. Singular Publishing Group, San Diego.

Tyler, R. S., Hall, J. W., Glasberg, B. R., Moore, B. C. J., and Patterson, R. D. (1984). Auditory filter asymmetry in the hearing impaired. *J. Acoust. Soc. Am.*, **76**, 1363–1368.

Tyler, R. S., Summerfield, A. Q., Wood, E. J., and Fernandes, M. A. (1982a). Psychoacoustic and phonetic temporal processing in normal and hearing-impaired listeners. *J. Acoust. Soc. Am.*, **72**, 740–752.

Tyler, R. S., Wood, E. J., and Fernandes, M. A. (1982b). Frequency resolution and hearing loss. *Brit. J. Audiol.*, **16**, 45–63.

Tyler, R. S., Wood, E. J., and Fernandes, M. A. (1983). Frequency resolution and discrimination of constant and dynamic tones in normal and hearing-impaired listeners. *J. Acoust. Soc. Am.*, **74**, 1190–1199.

van Dijkhuizen, J. N., Festen, J. M., and Plomp, R. (1991). The effect of frequency-selective attenuation on the speech-reception threshold of sentences in conditions of low-frequency noise. *J. Acoust. Soc. Am.*, **90**, 885–894.

van Rooij, J. C. G. M., and Plomp, R. (1990). Auditive and Cognitive factors in speech perception by elderly listeners.II: Multivariate analyses. *J. Acoust. Soc. Am.*, **88**, 2611–2624.

van Tasell, D. J., and Crain, T. R. (1992). Noise reduction hearing aids: Release from masking and release from distortion. *Ear Hear.*, **13**, 114–121.

van Tasell, D. J., Fabry, D. A., and Thibodeau, L. M. (1987). Vowel identification and vowel masking patterns of hearing-impaired subjects. *J. Acoust. Soc. Am.*, **81**, 1586–1597.

Verschuure, J. (1981a). Pulsation patterns and nonlinearity of auditory tuning. I. Psychophysical results. *Acustica*, **49**, 288–295.

Verschuure, J. (1981b). Pulsation patterns and nonlinearity of auditory tuning. II. Analysis of psychophysical results. *Acustica*, **49**, 296–306.

Verschuure, J., and van Meeteren, A. A. (1975). The effect of intensity on pitch. *Acustica*, **32**, 33–44.

Viemeister, N. F. (1972). Intensity discrimination of pulsed sinusoids: The effects of filtered noise. *J. Acoust. Soc. Am.*, **51**, 1265–1269.

Viemeister, N. F. (1979). Temporal modulation transfer functions based on modulation thresholds. *J. Acoust. Soc. Am.*, **66**, 1364–1380.

Viemeister, N. F., and Wakefield, G. H. (1991). Temporal integration and multiple looks. *J. Acoust. Soc. Am.*, **90**, 858–865.

Villchur, E. (1973). Signal processing to improve speech intelligibility in perceptive deafness. *J. Acoust. Soc. Am.*, **53**, 1646–1657.

Villchur, E. (1974). Simulation of the effect of recruitment on loudness relationships in speech. *J. Acoust. Soc. Am.*, **56**, 1601–1611.

Villchur, E. (1977). Electronic models to simulate the effect of sensory distortions on speech perception by the deaf. *J. Acoust. Soc. Am.*, **62**, 665–674.

Villchur, E. (1989). Comments on 'The negative effect of amplitude compression in multichannel hearing aids in the light of the modulation-transfer function'[J. Acoust. Soc. Am. 83, 2322-2327(1988)]. *J. Acoust. Soc. Am.*, **86**, 425–427.

von Békésy, G. (1947). The variations of phase along the basilar membrane with sinusoidal vibrations. *J. Acoust. Soc. Am.*, **19**, 452–460.

von Békésy, G. (1960). *Experiments in Hearing*. McGraw-Hill, New York.

Wakefield, G. H., and Nelson, D. A. (1985). Extension of a temporal model of frequency discrimination: intensity effects in normal and hearing-impaired listeners. *J. Acoust. Soc. Am.*, **77**, 613–619.

Walden, B. E., Schwartz, D. M., Montgomery, A. A., and Prosek, R. A. (1981). A comparison of the effects of hearing impairment and acoustic filtering on consonant recognition. *J. Speech Hear. Res.*, **24**, 32–43.

Wallach, H. (1940). The role of head movements and vestibular and visual cues in sound localization. *J. Exp. Psychol.*, **27**, 339–368.

Walliker, J. R., and Howard, I. S. (1990). The implementation of a real time speech fundamental period algorithm using multi-layer perceptrons. *Speech Comm.*, **9**, 63–71.

Ward, W. D. (1954). Subjective musical pitch. *J. Acoust. Soc. Am.*, **26**, 369–380.

Webster, J. C., and Schubert, E. D. (1954). Pitch shifts accompanying certain auditory threshold shifts. *J. Acoust. Soc. Am.*, **26**, 754–760.

Wegel, R. L., and Lane, C. E. (1924). The auditory masking of one sound by another and its probable relation to the dynamics of the inner ear. *Phys. Rev.*, **23**, 266–285.

Weiss, M. (1987). Use of an adaptive noise canceller as an input preprocessor for a hearing aid. *J. Rehab. Res. Devel.*, **24**, 93–102.

Wightman, F. L., and Kistler, D. J. (1989). Headphone simulation of free field listening I: Stimulus synthesis. *J. Acoust. Soc. Am.*, **85**, 858–867.

Wightman, F. L., McGee, T., and Kramer, M. (1977). Factors influencing frequency selectivity in normal and hearing-impaired listeners. In *Psychophysics and Physiology of Hearing*, (ed. E. F. Evans and J. P. Wilson), pp. 295–306. Academic Press, London.

Wilson, B. S., Finley, C. C., Lawson, D. T., Wolford, R. D., Eddington, D. K., and Rabinowitz, W. M. (1991). Better speech recognition with cochlear implants. *Nature*, **352**, 236–238.

Woolf, N. K., Ryan, A. F., and Bone, R. C. (1981). Neural phase-locking properties in the absence of outer hair cells. *Hear. Res.*, **4**, 335–346.

Yates, G. K. (1986). Frequency selectivity in the auditory periphery. In *Frequency Selectivity in Hearing*, (ed. B. C. J. Moore), pp. 1–50. Academic Press, London.

Yates, G. K. (1990). Basilar membrane nonlinearity and its influence on auditory nerve rate-intensity functions. *Hear. Res.*, **50**, 145–162.

Yost, W. A. (1974). Discrimination of interaural phase differences. *J. Acoust. Soc. Am.*, **55**, 1299–1303.

Yost, W. A., and Dye, R. (1988). Discrimination of interaural differences of level as a function of frequency. *J. Acoust. Soc. Am.*, **83**, 1846–1851.

Yost, W. A., Wightman, F. L., and Green, D. M. (1971). Lateralization of filtered clicks. *J. Acoust. Soc. Am.*, **50**, 1526–1531.

Young, E. D., and Sachs, M. B. (1979). Representation of steady-state vowels in the temporal aspects of the discharge patterns of populations of auditory-nerve fibres. *J. Acoust. Soc. Am.*, **66**, 1381–1403.

Zeng, F. G., and Turner, C. W. (1991). Binaural loudness matches in unilaterally impaired listeners. *Q. J. Exp. Psychol.*, **43A**, 565–583.

Zhou, B. (1995). Auditory filter shapes at high frequencies. *J. Acoust. Soc. Am.*, (in press).

Zurek, P. M. (1981). Spontaneous narrowband acoustical signals emitted by human ears. *J. Acoust. Soc. Am.*, **69**, 514–523.

Zurek, P. M., and Delhorne, L. A. (1987). Consonant reception in noise by listeners with mild and moderate sensorineural hearing impairment. *J. Acoust. Soc. Am.*, **82**, 1548–1559.

Zurek, P. M., and Formby, C. (1981). Frequency-discrimination ability of hearing-impaired listeners. *J. Speech Hear. Res.*, **24**, 108–112.

Zwicker, E. (1952). Die Grenzen der Hörbarkeit der Amplitudenmodulation und der Frequenzmodulation eines Tones. *Acustica*, **2**, 125–133.

Zwicker, E. (1956). Die elementaren Grundlagen zur Bestimmung der Informationskapazität des Gehörs. *Acustica*, **6**, 356–381.

Zwicker, E. (1958). Über pschologische und methodische Grundlagen der Lautheit. *Acustica*, **8**, 237–258.

Zwicker, E. (1970). Masking and psychological excitation as consequences of the ear's frequency analysis. In *Frequency Analysis and Periodicity Detection in Hearing*, (ed. R. Plomp and G. F. Smoorenburg), pp. 376–394. Sijthoff, Leiden.

Zwicker, E., Flottorp, G., and Stevens, S. S. (1957). Critical bandwidth in loudness summation. *J. Acoust. Soc. Am.*, **29**, 548–557.

Zwicker, E., and Scharf, B. (1965). A model of loudness summation. *Psychol. Rev.*, **72**, 3–26.

Zwicker, E., and Schorn, K. (1978). Psychoacoustical tuning curves in audiology. *Audiology*, **17**, 120–140.

Zwicker, E., and Terhardt, E. (1980). Analytical expressions for critical band rate and critical bandwidth as a function of frequency. *J. Acoust. Soc. Am.*, **68**, 1523–1525.

Zwislocki, J. (1953). Acoustic attenuation between ears. *J. Acoust. Soc. Am.*, **25**, 752–759.

Zwislocki, J. J. (1960). Theory of temporal auditory summation. *J. Acoust. Soc. Am.*, **32**, 1046–1060.

Zwislocki, J. J., and Jordan, H. N. (1986). On the relations of intensity jnds to loudness and neural noise. *J. Acoust. Soc. Am.*, **79**, 772–780.

Index